A SYNOPSIS OF CONTEMPORARY PSYCHIATRY

A SYNOPSIS OF
Contemporary psychiatry

GEORGE A. ULETT, M.D., Ph.D.

Director, Department of Neurology and Psychiatry
and Psychosomatic Research Laboratory,
Deaconess Hospital, St. Louis, Missouri;
formerly Professor and Chairman, Missouri Institute of
Psychiatry (St. Louis), University of Missouri School of Medicine;
Visiting Professor of Psychiatry,
University of Istanbul, Istanbul, Turkey;
Director, Division of Mental Health for the State of Missouri,
Jefferson City, Missouri

KATHLEEN SMITH, M.D.

Professor of Psychiatry,
Washington University School of Medicine;
Superintendent, Malcolm Bliss Mental Health Center,
St. Louis, Missouri

SIXTH EDITION

The C. V. Mosby Company

ST. LOUIS • TORONTO • LONDON   1979

SIXTH EDITION

Copyright © 1979 by The C. V. Mosby Company

All rights reserved. No part of this book may be reproduced in any manner without written permission of the publisher.

Previous editions copyrighted 1956, 1960, 1965, 1969, 1972

Printed in the United States of America

The C. V. Mosby Company
11830 Westline Industrial Drive, St. Louis, Missouri 63141

Library of Congress Cataloging in Publication Data

Ulett, George Andrew, 1918-
  A synopsis of contemporary psychiatry.

  Bibliography: p.
  Includes index.
  1. Psychiatry—Outlines, syllabi, etc.
I. Smith, Kathleen, 1922-   joint author.
II. Title. [DNLM: 1. Mental disorders.
WM100.3.U37s]
RC457.U4 1979   616.8'9   79-14554
ISBN 0-8016-5176-X

C/CB/CB 9 8 7 6 5 4 3 2 1   02/C/210

TO

Our inspiring teacher

the late

Dr. EDWIN F. GILDEA

Preface

What a challenge is presented by contemporary psychiatry!
New discoveries in the brain sciences continually bring us closer
to the causes of mental illnesses. Psychopharmacological agents
and behavioral techniques offer hope for recovery where previously there was none. United States Public Health Service statistics estimate 17% of the population have some form of mental illness, and some recent studies show up to 80% of persons with
troublesome psychiatric symptoms. While psychotropic drugs
continue to reduce overcrowding in state hospitals, a steady rise in
admissions and readmissions increases the work load. As the
length of hospital stay becomes ever shorter, more patients are followed or receive initial care in psychiatric units in general hospitals, community mental health centers, burgeoning outpatient
clinics, emergency rooms, rehabilitation facilities, halfway houses,
foster homes, boarding homes, and foster communities.

Today patient care moves steadily into the community,
while at the same time admissions to hospital inpatient services
continue to rise. Greater and greater numbers of people are becoming involved in the treatment and rehabilitation of mentally ill
persons. Thus, more than ever before, there is a need for a brief
outline to summarize the facts about mental illness simply and to
serve as an introduction to this complex field. This synopsis is designed for the beginning medical student, nurse, and mental
health worker. Previous editions of this book have found use as a
review for professional examinations for students in medicine,
nursing, psychology, and social work and as a concise pocket reference for busy general physicians and psychiatric residents.

George A. Ulett, M.D.
Kathleen Smith, M.D.

Contents

1   Introduction, 1

2   History of psychiatric thought, 4

PART I
HISTORY TAKING AND DIAGNOSTIC PROCEDURES

3   Examination of the psychiatric patient, 13

4   General physical and neurological examination, 21

5   Examining for agnosia, apraxia, and aphasia, 26

6   Electroencephalographic examination, 33

7   Psychological examination, 40

8   Psychodynamic concepts of personality development, 60

9   Symptoms of psychiatric disorders, 71

PART II
CLINICAL SYNDROMES

10 Problem of classification, 81

11 Standard nomenclature of mental disorders, 84

12 **Organic brain syndromes (O.B.S.),** 99

13 **Psychoses not attributed to known physical condition,** 141

14 **Neuroses,** 174

15 **Personality disorders and certain other nonpsychotic mental disorders,** 190

16 **Miscellaneous—psychiatric conditions not in standard nomenclature,** 210

17 **Psychophysiological disorders,** 214

18 **Transient situational disturbances and conditions without manifest psychiatric disorder,** 239

19 **Behavior disorders of childhood and adolescence,** 245

20 **Mental retardation,** 254

PART III
THERAPEUTIC MEASURES

21 **The psychiatric treatment team,** 263

22 **Individual psychotherapy,** 269

23 **Group therapy,** 302

24 **The physical therapies (ECT, insulin, sleep therapy, psychosurgery),** 308

25 **Chemotherapy in mental illness,** 324

26 **Management of suicidal patients,** 349

27 **Sleep disorders,** 354

28 Forensic psychiatry, 359

29 The psychiatrist and community mental health, 367

Contributors to psychiatric thought, 375

Glossary, 387

1

Introduction

The beginning student of psychiatry is confronted by a confusion of different diagnostic terminologies of the several schools of thought and nomenclatures within this medical specialty. He or she may be perplexed in attempting to define the limits of a psychiatry which now ranges from the microbiology of individual cells through anatomy, biochemistry, genetics, neurophysiology, clinical medicine, neurology, psychology, and sociology to include pronouncements in law, foreign relations, and religion. Psychiatry even includes an involvement in practical politics at the community level as groups of people seek fulfillment of the promises of a better society through the application of forces and facilities at the community level in their search for solutions to local public mental health problems.

In this synopsis the scope is less broad. Despite differences in classifications of mental illnesses, there exists considerable agreement on broad groupings of the major clinical entities and their management. In view of current limitations of knowledge it is obviously unwise for one who seeks for patients the best treatment method that is available to settle for psychoanalysis, behavior modification, or some chemotherapeutic agent as the single answer to the complex psychobiosocial problems of psychiatric illness. It is hoped, as a result of an increasingly rigorous application of research and statistical fact gathering to the methods and outcome of decision making in psychiatry, that treatment procedures for the mentally ill will be improved. In the meantime an increase in popular knowledge about the problems of mental illness and a more ready availability of existing treatment methods will be promoted through legislative and public action such as has produced the current community mental health center movement.

This book is organized to serve as a convenient, easy reference. It is divided into three sections: *diagnostic procedures, major disease entities,* and *therapeutics.* The topic headings of the current *Diagnostic and Statistical Manual of Mental Disorders (DSM II)** will be used. Where knowledge exists, the histological, physiological, or chemical pathology of the brain will be described. Little attempt will be made to present theoretical formulations of etiology except where they are widely used as a basis for a therapy of some demonstrated efficacy. Added evidence from the important research of recent years gives rise to the belief that the future of psychiatry may be more scientifically productive than its past.

Despite the promising advances of the past 50 years in the understanding of human brain function, personality development, and various therapeutic techniques, psychiatric disorders constitute a major public health problem. Since 1955 the overcrowded populations in state mental hospitals have been steadily decreasing, but the number of persons seeking treatment for mental illness has been increasing at a rate of over 5% per year. Obviously this is one of medicine's most challenging frontiers.

To increase knowledge in this field, we would like to emphasize the great need for application of the scientific method of collection and analysis of psychiatric data—to correct an almost universal failure in reports of clinical psychiatry, which filled our literature in the past with much confusing misinformation. It is our belief that an answer to many problems in this field can be found through well-planned comprehensive studies of human behavior, utilizing a multidimensional approach which includes observations by neurophysiologists, biochemists, geneticists, anthropologists, psychiatrists, sociologists, and a host of other workers. Evaluation of treatment procedures should include the use of adequate controls, statistical validation, and methods of handling data which will permit a ready acceptance of psychological observations into the general body of scientific knowledge.

With the current trend toward detailed encyclopedic compila-

---

*Washington, D.C., 1968, American Psychiatric Association.

tions which attempt to cover the total field of psychiatric schools, philosophies, and theories, the need appears even greater than before for a brief, factual, and eclectic introduction to the increasingly complex field of psychiatry.

SUGGESTED READINGS

Freedman, A. M., Kaplan, H. I., and Sadock, B. J.: Modern synopsis of comprehensive textbook of psychiatry/II, ed. 2, Baltimore, 1976, The Williams & Wilkins Co.

Kolb, L. C.: Modern clinical psychiatry, ed. 9, Philadelphia, 1977, W. B. Saunders Co.

Nicholi, A. M., Jr.: The Harvard guide to modern psychiatry, Cambridge, 1978, Belnap Press of Harvard University Press.

2

History of psychiatric thought

Man has always feared mental illness, and the tendency to ascribe its phenomena to supernatural causes is even yet extant. Progress in banishing these beliefs has been slow despite the fact that long before the Christian era enlightened Greeks treated their mentally sick by baths, music, exercise, drugs, venesection, and the surroundings of beautiful gardens. *Hippocrates* promulgated the concept of mental disease resulting from natural causes and included among his many keen descriptions the syndromes of mania, melancholia, and dementia. For 700 years, beginning with Hippocrates and ending with the death of *Galen* A.D. 200, patients with mental diseases were treated with some degree of humanitarianism. Then, with the fall of the Roman Empire and disintegration of classical civilizations, fifteen centuries of primitive attitudes of fear ensued, attitudes which were typified by the Inquisition with its accusation and persecution of the mentally ill as witches.

Philippe Pinel of France in 1792 started the era of "the moral treatment of the insane" by striking off the chains of patients in the Bicêtre. In England a similar role was played by *William Tuke,* representing the Quakers in the founding of the York Retreat. At this time in Philadelphia an energetic pioneer physician and signer of the Declaration of Independence, *Benjamin Rush,* was protesting against conditions and punishment of mental patients in the Pennsylvania Hospital.

During the early nineteenth century, *Jean-Etienne Esquirol,* a pupil of Pinel, applied statistical methods to his clinical studies. In

Germany *Wilhelm Griesinger* advocated nonrestraint, while other Germans created the first modern description of mental disease (*Hecker*—hebephrenia; *Kahlbaum*—catatonia and cyclothymia). In America in the years following 1824 numerous state hospitals were developed and men such as *Pliny Earle, Isaac Ray, Luther Bell, Amariah Brigham, John Butler,* and *Thomas Kirkbride* were prominent in plans, construction, and administration. *Samuel Woodward* was the first president (1844) of the Association of Medical Superintendents of American Institutions for the Insane—later to become the American Psychiatric Association. In 1841 *Dorothea Lynde Dix* began her courageous crusade to remove mental patients from the jails and almshouses into mental hospitals.

Early unsuccessful attempts to classify personality disorders in terms of will, emotions, and intellect were resolved by the classification of *Paul Moebius,* which divided the mental diseases into exogenous and endogenous types, and by *Emil Kraepelin* (1855-1926) whose work established the basis for the present clinical classification. Using concepts which originated with *Morel* in 1860, Kraepelin established the general form of both dementia praecox and manic-depressive psychosis. He believed that the outcome of mental disease is predetermined and laid great stress on the physical causation of these disorders. About this time an attempt was made by *Ernst Kretschmer* to relate manic-depressive disease and dementia praecox to body types, an effort which represented a further outgrowth of German psychiatry. Finally *Eugen Bleuler* (1857-1939), revising the Kraepelinian concept of dementia praecox, introduced the term "schizophrenia"; he conceived of schizophrenia not as a progressive deteriorative mental disease but rather as a group of psychotic reactions characterized by a basic disturbance in associative thought processes, accompanied by emotional irritability, indifference, and autistic symptoms. A foreshadowing of today's wide research interest in physiological-psychological correlates occurred with *William Falconer's* book entitled *The Influence of the Passions Upon the Disorders of the Body* (1796) and with *Johann Heinroth's* discussion of the psychosomatic determinants of insomnia (1818).

Paralleling this development of descriptive psychiatry, an increasing understanding of psychological mechanisms developed. Pursuing a path shown earlier by *Franz Anton Mesmer* (1734-

1815) in France and later by *James Braid* (1795-1850) in England, *August Liebault* and *Hippolyte-Marie Bernheim* (Nancy school) revived an interest in the use of hypnosis and treatment by suggestion. These methods flourished under the influence of such men as *Emil Coué* (new Nancy school), *Jean-Martin Charcot* Salpêtrière school), and *Josef Babinski.* It was in this atmosphere that *Pierre Janet,* a pupil of Charcot, studied and defined hysteria, described various automatisms, fixed ideas, and a syndrome characterized by obsessions, doubts, and phobias which he named psychasthenia. He also introduced (1889) the concepts of dissociation, the subconscious, and psychological tension.

Sigmund Freud (1856-1939) early studied with Charcot and Bernheim and then returned to Vienna to collaborate with *Joseph Breuer* in 1893 in the publication of a new method of investigation and treatment of hysteria. This technique of releasing repressed ideas and their associated affect (i.e., catharsis) led later to the development of techniques of free association and dream analysis, the hypothesis of the unconscious, studies of the stages of psychosexual development, studies of the psychopathology of everyday life, and the analysis of transference reactions. These concepts form the historical basis for modern psychotherapy. Additional significant contributions to psychiatric thought were made by several of Freud's collaborators who later diverged from the mainstream of analytic thought. *Carl Gustav Jung* (1875-1961) of Zurich, who earlier headed the psychoanalytic movement, made significant contributions to the study of word association techniques, schizophrenic processes, and personality types (introvert-extrovert); in addition, he wrote extensively of psychological aspects of man's religious and cultural strivings (the collective unconscious). *Alfred Adler,* an early supporter of Freud, later separated to form his own school which promulgated the theories of "individual psychology," including notably a theory of aggression (power instinct) producing neurotic symptoms and resulting from organ inferiority. His simple formulations, such as over-compensation, masculine protest, and inferiority complex, and the use of organ jargon ("pain in the neck," etc.) had great popular appeal. Another early collaborator of Freud's, *Otto Rank,* believed the cause of all neurosis lay in the individual's attempt to overcome the trauma of birth with its associated "primary" anxiety. His method (will therapy) involved a reexperiencing of separation from the mother figure (therapist) in an effort to strengthen the will.

Karl Abraham (1877-1925), a productive contributor to analytic theory, helped clarify the relation of the pregenital stages of personality development to character disorders. He observed a similarity between obsessive-compulsive neurotics and manic-depressive patients who are in remission. He contributed to the dynamic theories of depression by pointing out the basic ambivalence and increased oral eroticism. He gave clinical support to Freud's interpretation of the internalized struggle which results in the self-punishing desires and self-destructive behavior of depressed patients.

Wilhelm Reich published an outstanding paper entitled "On Character Analysis" (1933), presenting the theory of character defenses ("armor"), which he conceived of as habitual attitudes and ways of behavior that mask inner feelings and basic conflicts. He contributed to analytic technique by pointing out the necessity for dealing with such resistances early in the course of therapy. In her book *The Ego and Mechanisms of Defense* (1946), *Anna Freud* further described man's ways of making psychological adaptation to inner conflict.

Sandor Ferenczi's major contributions were in the realm of psychoanalytic technique and psychopathology. He early advocated active therapy as a way to heighten the emotions produced during the analytic hour but later, with an emphasis on the analyst's personality as the instrument of cure, he recommended an attitude of friendly acceptance on the part of the therapist.

Coincident with the development of psychoanalysis, other contributions to dynamic psychiatry appeared. Hysterical dissociative states were studied and described by *Morton Prince*, who used the method of hypnosis. A few years later the Dean of American psychiatry, *Adolph Meyer* (1866-1950), introduced the broad concepts of psychobiology (ergasiology). He focused the psychiatrist's attention upon the total context of social, emotional, and physical bases of personality. He introduced the life chart and distributive analysis. *Paul Schilder,* German neuropsychiatrist and later student of Meyer, is well known for his formulation of "body image" concepts. *Harry Stack Sullivan* taught that personality develops in response to family patterns of social interaction and that anxiety is most basically an aspect of a relationship rather than of an individual. The therapist's role as a participant-observer in the patient's system of disturbed relationships was stressed. Along with *Paul Federn, Frieda Fromm-Reichmann,* and others, Sullivan promoted the use of psychotherapy in the treatment of the psychoses. His concepts of interpersonal relations, like those of *Karen Horney,* have formed a basis for relating the social sciences to psychiatry.

The study of the developmental origins of personality began with *A. Kussmaul's* observations of the neonatal period (1859) and with *Charles Darwin's* biographical sketch of an infant (1877). A landmark in child development was the report by *Wilhelm Preyer* in 1882 of growth in his son over the first 4 years. *G. Stanley Hall's* research on childhood and on adolescence (1893) was followed by *Alfred Binet* and *J. Simon's* elaborate studies of the development of intelligence (1916). Measurements of infant and preschool development was stimulated by *Arnold Gesell's* standard scheme (1923) for classifying the phasic achievement of simple sensorimotor and locomotor skills. Of historic importance have been the voluminous and careful studies of the development of cognitive capacities carried out since 1929 by *Jean Piaget.*

The neurophysiological processes underlying behavior have yet to find their proper place in relation to these dynamic psychiatric concepts. Early work by *Ivan Pavlov* (1849-1936) in Russia focused on the potentialities of this approach and gave us the concept of the conditioned reflex. Behaviorism, an extension of this theoretical framework in the field of psychology, was developed by *John B. Watson* in the United States and forms the foundation for certain modern concepts of brief psychotherapy. Various physical methods of altering neurophysiological processes, and hence behavior, have been useful. *Julius Wagner von Jauregg* in Vienna in 1918 initiated the method of malarial fever therapy in the treatment of general paresis. *Manfred Sakel* in Vienna in 1937 introduced insulin coma therapy for schizophrenia. *Von Meduna* (1935) popularized Metrazol shock therapy. In 1938 *Ugo Cerletti* and *Bini* in Italy first systematically described the successful use of electroshock treatments in mental disorders (although a case report of electroconvulsive treatment had been published by Babinski in 1903 and electrical stimulation therapy had begun in the eighteenth century). Subsequent to this, modified forms of electrocerebral therapy were introduced in France by *P. Delmas-Marsolet,* who used continuous stimulation, and in the United States by *Friedman, Paul Wilcox,* and *Vladimir Liberson,* who used unidirectional currents.

The surgical treatment of mental disorders probably began with primitive man, skulls being trephined for the treatment of those who were "possessed." Knowledge of the function of the frontal lobes had been gleaned mostly from cases of accidental destruction as in *Harlow's* report (1868) of Phineas Gage, an efficient and capable railroad foreman who became profane, irreverent, capricious, and obstinate following destruction of the frontal lobes by an iron dynamite-tamping rod. *Burkhardt,* a Swiss, resected portions of the left hemisphere in 1888 for the relief of vivid hallucinations. In 1935 *C. F. Jacobsen* in the United States demonstrated that frustrated, anxious, and restless chimpanzees became calm and docile following lobectomy, and in the same year *Egaz Moniz* of Lisbon, Portugal, persuaded *Almeida Lima* to perform the first prefrontal lobotomies upon agitated patients refractory to other treatment. *Walter Freeman* and *J. W. Watts* popularized the method in the United States, and it is estimated that by 1955 more than 25,000 patients had been treated by this method.

The discovery of the behavioral effects of chlorpromazine by *Courvoisier* and associates and, from this, the development of important clinical studies by *Delay* and *Deniker* ushered in the new age of psychopharmacology. The availability and widespread use of potent psychotropic agents have resulted (since 1955) in a marked reduction of the chronic population of large public mental hospitals. This has been coupled with an increased emphasis upon rehabilitative techniques, which, according to *Maxwell Jones* (England), *Leighton, Caplan* (U.S.A.), and others, include the concepts of open ward, patient government, therapeutic milieu, and social and community aspects of psychiatry. In the United States the report of the Joint Commission on Mental Illness and Health, *Action for Mental Health* (1961), with ensuing community mental health center legislation (1963), represents attempts by an alerted public through legislative action to shift the emphasis from custodial care to active treatment. Although exciting and effective, these developments but presage the major attack which will be based upon research findings on the basic etiology of mental illnesses that must yet occur if we are ultimately to solve this grave and costly public health problem.

SUGGESTED READINGS

Ackerknecht, E.: Short history of psychiatry, New York, 1959, Hafner Publishing Co., Inc.

Alexander, F., and Selesnick, S.: The history of psychiatry, New York, 1966, Harper & Row, Publishers.

Deutsch, A.: The mentally ill in America, ed. 2, New York, 1949, Columbia University Press.

Ellenberger, R.: The discovery of the unconscious. The history and evolution of dynamic psychiatry, New York, 1970, Basic Books, Inc.

Hunter, R., and Macalpine, I.: Three hundred years of psychiatry 1535-1860, New York, 1963, Oxford University Press, Inc.

Jones, E.: The life and work of Sigmund Freud, vols. 1 through 3, New York, 1953-1957, Basic Books, Inc.

Zilboorg, G., and Henry, G. W.: A history of medical psychology, New York, 1941, W. W. Norton & Co., Inc.

I

HISTORY TAKING AND
DIAGNOSTIC PROCEDURES

3

Examination of the psychiatric patient

It has long been traditional in psychiatry that to obtain a *mental status* is synonymous with making a psychiatric examination. With the advent of a psychiatry more interested in the study of etiological factors, more emphasis is now placed on the *longitudinal case history* in order to assess personality development as it relates to current symptoms. The psychiatrist should learn to use the mental status (behavioral status) and case history in a complete and orderly fashion to gain an initial diagnostic impression and to formulate tentative plans for treatment. Repeating the behavioral examination at regular intervals can lead to *progress notes*, which will contribute to an objective basis for judging personality changes.

In his appraisal of the patient, the psychiatrist is aided by the instruments of the psychologist and neurologist. Through *intelligence tests* the psychologist furnishes a measure of present intellectual functioning as well as unrealized or damaged potentialities; by the use of *projective techniques* (which see behind the patient's psychological defenses) the psychologist forms an impression of habitual personality and areas of conflict.

It should not be forgotten that mentation and behavior are related to brain function and, although such theoretical concepts as id, superego, and ego may almost assume the proportions of tangible reality in some psychiatric formulations, it remains for the neurophysiologist and the biochemist to relate specific aspects of personality functioning to the topography of the neuraxis. At the present time, nevertheless, a clinical estimation of brain function obtained from neurological examination can give some useful clues to understanding the pathology of behavior. Psychiatric diseases such as pellagra, general paresis, and the senile psychoses have a recognized neuropathology; therefore, in these and in other mental diseases a careful *neurological examination* aided by the *electroencephalogram, spinal fluid studies,* and *roentgenography* can be of assistance to the psychiatrist.

INITIAL PSYCHIATRIC INTERVIEW

In psychiatry, therapy and history taking go hand in hand. Diagnosis and plans for treatment depend upon the results of appraisal of the *psychological functioning* of the patient. Initial immediate planning, working diagnoses, hospital orders, and instructions to aides and nurses must often be formulated after brief contact with the patient. This initial examination is also known as the mental or the behavioral status. To obtain significant diagnostic material, the patient's confidence must be won, and it should be remembered that the psychiatric patient is often initially less cooperative than are many medical patients. He may be frightened, anxious, hostile, agitated, or mute. He resents the implication that he is crazy and is brought to a mental hospital, or he fears that you may discover evidence to prove correct his apprehension that he is losing his mind.

The history-taking process may be expedited by a minute or two spent in getting acquainted, by discussing the patient's home town, occupation, or topics of some current interest. It is helpful to identify yourself and the purpose of the examination. Proceed slowly and ask questions about the mental state within as neutral a frame as possible—along with questions regarding other illness or habits of living, e.g.: "When you get 'nervous,' does it interfere with your thinking?" "Can you, for example, tell me the year you were born?" "Today's date?" Introduce the subject of delusions and hallucinations with care, e.g.: "Do you consider yourself a religious person?" "Some people say they have actually heard God's voice; has this happened to you?" "Do you hear other voices when no one is around?" "Have you ever felt that you are different from other people?" "In what way?" "Are others aware of this?" "Have they looked at you more than is usual?" "Do you believe in mental telepathy?" "Can others read your mind?" Approach with initial caution those areas about which many persons are reticent: suicide, sex, and hostile feelings. Always see the patient in private; his revelations may be embarrassing to him. Try to keep in tune with the patient's mood. Encourage him and let him know you are on his side by your warm understanding manner and nods of acknowledgement.

INITIAL EXAMINATION OF BEHAVIOR (BEHAVIORAL OR MENTAL STATUS)

GENERAL APPEARANCE AND ATTITUDES. We should observe the patient's behavior in the presence of the examiner. His ability to participate appropriately and peculiarities of physical appearance, facial expression, amount of activity, mannerisms, posture, dress, gait, and voice may suggest characteristic attitudes: denial, suspicion, irritability, fearfulness, and self-blame.

SPEECH ACTIVITY. An accurate description of the patient's speech activity is important for an understanding of underlying thought processes. One should note the rapidity, pauses, blocking, flight of associations, distractibility, relevance of associations, rhyming, punning, neologisms, circumstantiality, confabulation, tone, slurring, and stuttering, as well as the extent of vocabulary and peculiar usage of words. The particular topics which are accompanied by increased speech disturbance should be noted for future investigation.

EMOTIONAL REACTIONS. We should note whether the patient's predominant affect is depressed, euphoric, anxious, apathetic, hostile, or negativistic and the extent to which the mood is appropriate to the thought content.

PATHOLOGICAL THOUGHT CONTENT AND ADJUSTIVE TECHNIQUES. In this section we describe such symptoms as delusions, false beliefs ("How are you treated? Do you feel that your troubles are the result of actions being taken against you by others?"), ideas of reference ("Do people talk about you? Do you feel that items in the newspaper refer to you?"), illusions (misperception of objects), hallucinations (hearing voices, seeing visions, etc.), obsessions (ideas or notions that persist despite conscious attempts to remove them), compulsions (acts committed against the conscious will of the individual), and phobias (obsessive, unreasonable fears). Feelings of unreality, of uncanniness, of being controlled by others, or of previously having experienced the present (déjà vu) should be noted.

If possible, relate the occurrence of pathological behavior or thought content to the preceding situation. Try to answer this question about each symptom: *In response to what sort of interpersonal situation does his symptom appear or become aggravated?*

INTELLECTUAL FUNCTIONS. An estimation of memory function is easily obtained both as to remote events and as to recent events. (Can he tell you what he has had for breakfast? Can he remember the names of several objects for a period of two minutes?) Impression of the patient's judgment should be formed. (What would he do in a theater if someone called out "fire"? What would he do if he found a stamped, addressed envelope on the street?) General information (names of rivers, presidents, states, etc.) should be sampled. Attention and concentration powers can be tested by asking the patient to make change or to subtract sevens serially, and his capacity for abstract concepts by obtaining his interpretation of simple proverbs. Orientation for time (exact date, place, name of hospital and person) should be determined, with careful attention being paid to differentiation between experiential confusion and true organic impairment. It should be determined how much insight the patient has into his illness, what he feels is wrong, and what he feels the etiological factors may be.

COMPLETE CASE STUDY

The psychiatric case study is completed not from one but from several interviews. In fact, psychotherapeutic interviews extending over many months' time are, at least in part, elaboration and addition to the patient's history. Over the course of such interviews, we seek to characterize the patient in terms of finding repetitive patterns of behavior which frequently associate with significant life events. The stress precipitating a symptom may be in the present or lie in the past. We are not concerned with how statistically abnormal a trait is in the population at large but rather with how much it bothers or affects *this* individual patient.

The history obtained from the patient may be unreliable or lacking in detail. Relatives (who should be identified in the chart) may contribute additional history. Friends, employers, school records, etc. can all serve to round out the picture.

The following outline presents a form to follow in writing the complete history. Always remember that hospital records are public property and that even your notes may be subpoenaed; so state the problem in simple and safe terms. For example, the statement "difficulties in marital sexual adjustment" is adequate for the clinical record although it is of less interest to the curious than a story of sexual liberties which indiscreetly names the parties involved. Brevity, legibility, and good grammatical form mark the history written by a well-trained clinician. Longer, detailed psychotherapeutic notes may be kept in a separate research file for teaching or similar purposes. The complete psychiatric case study should include such data as the following.

Identifying data

This is the *(first, second, etc.)* hospital admission of this *(age)* year old *race) (religion) (sex) (occupation or civil status, such as escapee, prisoner, parolee)* of *(residence),* who was brought to the hospital by *relatives, police, self)*.

Informants

Name, address, telephone, relationship, length of time they have known patient, frankness and reliability, attitude toward patient's illness ("can snap out of it," "just putting on," "a disgrace") and his admission to the hospital (concerned about patient's welfare, glad to be rid of him, overly solicitous, not understanding admission at this particular time).

Chief complaint

Chief symptoms (quote the patient if possible) and duration; circumstances surrounding admission.

Present illness

Patient was well until (chronological account of development of *symptoms*). Was *onset* sudden or gradual? Is the illness episodic? Was there a *precipitating factor* (death, separation, loss, frightening experience, domestic trouble)? When did patient quit *work* or begin neglecting housework? What time of day do symptoms get better or worse? Have *physiological functions* changed (eating, sleeping, elimination, menses, potency)? Any loss of weight? Changes in memory, mood, or judgment? Behavior changes suggesting *hallucinations? Suicidal* or *homicidal* tendencies? Any ideas of sin, persecution, infidelity, or jealousy?

Family, social, and cultural background

Family history of disease. Mental illness (relation, symptoms, age at which breakdown occurred, length of hospitalization, treatment used), alcoholism, eccentricity, suicides, epilepsy, mental retardation, delinquency, syphilis, glandular disorders.

Family constellation. Father, mother, siblings, spouse, children, stepparents, or foster parents. Whether raised in an institution. Give sketch of each member—name, maiden name of mother, age, marital status, children, health, occupation, residence, personality characteristics, attitudes toward patient.

Socioeconomic background. Housing conditions, number of rooms, plumbing, neighborhood; debts, whether breadwinner is steady worker or ill, hospitalization, insurance; race, minority group, community attitudes and values; religion, sect, regular attendance, scrupulousness, conversion experiences.

Past medical history

In chronological order—*operations, illnesses, injuries,* with duration, severity, sequelae. Inquire specifically about *syphilis* (lumbar puncture?—how treated) *encephalitis, convulsions* (how controlled), *head injury* (how long unconscious, sequelae). Inquire as to all chronic diseases, allergies, neurotic symptoms, etc. List previous attacks of *mental illness* (symptoms, duration, treatment, where hospitalized, degree of health between episodes, suicidal or homicidal attempts). Ask about drugs, especially narcotics, barbiturates, bromides, patent medicines. Amount and kind of alcoholic intake. Occupational *poisoning* (lead, arsenic, mercury).

School and occupational history

Grade completed and *age* when patient stopped and why, ability to read and write, whether failed or especially bright, relationships with teachers and classmates; whether *behavior problem* hyperaggressive (truancy, cruelty, stealing, lying) or withdrawn. *Jobs,* how long, reasons for changing, idle periods, how got along with boss and fellow workers, reasons for getting fired, is job commensurate with ability. *Time spent in the service,* duties, kind of discharge, any time spent in guardhouse or hospital. Juvenile court, reformatory, welfare, or police records.

Sexual and marital history

Some care should be exercised in pursuing this material in order not to create too much anxiety. With some patients, if information is requested in a matter-of-fact manner, much can be learned in the first interview; with others, information is obtained only after a positive relationship is formed with the therapist. The *experiences* and *attitudes* centering around the patient's early feeding and toilet-training situations, the degree of adolescent anxiety concerning sexual functions and the present sexual habits are desirable to know. Important homosexual or heterosexual experiences in the past should be noted, with the patient's feelings about them.

Age *menses* began, how prepared for it by parents (gives idea of family attitude toward sex), whether frightened. Whether menopausal? Age, number and duration of marriages, with age of spouse, sexual adjustment, and length of courtship. Use of contraceptives and whether pregnancies were wanted or planned. Guilt over extramarital affairs, abortions, illegitimate children, masturbation, perversions (sodomy, homosexuality, child molestation, fellatio, rape).

Developmental history

Rejected child, overindulged, birth injury, breast-fed, colic, bowel and bladder training, enuresis, temper tantrums, stuttering, tics, excessive thumbsucking, phobias, night terrors, sleep-walking, rituals, whether ever ran away from home. Age of sitting, walking, talking, coordination. Eating habits, weight curve, fainting spells, convulsions. Handicap such as crippling or blindness. Which parent seemed concerned, and in what manner, with development at different ages?

Personality traits

Kinds of activities enjoyed, whether solitary or group, active or passive, whether leader or follower. Aggressive or sub-assertive toward authority. Inclined to blame others or self. Demonstrative or reserved. Sense of humor. Mood fluctuations.

Adjustive techniques

It is well to describe briefly the behavior of a patient with the physician, particularly as related to emotionally laden material brought out in the interviews. Patient's facial expression, appearance, affect, verbal content, motor and autonomic reactions should be noted, with specific examples given. The therapist should attempt to understand in what ways the patient's behavior toward him is related to his behavior toward other important figures in life.

Impression

Use a phrase which fits the official psychiatric nomenclautre and which indicates succinctly the principal types of pathology.

Recommendations

Diagnostic. For example—"further history from spouse by social worker, lumbar puncture, EEG, and skull films."

Therapeutic. These include *medical treatment*, current *milieu therapy*, and *rehabilitation planning*. For example—"hydrotherapy, electroshock, supportive psychotherapy; stay on locked ward, simple activities, no visiting; introduce vocational counselor for later planning when patient improves," or "intensive psychotherapy; hospital privileges, give patient ward jobs, family visit any time, encourage to occupational therapy; social worker to see wife."

Prognosis

Results to be expected and just how many months' hospitalization will be required. Whether patient will likely be able to return to old job, and living arrangements to be made. Note any important factors likely to be crucial in determining outcome.

SUGGESTED READINGS

Climent, E. C., Plutchik, R., Estrada, H., Gavina, L., and Arevalo, W.: A comparison of traditional and symptom checklist based histories, Am. J. Psychiatry **132**:450, 1975.

Lazare, A.: The psychiatric examination in the walk-in clinic, Arch. Gen. Psychiatry **33**:96, 1976.

MacKinnon, R. A., and Micheis, R.: The psychiatric interview in clinical practice, Philadelphia, 1971, W. B. Saunders, Co.

Mickle, S., and Gerrital, R.: A comparison of psychiatric symptom frequency under narrative and checklist conditions, Am. J. Psychiatry **127**:379, 1970.

Schloss, A. P., and Mendels, J.: The value of interviewing family and friends in assessing life stressors, Arch. Gen. Psychiatry **35**:565, 1978.

Stevenson, I.: The diagnostic interview, New York, 1971, Harper & Row, Publishers.

Strub, R. L., and Black, F. W.: The mental status examination in neurology, Philadelphia, 1977, F. A. Davis Co.

4

General physical and neurological examination

GENERAL PHYSICAL EXAMINATION

The physical examination of the psychiatric patient is no less important than that of any other sick person. In one-third of unselected psychiatric hospital admissions physical morbidity has been observed. Also, it is of special importance to remember that certain conditions, such as carcinoma of the pancreas, etc., may masquerade as psychiatric disorders, and that patients with surgically treatable brain tumors have died in mental hospitals with their pathology unsuspected. The medical examination of the patient is one of the contractual duties and responsibilities of the psychiatric physician. And the firsthand assurance of physical good health is often a strong initial step in the treatment of persons with anxiety reaction and other psychiatric disturbances. The technique will not be described here, as it is known to every physician and does not differ for psychiatric patients except that in very disturbed individuals some portions of it may, of necessity, be postponed. Particular attention should be paid to adequate chaperoning during rectal and vaginal examinations. A neurological examination is a necessary part of every complete psychiatric work-up because, after all, the symptoms of mental disease are mediated through the central nervous system. As elsewhere in physical diagnosis, the most common sins are those of omission. To interpret correctly the findings of the neurological examination requires the skill of specialized neurological training, but to suspect brain pathology requires only that the neurological examination be complete. "The neurologist differs from other physicians in that he tests *all* the cranial nerves." To aid in the performance of a complete neurological examination, the following outline is included.

EXAMINATION OF THE NERVOUS SYSTEM

GENERAL OBSERVATIONS

Position of body, head, extremities
Shape, tenderness, percussion of head
Tenderness and rigidity of neck

CRANIAL NERVES

I. Olfactory
   SUBJECTIVE—Hallucinations of smell, loss or impairment of function
   OBJECTIVE—Response to test odors

II. Optic
   SUBJECTIVE—Failing vision, limitation of fields, hallucinations of light
   OBJECTIVE—Visual acuity, perimetry. Fundi—shape, size, color of disc, lamina cribrosa, physiological cupping, engorged or tortuous veins, constriction or streaking of arteries, exudate, hemorrhage, choking

III. Oculomotor   SUBJECTIVE—Diplopia
                        OBJECTIVE—External ocular movements, nystagmus, ptosis, palpebral fissures. Pupils—size,
IV. Trochlear   equality, regularity, reaction to light, accommodation
VI. Abducens

V. Trigeminus
   SUBJECTIVE—Pain, paresthesia, numbness
   OBJECTIVE
      1. Sensory—anesthesia, hypesthesia, hyperesthesia, corneal reflex
      2. Motor—deviation of jaw, paralysis of temporal and masseter muscles

VII. Facial
   SUBJECTIVE—Hyperacusis, taste disturbance, spasmodic contractions of facial muscles, disturbance of lacrimal and salivary secretions, assymmetry of face

OBJECTIVE
1. Motor—facial expression, nasolabial folds, inability to retract corner of mouth, to close eye completely, to wrinkle forehead
2. Sensory—taste on anterior two-thirds of tongue
3. Secretory—lacrimal and salivary secretions

VIII. Acoustic

Cochlear

SUBJECTIVE—Impairment of auditory acuity, tinnitus
OBJECTIVE
1. Tick of watch
2. Tuning fork test—Rinné or Weber
3. Otoscopic examination

Vestibular

SUBJECTIVE—Dizziness, unsteadiness of gait
OBJECTIVE
1. Bárány test
2. Items listed under cerebellum

IX. Glossopharyngeal

SUBJECTIVE—Dysphagia

OBJECTIVE—Taste on posterior one-third of tongue, pharyngeal reflex

X. Vagus

SUBJECTIVE—Regurgitation of fluids, difficulty of speech, projectile vomiting

OBJECTIVE—Deviation of soft palate, pulse, laryngeal paralysis

XI. Spinal accessory

Paralysis of sternocleidomastoid and trapezius muscles

XII. Hypoglossal

Paralysis of tongue

CORPUS STRIATUM

Muscular rigidity, tremors, slowness of voluntary movements, change of emotional expression

CEREBELLUM

Station, Romberg sign, gait, hypotonicity, nystagmus, dysarthria

Finger-to-finger
Finger-to-thumb
Finger-to-nose
Heel-to-knee
Past-pointing
Adiadokokinesis
} Ataxia, asynergy

SPINAL CORD AND BODY SEGMENTAL REPRESENTATION OF SENSORY AND MOTOR FUNCTIONS—REFLEXES

Proceed in this examination so that neck, shoulders, upper extremities, trunk, abdomen, and finally lower extremities are covered in systematic manner.

SUBJECTIVE
1. Muscular weakness (local or general), difficulty in walking, dragging toe of shoe, stumbling or falling, sphincteric disturbances
2. Changes in sensation (local or general), pain (fixed or radiating)
3. Abnormal sweating

OBJECTIVE
1. Motor—range of muscular movement, contractures, atrophy, strength of muscles against resistance, tremors
2. Sensory—segmental sensory level: pain, temperature, light touch, tactile discrimination, deep sensation (muscle, bone, joint, and vibratory sense)
3. Reflexes, superficial—abdominal, cremasteric, Babinski, Chaddock, Oppenheim, Gordon
4. Reflexes, deep—biceps, triceps, knee and ankle jerks, radial, periosteal, ankle clonus (indicate strength and equality by means of x's as on chart below)

NEUROLOGICAL SUMMARY

Cranial nerves	Done	Abnormality
I	√	_____
II	√	_____
III, IV, VI	√	_____
V	√	_____
VII	√	_____
VIII	√	_____
IX	√	_____
X	√	_____
XI	√	_____
XII	√	_____
Motor	√	_____
Sensory	√	_____
Gait	√	_____
Other	√	_____

SUGGESTED READINGS

Baker, A. B.: An outline of clinical neurology, Dubuque, Iowa, 1958, Kendall/Hunt Publishing Co.

Clark, R. C.: Clinical neuroanatomy and neurophysiology, ed. 5, Philadelphia, 1975, F. A. Davis Co.

Freeman, F. R.: Evaluation of patients with progressive intellectual deterioration, Arch. Neurol. **33:**658, 1976.

Kampmeier, R. N.: Diagnosis and treatment of physical illness in the mentally ill, Ann. Intern. Med. **85:**637, 1977.

Peele, T. L.: The neuroanatomic basis for clinical neurology, ed. 3, New York, 1977, McGraw-Hill Book Co.

Strub, R. L., and Black, E. W.: The mental status examination in neurology, Philadelphia, 1977, F. A. Davis Co.

Weiner, H. L., and Levitt, L. P.: Neurology for the house officer, ed. 2, Baltimore, 1978, The Williams & Wilkins Co.

5

Examining for agnosia, apraxia, and aphasia

The current state of knowledge about the anatomy and physiology of thinking should command the attention of every serious student of psychiatry. Ultimately all psychological theory must be tested for its compatibility with the facts of cortical and subcortical functioning. The study of language disorder, in its broadest concept, should furnish the psychiatric researcher some help in the search for a model of thinking disorder. The careful clinician will consider aphasia in the differential diagnosis of the thought disorder seen in a variety of psychiatric conditions. A minimal brain lesion lying posterior to the motor area may produce only jargon aphasia and a clinical picture without other neurological signs, which could well be mistaken for schizophrenia with "word salad."

Although the physical basis of mind has puzzled thinkers from Hippocrates to Descartes, there has in the last quarter century appeared new and exciting information from biochemistry and neurophysiology. Evidence from histological studies of cell structure, from the chemistry of the synapse, and from brain stimulation in the intact, awake human patient continues to strengthen the belief that the basis of all memory, the permanent patterning of thoughts must be located at the synapse. Here, where the branches of one nerve cell join the body of another, some physical-chemical alteration is produced by the passing stream of electrical potentials subsequent to sensory stimulation. Of such stuff are formed thinking and memory—the elusive engram pattern. The mechanism of recall has been succinctly described by Penfield. He suggests that the patient, upon seeing an old friend after many years, recognizes him through a memory flashback record of the past. By such a cerebral mechanism he is able to compare the present sensory picture with the old memory image, which is so vivid that small changes in the friend's mien are detectable. In order to produce such an experiential response a ganglionic record is activated. This engram is stored not in the cortex but rather, more likely, in the hippocampus. Such ganglionic patterns clearly formed by single exposures in earlier life, even when they have been forgotten for many years, can be immediately elicited by focal electrical stimulation or sometimes by hypnosis or by the free associational methods of psychoanalysis.

Attempts to localize language functions in the brain by *post hoc* case reconstructions of autopsy specimens have produced a voluminous, confused, and controversial literature. At best it appears that language function in most individuals resides in a dominant left hemisphere. This is regardless of handedness. Cerebral injuries early in life can reverse such dominance. Evidence from the work of Penfield and his collaborators at the Montreal Neurological Institute indicates clearly that the speech mechanism must function as a whole and is not, as the early phrenologists believed, divided into discrete areas of functioning. Man in his thinking may utilize several sets of neuronal patterns in his ideational speech mechanism, but the foci are only regions of a total network and not discrete localizations. On the sensory side, neuronal patterns are concerned with the sound of the word in listening and the visual units of the word in reading. On the motor side, the verbal units of speech and manual units for writing all contribute to language formulation. Three basic cortical areas have been outlined as utilized in the ideational elaboration of speech: (1) a large area in the posterior temporal and the posteroinferior parietal regions, (2) a small area in the posterior part of the third frontal convolution, and (3) part of the supplementary motor area within the midsagittal fissure. Motor mechanisms of speech, including voice control, articulating movements, and vocalization, and the mechanism for writing lie in the supplementary motor areas of either side. These areas are situated close to and between the principal areas for ideational speech. (See Fig. 1.)

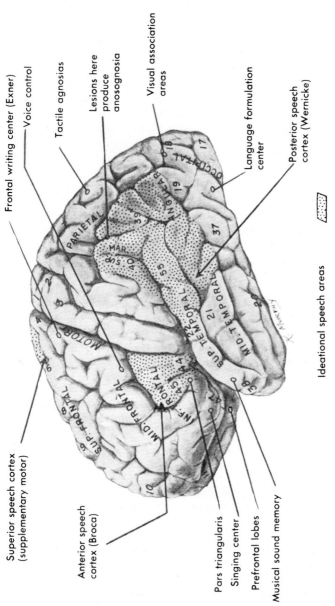

Fig. 1. The human cerebral cortex, illustrating major anatomical divisions, important physiologically delineated areas, and regions designated as important for language function. (Adapted from Penfield, W., and Roberts, L.: Speech and brain mechanisms, Princeton, N.J., 1959, Princeton University Press.)

The functions of the cortical speech areas in man are coordinated by projections of the thalamus. It is obvious that the unilateral cortical speech mechanism must be integrated into the functional mechanisms of the whole brain. It has been hypothesized that nonspecific connections are made through a coordinating mechanism of the centrencephalic system.

Language is a function of human life that results from the dynamic interplay of several brain areas. It is concerned with more than just sensory (receiving) and motor (expressing) functions. Direct contact of sensory and motor neurons would result only in stereotyped, automatic, or mechanical responses. The richness of human speech, thought, and imagination is a result of the rich neural association network which intervenes. Recollection (reminiscence), which includes recall of experiential (detailed memory) and of conceptual (generalizing) images, is part of the stream of consciousness whose level of activity is controlled by the centrencephalon and inflow of the total reticular activating system.

The very complexity of this dynamic organization makes it highly unlikely that pure types of aphasia exist. When, however, the pathway is broken at any of several points, but the rest of the dominant hemisphere and its subcortical connections are intact, the subject is no longer able to find words though he knows what he wishes to say.

Rarely if ever is the aphasic patient perfect in any department of speech. However, his defect may be predominantly more in one area than another. If his difficulty appears greatest in understanding spoken language, he is said to be suffering from *sensory aphasia;* if, on the other hand, his difficulty is in expressing thoughts, it has been called *motor aphasia;* if in reading, *alexia;* or if in writing, *agraphia.*

The closer the lesion is to Broca's area (posterior part of third frontal convolution) and the adjacent precentral face area, the more the motor components of speech are involved. The nearer the lesion is to the junction of the parietal, temporal, and occipital lobes, the more are reading and writing affected; and the more the posterosuperior temporal region is involved, the greater is the difficulty in the comprehension of spoken words.

The patient-centered concepts of Wepman, which focus on aphasia testing as a means for planning therapy, are an important addition to the older writings in this field. Until the final clear answer becomes known, theories must guide the development of further knowledge. Admittedly such terms as "agnosia" and "aphasia" have their limitations, but wide usage necessitates some acquaintance with their commonly accepted definitions.

AGNOSIA

The term "agnosia" refers to loss of function through failure of recognition resulting from an organic cerebral lesion. Distinction must be made as to the sensory modality concerned, and merely to say visual agnosia is not enough. The type of visual agnosia can be further specified as the loss can be specific for animate or for inanimate objects, for their color, for distance, etc. Lesions may produce visual agnosia for various parts of the body (anosognosia, visual finger agnosia) or for the whole body (autotopagnosia).

Lesions causing agnosias in the sphere of language are more complex, but in general the area of cortex essential to visual recognition of letters, syllables, words, and musical notes is the angular gyrus. The terms "cortical" and "subcortical" were used to designate types of language agnosia occurring with lesions of the angular gyrus. "Cortical" was used by some to indicate the occurrence of agraphia in conjunction with the visual defect, whereas when agraphia was absent the term "subcortical" was applied.

Auditory agnosia occurs with involvement of the temporal lobe, and the patient may show paraphasia or senseless repetition of sounds heard (imperfect performance of the minor side).

Tactile agnosia (astereognosis) may result with parietal lesions. Such lesions, involving the gyri of Gratiolet, can produce disturbance in the tactile recognitions of one's own body.

EXAMINING FOR AGNOSIA. Test the patient's position sense, light touch, vibration sense, two-point discrimination, tactile recognition of objects, recognition of digits written on the palm by a dull instrument, and general visual, olfactory, and auditory recognition.

APRAXIA

The term "apraxia" refers to motor disturbances and therefore need not concern language function at all. However, "apractic (motor) aphasia" concerns disturbance of motor speech patterns as, for example, those located in the convolution of Broca. Similarly, apraxia of the cortical motor patterns used in writing may produce agraphia. Thus apraxia is a disturbance in which a patient without dementia, incoordination, or paralysis is nevertheless, because of a motor incapacity affecting association neurons, unable to apply his voluntary motor powers for parts of the body which are involved in a given purposive movement.

EXAMINING FOR DYSPRAXIA. A simple test routine might include such commands as "Show me how you would use these objects (scissors, comb, or toothbrush—give each object to the patient), how you would light a cigarette, make a fist, clap hands, put out your tongue, put out tongue and scratch head at the same time, wink, blow a kiss, knock on a door, count money," etc.

It is important to ascertain whether the patient may be capable of executing a given movement spontaneously but will fail to carry out the same movement in response to a command. Failures may be due to inability to comprehend the command when there is sensory aphasia or when the movement involves manipulation of an object not recognized (dysgnosia). Perseveration may cause the patient to carry out a movement appropriate to a previous command. The patient's powers of imitation as well as response may be tested. Check for confusion. Check history of various motor incapacities and the patient's awareness of them and of the complexities of tasks involved.

APHASIA

Aphasia consists of an organic disease of the cerebral memory engrams for language (i.e., embraces those agnosias and apraxias that have to do with language). The term "aphasia" means loss of power to associate the sensory images of speech with the motor speech functions. Formulation aphasia (paraphasia, jargon aphasia) is the inability to formulate language.

When the power to determine the significance of the symbol is lost as well, the adjective *semantic* is added. Thus one might recognize and repeat a word but be totally unaware of its significance. As pointed out by Head, an element of semantic aphasia (i.e., a quantitative reduction in speech comprehension or capacity) can occur with many types of diffuse brain damage, as well as with a focal lesion to speech centers. No portion of brain can be impaired functionally without affecting the function of the brain as a whole.

EXAMINING FOR APHASIA. Test the ability of the patient to pay attention, to see, to hear, and to act. If there is confusion, it is difficult to decide whether the amount present is sufficient to account for the aphasia observed. These patients fatigue easily, so examine for only 15 to 20 minutes at a time. Gain rapport, explain procedures, and gloss over failures with sympathy and encouragement. If the patient can write well, he probably does not have aphasia of any kind. (Writing one's own name is not an adequate test for aphasia.) It is worth knowing how well the patient could formerly speak, read, and write. Follow the testing with logical thinking on your own part. "If the patient cannot recognize an object by sight (visual-occipital), can he by feel (touch-parietal)?" "If he cannot get the words by vision or sound, can he recognize them by feeling wooden letters?" A simple test routine includes measures of (1) ability to understand spoken words, such as "close your eyes, touch your right ear with your left hand," (2) ability to understand written words, (3) ability to express oneself in speech (note defective grammar and syntax), (4) ability to express oneself in writing, (5) ability to name objects (patient is asked to name a series of common objects shown to him, such as a penny, a button, a fountain pen, etc.—for tactile agnosia) to see if he can recognize objects in hand with the eyes closed, and (6) ability to read aloud.

SUGGESTED READINGS

Agranowitz, A., and McKeown, M. R.: Aphasia handbook, Springfield, Ill., 1969, Charles C Thomas, Publisher.

Dimond, S. J., and Beaumont, J. G.: Hemispheric function in the human brain, New York, 1974, John Wiley & Sons, Inc.

Freud, S.: On aphasia, a critical study, 1891 (translated by E. Stengel), New York, 1953, International Universities Press, Inc.

Geschwind, N.: The organization of language and the brain, Science **170:**940, 1970.

Geschwind, N.: Current concepts of aphasia, N. Engl. J. Med. **284:**654, 1971.

Goldstein, K.: Language and language disturbances, New York, 1948, Grune & Stratton, Inc.

Kertesz, A., and McCabe, P.: Recovery patterns and prognosis in aphasia, Brain **100:**1, 1977.

Schuell, H., Jenkins, J., and Jimenez-Pabon, E.: Aphasia in adults: diagnosis, prognosis, and treatment, New York, 1964, Harper & Row, Publishers.

Wepman, J. M.: Aphasia and the "whole-person" concept, Am. Arch. Rehab. Ther. **6:**1, 1958.

6

Electroencephalographic examination

The electroencephalogram (EEG) is a recording of the electrical activity of the brain. Unlike the EKG, which periodically repeats a characteristic cycle accompanying the activity of the heart, the EEG records brain waves, which are continually varying in form, frequency, and amplitude. The overall tracing, however, may demonstrate a pattern that is quite characteristic for a given individual. Different anatomical regions of the brain produce somewhat different patterns of resting activity. Thus, for example, the resting alpha rhythm of normal individuals is seen most clearly from parieto-occipital leads when the subject is at rest with eyes closed. Electroencephalograms are altered by attention, sensory stimulation, sleep or other disturbances of consciousness, central nervous system disease, and toxic and metabolic changes in the brain cells. Therefore similar EEG changes may be seen with morphological (anatomical) injury and with physiological (biochemical) insult.

By means of small silver or gold disks or needles attached to the scalp, the brain potentials (measured in millionths of a volt) are led by wires to a powerful amplifier. The brain patterns are then permanently recorded on moving paper by an ink-writing oscillograph. With proper spacing, a few pairs of electrodes provide a sampling of the activity from representative anatomical divisions of the brain and permit a comparison of homologous areas (left and right) which should show similar activity. The array of electrodes on the scalp may vary from one laboratory to another; however, the international (ten-twenty) electrode placement, or some modification, is becoming as extensively used here as it is abroad. The brain wave activity from each electrode pair is fed into a separate amplifier and activates its own pen writer. Each unit is called a channel. Modern machines with eight or more channels permit the simultaneous recording of many separate brain areas at one time. The pens write upon paper which moves at the rate of 3 cm./ sec. Such paper is commonly ruled into 1-second and $^1/_5$-second divisions for ease in determining the frequency of waves in cycles per second. The average amplitude of normal activity is 20 to 75 microvolts, and calibration markings on the graph indicate the value in microvolts of the amount of pen deflection (usually 6 to 7 mm. = $50\mu v$).

The brain waves as conventionally recorded vary from 1 to 50 cycles per second (c.p.s.) or hertz (Hz), although frequencies above and below this range exist. The most conspicuous activity in a normal recording is the *alpha* pattern, 8 through 13 c.p.s. (Fig. 2), seen predominantly in the occipital region in about 75% of a control population either as occasional bursts or as a continuous pattern of varying amplitude. The alpha rhythm tends to disappear when the eyes are opened and when the subject is tense and, in many persons, with mental activity, attention, or anxiety. In about 10% of a control population no recognizable alpha is seen and the low-voltage background activity that predominates is called low-voltage fast (LVF). This is usually considered normal, although it frequently indicates some tension in the subject. Similar low-voltage fast activity is usual in the frontal and temporal areas of the head and in the occipital area when the eyes are open.

A moderate amount of activity below 8 c.p.s. is seen in some 10% to 15% of a control population. Activity in the range of 4 through 7 c.p.s. is called *theta* activity, and records containing it in any significant amount are considered to show a borderline disorder. In the Gibbs classification these are termed "S_1" records, the term "S_2" being reserved for records containing a large amount of slow or *delta* activity (under 4 c.p.s.) S_2 records are considered disordered or pathological and are seen in only 1% to 2% of a control population. Disordered records containing fast or *beta* activity (above 13 c.p.s.) are termed, "F_1" or "F_2" records, depending upon the amount and voltage of the fast activity present.

In an epileptic population 50% show diagnostically severe abnormality (Fig. 2). Many of these records are paroxysmal in nature (i.e., have sudden bursts of high-voltage disordered activity differing in character from the background rhythm). Thirty percent of the remainder of the records show borderline disorder. The pat-

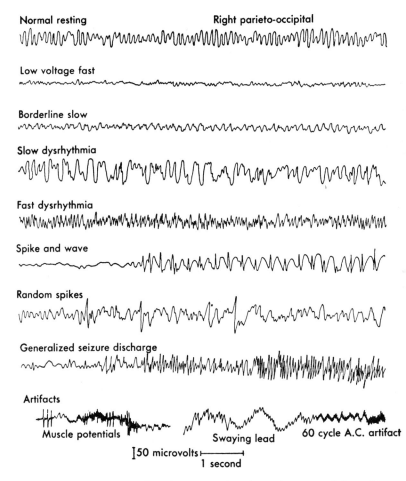

Fig. 2. Representative samples of tracings taken from electroencephalographic recordings.

tern of the EEG may even suggest the type of seizure (e.g., the 3/sec. spike and wave as seen with petit mal). Variants of this pattern occur in akinetic and myoclonic seizures. Although rapid activity (F_2) occurs with grand mal seizures, the interseizure records of persons with such disorder may show a paroxysmal slow dysrhythmia or even be entirely normal. A spike pattern or other paroxysmal abnormality occurring from a single pair of electrodes points to the location of abnormal brain tissue responsible for a focal seizure (e.g., temporal lobe spike of psychomotor epilepsy). In a similar fashion, a slow wave focus of 2 to 3/sec. activity may either lateralize or localize a brain tumor, abscess, or other focal encephalopathy.

As with other laboratory procedures, the EEG is to be interpreted in the light of clinical data. Its diagnostic suggestions are more often presumptive than positive. A single EEG tracing is of less worth than a series of tracings, which permits better evaluation of possible artifacts, the patient's stage of apprehension, and his drowsiness. The series should include such techniques as hyperventilation and sleep recording.

It has been stated that the EEG is of little value in psychiatry. It is, however, becoming increasingly evident that disordered brain patterns occur in psychiatric disease and that with psychiatric screening of a control group the amount of electroencephalographic disorder found decreases. Abnormal EEG activity in an otherwise normal subject may well be evidence of some disturbance involving the central nervous system. Investigations using depth electrodes have demonstrated EEG abnormality not seen from scalp electrodes during strong emotion and in schizophrenics and other psychotic patients.

In the broad category of psychoneurosis, one third of patients show definite disorder and an almost equal number show borderline records. The abnormalities seen are usually of mild degree, such as 4 to 7/sec. activity or an increase in activity at fast frequencies. Mild slowing has been found in some obsessive-compulsive neurotics, whereas poor alpha organization and rapid activity are reported in patients with symptoms of anxiety.

Studies of intercorrelations between the EEG and personality type are of considerable interest, but as yet the findings are inconclusive.

For patients in hysterical trance states and under hypnosis the

EEG is reported as but little altered, and arrest of alpha upon opening the eyes has been used as a test for hysterical blindness.

There is no relationship between the EEG and intelligence, although of course brain damage or anomalies that are associated with mental deficiency will account for some EEG disorder.

In neurosyphilis, as with other infectious diseases of the nervous system, the EEG abnormality may follow the course of the disease. In early untreated cases an increase in fast and slow activity is seen. High-voltage slow activity occurs in patients showing confusion, disorientation, and profound memory loss. Fast rhythms are seen in patients with mood change or thought disorder without mental confusion. The clinical improvement of paresis by treatment with penicillin is paralleled by improvement in the EEG. The EEG may be useful in evaluation and diagnosis of psychosis with epilepsy, or with drug or toxic encephalopathy, and corresponds in abnormality to the underlying pathology in organic psychoses. Abnormal EEG findings in children of patients with Huntington's chorea may identify carriers of the dominant mutant gene and indicate which offspring are more than likely to have the disease in at least incomplete expression.

Studies of the EEG in cases of psychopathic personality have been made difficult by a lack of accepted criteria for the clinical diagnosis of this condition. A review of studies in this field reported that nearly 50% of the subjects showed disorder, with the most characteristic finding being an increase of activity in the 5 to 7/sec. range. These EEG changes are nonspecific, neither focal nor paroxysmal. The more severe the clinical disorder, the greater the percentage of EEG abnormality. In general these are viewed as signs of immaturity.

EEG studies of the major psychoses have been disappointing. No consistent diagnostic patterns have been described for manic-depressive disorder or schizophrenia. In the latter condition, however, the brain activity may be poorly organized with diffuse slow activity, and occasional paroxysmal rhythms have been reported in the catatonic phase.

To increase the diagnostic usefulness of the EEG, a number of activation techniques have been introduced. Such methods include hyperventilation, the intravenous introduction of repeated small doses of Metrazol or Megimide, exposure to a light flashing at different frequencies (photic stimulation), and the use of such photic stimulation in conjunction with Metrazol (pho-mac), hexazole, or other convulsant drugs.

These methods occasionally are successful in producing transient seizure discharges in the EEG. Such abnormal rhythms are often evoked more readily in the epileptic than in the nonepileptic, but there is such an overlap of the two groups that unless the findings are specific and focal the procedure may have little clinical value. Other activation techniques include intracarotid Amytal injection, carotid compression, and overhydration from antidiuretic. Sodium Amytal injection is helpful in determining the location of a primary epileptogenic focus and also the side of cerebral dominance. Bilateral epileptic activity is reduced or stopped with injection on the side of the focus and ipsilaterally abolished when there is a contralateral focus. Diffuse slow activity may be brought about when there is significant occlusion of the opposite carotid artery and the normal one is compressed.

The use of sleep, both natural and induced, has served as an activation method of particular value in detecting focal temporal lobe pathology in patients with psychomotor seizures. Considerable attention has been given to the occurrence of positive spikes in the general frequency ranges of 14 and 6 c.p.s. appearing maximally over the posterior temporal area during light sleep. This pattern has been reported to relate to recurrent autonomic symptoms and to aggressive behavior but is also seen in the records of many apparently normal persons. Almost continuous high-voltage spindles have been found in the sleep records of some mentally retarded children.

In summary it can be stated that, at the present time, neither studies of the resting EEG pattern nor studies of records taken with activation techniques have presented substantial evidence of specific EEG patterns that relate to psychiatric diagnostic classifications. EEG findings of focal disturbances in temporal and diencephalic areas reported in patients previously classified as neurotic, behavior disorder, etc., may point to an overlap between diagnoses formerly considered purely psychiatric and certain of the seizure disorders. The interpretation of the EEG's of psychiatric patients is becoming increasingly complicated because the majority of such patients are now on psychotropic drugs, and these, almost without exception, can produce marked alterations in the EEG which may persist for weeks after medication has been withdrawn.

SUGGESTED READINGS

Anderson, P.: Physiological basis of alpha rhythm, New York, 1968, Appleton-Century-Crofts.

Berger, H.: The electroencephalogram of man, Amsterdam, 1969, Elsevier Publishing Co.

Brazier, M. A. B.: A history of the electrical activity of the brain, New York, 1961, The Macmillan Co.

Fois, A.: The electroencephalogram of the normal child (translated by N. L. Low), Springfield, Ill., 1961, Charles C Thomas, Publisher.

Fois, A.: Clinical EEG in epilepsy and related conditions in children, Springfield, Ill., 1963, Charles C Thomas, Publisher.

Gibbs, F. A., and Gibbs, E. L.: Atlas of electroencephalography, ed. 2, Reading, Mass., 1950, 1952, 1964, Addison-Wesley Publishing Co., Inc., vols. 1 to 3.

Gibbs, F. A., and Gibbs, E. L.: Fourteen and six per second positive spikes, Electroenceph. Clin. Neurophysiol. **15:**553, 1963.

Laidlaw, J., and Stanton, J. B.: The EEG in clinical practice, Edinburgh, 1966, E. & S. Livingstone, Ltd.

Magoun, H. W.: The waking brain, Springfield, Ill., 1963, Charles C Thomas , Publisher.

Rémond, A., editor: Handbook of electroencephalography and clinical neurophysiology; the "EEG Handbook," vols. 1 to 16, Amsterdam, 1978, Elsevier Publishing Co.

Stewart, L. F.: Introduction to the principles of electroencephalography, Springfield, Ill., 1962, Charles C Thomas, Publisher

Ulett, G. A., Heusler, A., and Word, V.: The effect of psychotropic drugs on the EEG of the chronic psychotic patient. In Wilson, W., editor: Applications of electroencephalography in psychiatry: a symposium, Durham, N.C., 1965, Duke University Press.

Walter, W. G.: The living brain, New York, 1953, W. W. Norton & Co., Inc.

Wiener, N.: Cybernetics, ed. 2, Cambridge, 1961, Massachusetts Institute of Technology.

Wilson, W. P., Musella, L., and Shot, M. J.: The electroencephalogram dementia. In Weils, C. E., editor: Dementia, ed. 2, Philadelphia, 1977, F. A. Davis Co.

Wilson, W. P., and Johnson, P. E.: Thyroid hormone and brain function, Electroenceph. Clin. Neurophysiol. **16:**321, 1964.

7

Psychological examination

On the psychiatric team the psychologist often functions as an expert on research design, a psychological theoretician, or even as a therapist. Originally his unique contribution to clinical psychiatry was in the realm of diagnostic testing. When prolonged observation of the patient is not feasible or it is desirable to quickly pick up clues to covert symptomatology, the psychological test battery can be of great value.

The psychologist gathers his data from the patient's test responses and from observations of the patient functioning within the framework of a standardized test situation. His battery of psychological tests is carefully planned with a series of specific questions in mind intended to assess the patient's assets, conflicts, major defenses against anxiety, and amenability to various forms of treatment. The report of psychological findings usually includes a descriptive summary of the patient's personality problems. In order to obtain the greatest value from the psychologist's report, however, the psychiatrist should have some familiarity with the test instruments used. The following tests are commonly included in the diagnostic psychological battery. They are discussed briefly in this chapter and some mention is made of their component parts and scoring scales, but for further details the reader is referred to the list of suggested readings.

Tests of intellectual functions
    Tests of general intelligence
        Wechsler Adult Intelligence Scale (WAIS)
        Revised Stanford-Binet Scale

Wechsler Intelligence Scale for Children (WISC)
Bayley Infant Scales of Development
Tests of specific areas of function
Bender Visual-Motor Gestalt Test
Tests of abstract and concrete thinking

Projective tests
Thematic Apperception Test (TAT)
Rorschach Psychodiagnostic Technique
Sentence Completion Test
Draw-A-Person Test
Word Association Test
Rosenzweig Picture-Frustration Test

Inventories
General personality scales
Minnesota Multiphasic Personality Inventory (MMPI)
Guilford-Martin Temperament Profile
Symptom check lists
Saslow Screening Test
Cornell Index
Behavior rating scales
Evaluation of development or social performance
Vineland Social Maturity Scale, Revised

Brief tests
Proverbs
Comprehension and Similarities
Subtracting Serial Sevens
General Information
Memory for Digits
Kent E-G-Y Test

TESTS OF INTELLECTUAL FUNCTIONS
Tests of general intelligence

The oldest and most carefully standardized portion of the psychological examination is the assessment of intelligence. In these testing situations a number of perceptual, conceptual, memory, and performance abilities are judged. Although the results of these tests are quite easily interpreted and fairly consistent under standard conditions, the tests are affected by cultural and personality variables. Furthermore, it is now known that a large number of individuals vary from 15 to 30 points in functioning at different stages of maturity. Corrections must be made in scoring to account for the decline in intellectual function occurring in the senium.

WECHSLER ADULT INTELLIGENCE SCALE (WAIS). Most commonly utilized by pschologists to measure adult intellectual functioning is the Wechsler Adult Intelligence Test. From scores obtained on eleven subtests (vocabulary, comprehension, information, similarities, digit span, arithmetic, picture arrangement, picture completion, object assembly, block design, and digit symbol) the intelligence quotient (I.Q.) is computed. On the basis of the I.Q. the population has been divided into seven groups: defective (69 and below, 2.2%), borderline 70 to 79, 6.7%), dull normal (80 to 90, 16.1%), average (90 to 109, 50.0%), bright normal (110 to 119, 16.1%), superior (120 to 129, 6.7%), and very superior 130 and over 2.2%). Although all subtests within this scale reflect certain aspects of intellectual functioning, there are interesting differences in the subtests, which are useful clinically.

The *Information* and *Vocabulary* subtests measure the subject's general intelligence, learning ability, and alertness to the world around him. In defining words a person tells much about his personality as well as his cultural background. Wechsler states that vocabulary scores decline least with age. *Comprehension* may be called a test of common sense and ability to evaluate past experience. Responses to this portion reveal much about personality or may provide clues to diagnosis of psychopathic personality or schizophrenia. The *Arithmetical Reasoning* subtest, while influenced by education, age, anxiety, and lapses of attention, seems to correlate reasonably well with intellectual capacity. The *Memory Span for Digits* subtest measures retentiveness. Decrease in memory span for digits, particularly in repeating digits backward, often reflects defects in attention and concentration and may be a sign of organic impairment. However, a low digit span score can also reflect marked manifest anxiety.

The *Similarities* subtest throws light upon the way a person reasons and his capacity for abstraction. The *Picture Arrangement* subtest measures an individual's grasp of a situation, his ability to size up what is going on socially; it seems to reflect general intelligence as applied in social situations. *Picture Completion* is useful for testing lower levels of intelligence and taps the ability to distinguish unessential from essential details. *Block Design* enables the examiner to observe how a person goes about discovering patterns and analyzing form. Success depends upon the ability to perceive the relations of the whole to its parts. It is a useful indicator of organic defect. On the *Digit Symbol* test the subject must speedily associate certain symbols with other symbols. Although this performance subtest measures intelligence, it is adversely affected by poor schooling as well as by the associative rigidity or the difficulty in concentration common in emotionally unstable patients. Another chance to observe a patient's intellectual approach to an unfamiliar task is provided by *Object Assembly*, which seems to reflect creative, mechanical, and conceptual abilities.

REVISED STANFORD-BINET SCALE. For a number of years the Stanford-Binet has been widely applied in assessing the intellectual development of children from preschool years to adulthood. Unlike the Wechsler-Bellevue, the same items are not administered to and scored for all subjects; each age level is defined by a series of items which measure various intellectual capacities. The score is expressed in terms of both I.Q. and the mental age attained over all the test items.

WECHSLER INTELLIGENCE SCALE FOR CHILDREN (WISC). Popular with clinicians since its publication in 1949, the Wechsler Intelligence Scale for Children is constructed similarly to the WAIS and expresses the position of a child 5 through 15 years old in relation to others within his own age group.

BAYLEY INFANT SCALES OF DEVELOPMENT. In recent years reliable tests of mental, motor, and behavior development have been developed for ages 6 months to 3 years. These items have been standardized for infants from different cultures and ethnic groups. The relationship of these scales to later intelligence measurement begins to appear after the age of 15 months.

Tests of specific areas of function

BENDER-GESTALT TEST. This test consists of nine designs which the subject is asked to copy. The manner employed in reproducing this series of perceptual tasks reflects the patient's habitual ways of dealing with outer realities. For example, extreme embellishments of the original design may suggest a manic condition; overaccuracy can indicate compulsive trends. This test is often used to detect organic deficit, arrests, and regressions, shown through impairment of visual-motor function.

TESTS OF ABSTRACT AND CONCRETE THINKING. A group of tests have been designed to explore the ways a patient has of seeing relationships between objects in the environment. Can he relate things only by their appearance in a very concrete way (as in in organic brain damage)? Can he see different types of relationships in terms of function, connotation, etc.? The *Goldstein-Scheerer Tests of Abstract and Concrete Thinking* may be mentioned as well as the *Concept Formation Test* (by Hanfmann and Kasanin).

PROJECTIVE TESTS

THEMATIC APPERCEPTION TEST (TAT). This test, developed by Morgan and Murray, is typical of the group. From ten to twenty of a series of thirty pictures are shown. These are designed to permit identification with persons of both sexes and of different age levels; in some the details are quite indefinite and ambiguous. The subject projects his personality into the situation by building stories about each picture. The interpretation of the test depends upon the figures with which the subject seems to identify, the characteristic mood prevalent in the stories, endings, formal features, topical generalizations, and other dynamic clues. More so than many projective devices, the TAT reveals the content of the patient's fantasies.

RORSCHACH TEST. The Rorschach is the best known of the projective techniques. Introduced by the Swiss psychiatrist Hermann Rorschach (1884-1922), it has been complexly elaborated. The test consists of a standard series of ten ink blots, some in black and white and some colored. These are shown, one at a time, to a subject who is instructed to state what the blot looks like to him or of what it reminds him. Responses are recorded verbatim.

When all cards have been presented, the examiner scores the test, using a system of symbols (Table 1). Each response is examined with the following questions in mind: (1) Where on the blot area was the response object seen? *(Location.)* (2) What was seen? *(Content.)* (3) What characteristic of the blot suggested the response or why was it seen? *(Determinant.)* (4) How well did the response correspond to the contour of the blot area used? *(Form-level.)* (5) How commonly is this response given by other persons? *(Originality.)* The appropriate answer to each of these questions with reference to the subject's response is the Rorschach scoring category that best describes the perceptual processes used. For example, if the subject's reaction to the whole of a large butterfly-shaped ink blot is the popular response "flying bat," the scoring would be W, A, FM, +, P (i.e., whole blot, animal, moving animal, good form, and popular response).

The most difficult step in Rorschach technique is the interpretation of personality characteristics from the assembled totals of scoring symbols and analysis of content. An extremely oversimplified approach to this is seen in Table 1, in which general interpretation areas are suggested for the various facets of personality that are related to the scoring categories. One cannot, however, make interpretative statements by simply noting that a subject's responses fall in certain scoring areas which in turn have some correspondence to a given characteristic of personality. The amount of scoring in any area must be interpreted in the light of the total number of replies given by the subject, in terms of accepted norms for each symbol category, and with modification by interrelationships among several separate categories.

Form, color, and *movement* scoring indicate three important interacting spheres of personality determination: *intellect, affect,* and *creative imagination.* Other symbol categories are listed in similar manner. These are not just arbitrary descriptions but arise from a consideration of the ink blot material as follows:

Form answers suggested by the contour of the blot area used are most frequently given. Such answers result from associative and reasoning processes that select or recall previously laid down "engram" patterns in the brain; hence these may be considered to give some measure of intellectual processes. The form level (+ or −) relates to the quality of such associative processes.

The ink blots do not move. Therefore, to see *movement,* as in "bat flying" implies the use of creative imagination.

Color has long been known to portray emotion in everyday life. The color on the cards seems to stimulate the subject. Some patients completely block on colored cards, with great show of emotion. Others use the color in a productive artistic way, indicating good constructive control of the emotions.

Shading responses to the black and white cards have, for want of a better term, been labeled "deep inner feelings." Such responses can indicate anxiety, oversensitiveness, or dysphoric feelings of depression. *Fc* and *c* responses seem to indicate sensitivity and desire for affection. The subject may actually run his hand across the design in giving a response such as

Table 1. Typical Rorschach scoring symbols and meanings

Scoring		Meaning
Location *(where it is seen)*		Approach to problems and to life
W	Use of whole blot	Usual, popular
Z	Organization toward whole	Ability to organize
D	Usual detail of blot	} Critical
Dd	Rare or unusual area	
S	White space	Oppositional
DW and Do	Abnormal responses	Pathological
Content *(what is seen)*		
H	Living human being	} Identifies easily with other people
Hd	Detail of human figure	
A	Animal	} Immature identifications
Ad	Detail of animal	
At	Anatomy (x-rays, surgical specimens, etc.)	Over-concern with illness
Obj	Objects	} Wealth of associational material
N	Nature (landscape, trees, etc.)	
T	Topical (fire, blood, sex, etc.)	Overvalent preoccupation
Form-level *(how well it is seen)*		
+	Superior form	Stability, good intellectual control
−	Poor form	Distorted, conceptual thinking
Originality *(how commonly it is seen by others)*		
P	Popular, seen by 1 of 5 persons	Conforming

"hairy." C' responses are given when black and white colors imply "gloom," "coldness," or somber moods. The K type responses, on the other hand, are more often said to represent anxiety. These (as depth or vista responses) may show insecurity within the self, a three-dimensional "how do I stand in relation to?" sort of feeling.

Another category, *apperception,* demonstrates the patient's approach to a new situation or shows how he organizes new knowledge in relation to old.

Study of the subject's associations (*content* analysis) can discover areas of preoccupation, reveal hostility, etc.

Table 1. Typical Rorschach scoring symbols and meanings—cont'd

	Scoring	Meaning
O+	Good original responses (1 of 100 records)	Superior, original thinking
O−	Poor original response	Bizarre thinking

Determinant *(how or why it is seen)*

Form
F	Responses on the basis of contour or form alone	Intellectual control

Movement
M	Human-like action	Creative imagination
FM	Animal-like action	Instinctual drives, immature
m	Inanimate movement or force	Inner tensions

Color
FC	Colored object with form	Good emotional control
CF	Color with indefinite form	Affective lability
C	Color only, form disregarded	Uncontrolled emotion

Shading and surface
FK	Shading suggesting three dimensions or vista	Self-awareness
K	Shading as diffusion (smoke, clouds, etc.)	Anxiety
Fc	Surface shading (hairy, fur rug, etc.)	Sensitivity
c	Shading as texture (furry shiny, etc.)	Oversensitive, sensuous
C′	White or black as a color	Dysphoria, depression

Score for *originality* indicates superior performance (+) or bizarre fantasy (−); *popular* responses indicate ability to think as other persons do.

This brief portrayal of Rorschach symbols and their approximate meanings enables one to see at a glance the main personality facets explored in this test procedure and to gain some immediate idea of their interrelationships.*

*From Ulett, G. A.: Rorschach introductory manual, St. Louis, 1960, Bardgett Printing & Publishing Co.

The picture of the subject revealed by the test is said to show those basic elements of personality structure which, for the most part, remain fixed. It is possible to corroborate or suspect the diagnosis of psychiatric disease entities by the patterns of response to this test.

The validity of the Rorschach Test as a scientific method is still questioned and Rorschach experts admittedly lean heavily upon clinical experience. However, the test has gained wide acceptance and is often worthwhile to administer if only because of its ability to lower defenses, put the patient "off guard," and hence bring to light material that might otherwise have been seen only after weeks of clinical interviewing.

SENTENCE COMPLETION TEST. Various tests have been devised which require that the patient complete sentences beginning in some such way as "I become very angry when . . . " or "Other people think I. . . ." Although this type of test is more transparent than most projective tests and generally does not utilize uniform scoring instructions, it is a useful supplementary source of data on how the patient wishes to present his attitudes about himself and toward others. Both mood and content are noted in relation to such areas as home, work, sickness, immediate family, etc.

THE DRAW-A-PERSON TEST. This test, originated by Goodenough and further explored by Machover, is believed to provide data about the patient's feelings and perceptions of bodily image. The subject is asked to "draw a person" and later to draw the opposite sex. Intuitive analysis is carried out concerning structural factors (placement of figure on the page, etc.) and content factors (parts of body used, emphasized or de-emphasized, etc).

WORD ASSOCIATION TEST. The word association test popularized by Jung consists of a series of 50 or more words which are presented to the subject one at a time. Mixed in the list are words assumed to be related to conflicts of this patient or words which generally produce emotional reaction. The type of association given to these words, together with signs of emotional disturbance such as delayed responses, suggests that the key word is related to a hidden complex.

PICTURE-FRUSTRATION STUDY (P-F). This test, developed by Rosenzweig, consists of 24 cartoonlike pictures, each representing two persons who are involved in a mildly frustrating situation of common occurrence. One figure in each picture is shown saying certain words which either frustrate the other individual or help to describe what is frustrating him. After examining the picture the subject writes in the blank space the first reply that enters his mind. The answers are scored in terms of the direction and type of aggression (i.e., *extrapunitive* if directed out upon the environment, *intrapunitive* if directed upon himself, or *impunitive* if the aggression is turned off). Similarly the responses are scored in terms of whether the patient is concerned more with the nature of the frustrating situation *(obstacle-dominant)*, with protecting himself *(ego-defensive)*, or with which solution of the problem is most important *(need-persistive)*. Interpretation is in relation to group norms and is suggested as giving some indication of the patient's usual behavior when under frustration.

INVENTORIES

In addition to tests of intellectual functions and projective tests, various self-administered inventories may be helpful. Not only are such paper-and-pencil tests economical in time but, because of their structure, they are also more reliable sources of personality data with many patients than are projective tests.

General personality scales

Two examples will be cited here of the large number of general personality inventories available to the psychologist.

MINNESOTA MULTIPHASIC PERSONALITY INVENTORY (MMPI). The patient is asked to consider 566 statements about himself and to answer, if possible, whether each statement seems "true" or "false." ("Cannot say" is also available.) In the analysis a variety of scales are applied to the items. These include four validity scales: the L (lie), the F (failure of normal response), the K (test-taking attitude), and the ? (evasiveness) scale. The clinical scales include the Hs (hypochondriacal), D (depression), Hy (hysteria), Pd (psychopath), Ma (mania), Mf (masculinity-femininity), Pa (paranoid), Pt (psychasthenic), and Sc (schizophrenic). An Si (social introversion) scale is also available. The patient's score on all of these composes the MMPI profile. The experienced psychologist makes his diagnoses by scanning the profile and giving weight to the various scoring combinations that occur. Overall, the Minnesota Multiphasic Personality Inventory

Table 2. Psychological test characteristics of psychiatric patients*

Wechsler Intelligence scales	MMPI	Rorschach	TAT
Depression			
Performance scales lower than Verbal scales; difficulty in maintaining concentrated effort; Comprehension and Similarity tests generally low; low Digit Span; verbal productions frequently short; distorted and morbid Picture Arrangement stories	High D scale; high Pt scales; high F scale; low Ma scale; difficulty in completing tests	Few responses; prolonged reaction time; low or absent M responses; low or absent color responses; high F+%; emphasis on D and Dd; few W responses; A% high; uncertainty, self-correction, self-depreciation, and qualification of responses	Themes of despair, lack of success, failure, loss of love, and death are frequent; stories usually short and pessimistic in attitude; outcomes bleak; picture may cause patient to cry
Schizophrenia			
Vocabulary and Information subtests generally hold up well; other subtests fall below; Comprehension and Arithmetic both impaired; Performance scales with greatest impairment are Picture Arrangement, Picture Completion, and Object Assembly; qualitatively, re-	Neutral to positive slope; bimodal curve; high F; low K; elevated neurotic triad (Hs, D, Hy) with Pt, Sc, and Pa higher than the neurotic triad	Abnormal responses (contamination, position responses, confabulation, perseveration, queer verbalization, personal references, descriptions, edging); many W responses, poor quality; bizarre and unusual details (Dd); M below normal; C and CF high; color naming (Cn);	Themes range from peculiar to bizarre, with private, cryptic meanings, sudden shifts in story, and lack of consistency or guiding story in the plot; sexual references common; length of story tends to be average but rarely may consist of several pages

sponses to any subtest may be peculiar, revealing distortion of thought and perceptual processes; interest scatter is wide

Manic-excitement

It may not be possible to obtain test results due to the patient's easy distractibility, flight of ideas, and disruption of productive effort because of stimulation of the test; qualitative signs are most predominant, with patient associating to various test stimuli; tests calling for prolonged and concentrated effort pose greatest difficulty

Doubtful that such a patient could focus energy and attention long enough to complete the test; high F; all other scales may be irregularly elevated with a solitary peak of 80 or more on Ma

Poor quality (F−); poor W responses (confabulatory DW); increase in M and color responses; decrease in D responses; A% high with FM

few popular responses; blocking; increased original (O+ and O−); stereotypy; increased A%

Possibility of obtaining protocol may be doubtful; stories may ramble on and on as both the picture and the patient's own story serve as a stimulus; stories thus disjointed and contain references to sexual prowess, business success, conquests, and other ego-inflating experiences, many of which are drawn from patient's life, real or imagined

Continued.

*This table was prepared by Richard B. Cravens, Ph.D. Like any other tests or laboratory findings used in clinical medicine, these patterns and signs are suggestive but not absolute diagnostic indicators. Particularly, the individual signs may not be meaningful in themselves but only when seen in patterns or in conjunction with other findings and observations. As such, they may give valuable and helpful clues in the diagnosis and management of patients with a mental disorder.

Table 2. Psychological test characteristics of psychiatric patients—cont'd

Wechsler Intelligence scales	MMPI	Rorschach	TAT
Paranoid			
Patterning is similar to protocol produced by schizophrenic patient; Information and Vocabulary hold up well; Comprehension also fairly well maintained; Digit Span suffers, as does Picture Arrangement and Object Assembly; may be close attention paid to irrelevant parts of test stimuli and meaning ascribed to purpose of the test	Neutral or positive slope, bimodal curve, high F; low K; Pa 75; Sc and Pt 58; elevation on Ma	Introversive Erlebnistypus with high M; high F%; and F+ %; high circumstantial elaboration of relationship of cards (similarities and differences); abstract personal references	Stories short; frequent questioning as to purpose of test; some pictures reacted to in highly personal way; patient questions source of picture or in some way relates picture to an aspect of his life; stories guarded, full of suspicion and distrust of motives of others; reference to people not viewed in picture; things may be happening to person that are beyond his control
Psychoneurosis			
Different neurotic conditions produce different patternings; in obsessive-compulsive conditions Information, Similarities, and Vocabulary tend to remain high, with Comprehension falling less	Validity scales within limits; negative slope; elevated neurotic triad peaking at D (Hs, D, Hy); inverted neurotic triad (high Hs, low D, high Hy) suggests psychosomatic symptoms	Rejection; no FC; shading shock; not over 1 M; color shock; high F%; over 50% animal or anatomical; not over 25 responses, Fm greater than M; (in anxiety: shading; preoccupation,	Stories range in length from below average for hysteric to usually above average for obsessive-compulsive; stories free of bizarre elements and tend to be complete, having plot and ending;

than Information; Verbal Scale elevated over Performance Scale; hysterics generally show Comprehension elevated over Information; lower Vocabulary; Performance Scale score higher than Verbal Scale; depressive reactions show long reaction time; Verbal Scale elevated over Performance Scale; lowered Arithmetic Digit Span		K, k, c); increase in m; overawareness of symmetry; increase in details, Hd, and Ad	may be precise and detailed description of picture per se as in case of obsessive-compulsive; gloomy, sad themes as in depressive reaction, or unsophisticated naive plots as created by hysteric

Character disorders

Test-taking attitude important as diagnostic indicator; attitude may be breezy, all knowing, but without depth, cavalier; impression created that patient could tell more about a subject (answer to a test question) if time permitted; Performance Scale significantly elevated over Verbal Scale; low along with Arithme-	Typical profile is double spike curve peaking first at Pd and the Ma; neurotic triad (Hs, D, Hy) low	Low number of responses; Erlebnistypus constrictive; high F%; poor form level (low F+%); FM greater than M; CF greater than FC; C/F and C; may have difficulty with cards VIII, IX, and X; few original responses; easy W and popular Anatomical, with crude sexual preoccupation); S responses; rejec-	Stories short, uncomplicated, and without depth; breezy quality; reference to alcohol, drugs, or criminal activities of major or minor nature, with hero escaping punishment; stories may consist of few lines (description); refusal to tell story and questioning purpose of the test

Continued.

Table 2. Psychological test characteristics of psychiatric patients—cont'd

Wechsler Intelligence scales	MMPI	Rorschach	TAT
Character disorders—cont'd tic and Similarities, although all Verbal scales may be low; Picture Arrangement and Object Assembly elevated'		tion of cards; suspicious inquiry; antisocial trends (few H); sadomasochistic coloring; egocentricity	
Organic psychoses Tests most sensitive to organic conditions are Digit Span, Similarities, Arithmetic, Digit Symbol and Block Design (all low); Vocabulary may remain high along with Information; Verbal Scale higher than Performance Scale; may be statements of perplexity and impotence; evidence of confusion and perseveration; fatigue frequently in the picture	This profile similar to neurotic profile but may contain secondary peak at Sc; Mf, Pa, and Ma are low; profile may also be sawtooth in appearance, with peaks at F, D, Pd, Pa, and Sc	Impotence (gives inadequate responses, unable to correct); perplexity (indecisive, seeks reassurance); automatic phrases, repetition, color naming (Cn); F+ % low; total responses low- prolonged reaction time; M low	Themes short, frequently limited to picture description with no story or plot; uncertainty expressed as to outcome; confusion, fatigue, and perseveration from one picture to next; illness common theme; reference to loss of ability or functioning

is a useful adjunct to other diagnostic techniques in defining self-attitudes, certain aspects of ego functioning, and types of symptomatology.

GUILFORD-MARTIN TEMPERAMENT PROFILE. This is a more recent inventory, not dissimilar to the MMPI and aimed at predicting various types of job and social performances as well as uncovering tendencies toward self-preoccupation, shyness, depression, emotional lability, leadership potential, inferiority feelings, etc.

Symptom checklists

If the psychiatrist is faced with the need to screen rapidly a large number of reasonably cooperative patients, for the presence or absence of psychiatric disorder, a symptom checklist may be useful. The following two instruments are but illustrations from a large group which have been designed for use under a variety of special circumstances.

SASLOW SCREENING TEST. This test differentiates with reasonable reliability between the psychoneurotic-psychophysiological group of patients and normal persons.

CORNELL INDEX. This is a similar but longer test that has been used with large numbers of persons.

Behavior rating scales

Another method of measuring the patient's psychological and social performance is the behavior rating scale. Hospital personnel often find this is a convenient way of following simple changes in the patient through time. On occasion it may be used by psychiatrists or psychologists as a concrete way of describing major disturbed behaviors and of following surface manifestations of improvement or relapse.

Currently used scales for rating the behavior of hospitalized patients include (1) the *Social Ineffectiveness Scale* by Parloff, Kelman, and Frank, (2) *L-M Fergus Falls Behavior Rating Scale* by Lucero and Meyer, (3) Cutler and Kurland's *Clinical Quantification of Depressive Reactions*, (4) *Ward Behavior Rating Scale* by Burdock et al., (5) Ellsworth's *MACC Behavioral Adjustment Scale (Form II)*, (6) *Normative Social Adjustment Scale* by Barrabee, Barrabee, and Finesinger, (7) Malamud and Sands' *Psychiatric Rating Scale*, (8) Wittenborn's *Psychiatric Rating*

Scales, (9) *Phenomena of Depressions* by Grinker et al., (10) *Brief Psychiatric Rating Scale* by Overall and Gorham, (11) Hamilton's *Rating Scale for Depression,* (12) Lorr's *Inpatient Multidimensional Psychiatric Scale,* (13) *Symptom and Adjustment Index* by Gross et al., (14) *Katz Adjustment Scales,* (15) *Clyde Mood Scale,* (16) Lorr's *Psychotic Reaction Profile,* (17) the *MMHC Depression Rating Scale* by Greenblatt, Grosser, and Wechsler, (18) *Psychiatric Judgment Depression Scale* by Overall et al., and (19) the *Hospital Adjustment Scale* by Ferguson, McReynolds and Ballachey.

Measures of social performance

Particularly in dealing with more seriously disturbed patients, when one is planning treatment, it is helpful to decide the degree to which the patient's illness has interfered with economic self-sufficiency and with effectiveness on the job, in the immediate family, with spouse, and with friends. At the present time no scales for measuring social performance have found wide employment. Perhaps the clinically most useful hypotheses in defining the social performance expected at various levels of maturity have been developed by Erikson.

VINELAND SOCIAL MATURITY SCALE, REVISED. This scale, devised by E. A. Doll, consists of a graduated series of item clusters, each of which expresses a slightly higher level of social maturity. These are rated from data derived from a stuctured interview situation held with someone close to the patient. The scale was constructed primarily for assessing severity of mental deficiency but may be used to express gross social performance in any child or adolescent.

BRIEF TESTS

If time does not permit the psychiatrist recourse to psychological consultation, he may himself employ selected items from tests to obtain a "thumbnail impression" of certain personality functions. For example, in searching for evidences of the schizophrenic's tendency toward loose associations, overgeneralized patterning of concepts, and defects in abstract thinking, questions borrowed from the *Comprehension and Similarities* subtests of the WAIS are clinically useful. If the patient is asked how a bicycle is like a wagon, a good reply would be in terms of function (i.e., they are both means of transportation). An answer which may indicate a tendency toward concrete thinking would be in terms of structure (i.e., they both have wheels). A poor answer would be either a failure to see any similarity or the use of bizarre or overinclusive type of similarity (i.e., they are both used outside the home).

PROVERBS. In addition to the above, proverbs are commonly employed by clinicians to test for evidences both of schizophrenic distortions and of concretization or sterility of associations found in the patient with organic brain damage. If, upon being asked to explain the proverbs "A rolling stone gathers no moss," "All that glitters is not gold," and "A bird in the hand is worth two in the bush," a patient with normal I.Q. replies only in terms of stones, gold, and birds and he cannot comprehend the application of these proverbs to human affairs, abstract thinking may be assumed to be impaired.

SUBTRACTING SERIAL SEVENS. A brief method of measuring attention and concentration abilities is to ask the patient to subtract 7's serially, starting from 100. Most persons can complete the task with no more than two errors in sixty seconds.

GENERAL INFORMATION Questions testing general information (e.g., "How far is it from San Francisco to New York?" "Who is governor of your state?") are useful indicators of both cultural and intellectual factors.

MEMORY FOR DIGITS. Having the patient repeat after the examiner a series of unrelated digits is a brief test of attention and memory. Most individuals should be able to do this forward up to six or seven digits and backward up to four or five digits.

KENT E-G-Y TEST. A number of brief tests of personality function have been devised. An example of a brief adult intelligence scale giving a simple, rough indication of both mental age and quality of thinking is the Kent E-G-Y Test.

Kent E-G-Y questions	Points
1. What are houses made of? (Any material you can think of.)	1-4
2. What is sand used for?	1, 2, or 4
3. If the flag blows to the south, where is the wind coming from?	3
4. Tell me the names of some fishes.	1-4
5. At what time of day is your shadow shortest?	3
6. Give the names of some large cities.	1-4
7. Why does the moon look larger than the stars?	2, 3, or 4

	Kent E-G-Y questions—cont'd	**Points**

8. What metal does a magnet pick up?   2 or 4
9. If your shadow points to the northeast, which way is the   4
   sun?
10. How many stripes in the American flag?   2

Points assigned in scoring:

Total points	"Mental age" rating	Total points	"Mental age" rating
10-13	8	21-23	12
14-16	9	24-27	13
17-18	10	28-31	14
19-20	11	32-36	14+

1. One point for each item up to four.
2. One point for "play" or "scrubbing." Two points for any construction use. Four points for "glass."
3. Three points for "north"; no partial credits.
4. One point each, up to four.
5. Three points for "noon."
6. One point each, up to four. "New York is counted as a city unless another state has been mentioned.
7. Two points for "moon is lower down." Three points for "nearer" or "closer." Four points for generalized statement that nearer objects look larger than distant objects.
8. Two points for "steel." Four points for "iron."
9. Four points for "southwest"; no partial credits.
10. Two points for "13." Anyone who responds "50" should have his attention called to his mistake and should be permitted to try again. If he responds "7," it should be made clear that both red and white stripes are included.

SUGGESTED READINGS

Ames, L. B., Metraux, R. W., and Walker, R. N.: Adolescent Rorschach responses; developmental trends from 10 to 16 years, New York, 1959, Paul B. Hoeber, Inc., Medical Book Department of Harper & Bros.

Ascough, J. C., Strouf, M. J., Cohn, C. S., and Smith, R. E.: Differential diagnosis of brain damage and schizophrenia by the Memory-for-Designs test, J. Clin. Psychol. **27:**471, 1971.

Barnes, G. W., and Lucas, G. J.: Cerebral dysfunction vs. psychogenesis in Halstead-Reitan tests, J. Nerv. Ment. Dis. **158:**50, 1974.

Beck, S. J.: Rorschach's test, ed. 3, New York, 1961, Grune & Stratton, Inc., vols. 1 to 3.

Clyde, D. J.: Clyde Mood Scale manual, Coral Gables, Fla., 1963, University of Miami Biometric Laboratory.

Hathaway, S., and Meehl, P.: An atlas for clinical use of the MMPI, Minneapolis, 1951, University of Minnesota Press.

Knesevich, J. W., Biggs, J. T., Clayton, P. J., and others: Validity of the Hamilton Rating Scale for Depression, Br. J. Psychiatry **131**:49, 1977.

Lanyon, R.: A handbook of MMPI group profiles, Minneapolis, 1968, University of Minnesota Press.

Lorr, M., and others: Inpatient multidimensional psychiatric scale, Palo Alto, Calif., 1963, Consulting Psychologist Press.

Pascal, G., and Suttell, B.:. The Bender-Gestalt test, New York, 1951, Grune & Stratton, Inc.

Terman, L., and Merrill, M.: Measuring intelligence, New York, 1937, Houghton Mifflin Co.

Ulett, G. A.: Rorschach introductory manual, St. Louis, 1960, Bardgett Printing & Publishing Co.

Wechsler, D.: The measurement and appraisal of adult intelligence, ed. 4, Baltimore, 1958, The Williams & Wilkins Co.

Williams, R. L., editor: Testing, measurements and Afro-Americans, Afro-American Issues 3(1): Winter 1975, Washington, D.C., 1975, Educational and Community Counselors Associates, Inc.

Wolff, H. G.: Non-projective personality tests; Cornell Indices and Cornell Word Form Application, Ann. N. Y. Acad. Sci. **46**:589, 1946.

8

Psychodynamic concepts of personality development

The term *psychodynamic* ("dynamic") refers to the study of the causative factors and motivations of human interpersonal behavior. It stresses the importance of past and current interhuman relationships as opposed to organic (anatomical and physiological) factors as most important in determining the variables of personality in mental illness. Originally almost synonymous with "psychoanalytic," the term is currently more broadly conceived. In this section will be mentioned briefly a few common psychodynamic concepts which psychiatrists find useful in relating patients' childhood experiences to their adult emotional illnesses. Often it seems clear not only that constitutional factors and immediate life stresses have operated as possible causes but also that the groundwork for later illness was laid in chronically maladaptive attitudes and behaviors unwittingly fostered by the human environment of childhood.

By means of a series of systematic changes, personality develops stepwise from the neonatal period through the stages of adult life. Each period of adaptation contains fairly uniform biological and social conditions that challenge the individual to learn new behaviors and roles and to give up former expressions and identifications appropriate to an earlier life stage. The infant-mother tie in the first week involves different issues from those of the infant-mother tie in the third month of life, just as the adolescent-parent relationship involves different problems at 14 years of age than those at age 19. The study of personality development consists in defining these stage-specific challenges and in trying to understand how the genes, the brain, the previous experience of the person, and the environment have influenced adaptation by setting limits to change and by providing alternative possibilities for new behaviors and experiences.

At present there is no coherent theory of personality. A variety of incomplete theoretical positions exist, each of which clarifies limited problems. Neurophysiology, theories of c conditioning and reinforcement, psychoanalysis, concepts of social role, ideas about ecological and cultural influences, and concerns with each person's uniqueness and essential moral potentials all attest to different aspects of personality. In our ignorance we are like the proverbial six blind men, each examining a different part of an elephant—no one has the imagination or the facts to construct a balanced picture of the whole.

The psychoanalytic philosophy of human functioning puts the patient's wishes in the center of theoretical focus. Within Freud's study of dreams as well as within his psychotherapeutic technique, the patient's frustrated yearnings and hopes were the starting point for understanding the illness. Whether intentionality is conceived in terms of biologically stuctured *instincts,* conditioned secondary *drives,* psychic *needs,* socialized *role functions,* or moral *requirements,* using any view of personality, the psychiatrist understands the patient's symptoms as by-products of maladaptive, inappropriate patterns of goal-directed behavior. Therefore, a person's health or illness is linked to (1) the nature of his goals (realistic or unrealistic, infantile or stage-appropriate), (2) his repertoire of interpersonal behaviors for pursuing these goals (coping or defense mechanisms), and (3) his available modes of experiencing relationships and situations. Following are two pathological illustrations of this connection: (1) Depressive illnesses are said to occur in depressive personalities who, since childhood, have tended to set unreliable perfectionistic goals followed by withdrawn behavior and with hopelessness, envy, and repressed rage; (2) schizophrenic illnesses are reported to occur in disorganized personalities who, since childhood, have lacked clarity and conviction about inner needs and realistic goals, who too quickly have experienced confusion in the face of the unexpected, and who have used unworkable behaviors to meet daily situations. In a number of experimental studies developmental psychologists have shown that children function best when environmental stimuli conform to the child's expectations and when the child is encouraged to have aspirations that are, in fact, capable of being fulfilled. In several studies parents of disturbed offspring have been found to have disorders of thinking, perception, and attention which may make it difficult for them to present meaningful and consistent views of experience to their children.

PERSONALITY DEVELOPMENT

The outer limits of personal capabilities and sensitivities as well as certain general temperamental tendencies (energy level, degree of passivity or activity in relationships, intellectual power, sensitivity to emotional arousal, and so on) are assumed to be set-

Table 3. Stages of personality development

Age	Stage	Developmental issues*
0-3 mo.	Neonatal	Psychophysiological patterning and maternal management of infant's tension; basis for autonomic stability or instability
3-6 mo.	Preattachment	Visual and auditory recognition; familiarity responses and strangeness anxiety begin; sociability and smiling; basis for trust or distrust
6-12 mo.	Attachment	Interpersonal vocalization; selective demand for mother; separation anxiety begins; basis for hope or hopelessness
1-2½ yr.	Early individuation (anal)	Walking, toilet training, exploration, verbalization, self-assertiveness, anxiety over self-control; basis for autonomy or doubt
2½-4 yr.	Late individuation (phallic)	Mastery of own body, communication, imaginative production; basis for socialized conscience or punitive and defective superego formation

*The terms listed are intended to indicate only in a general way a few salient intrapsychic, behavioral, and psychosocial changes characteristic of but not limited to each stage.

tled by the arrangement of genes at the moment of conception. Predisposition to inherited disorders is also settled or influenced at this time. During fetal life it is known that certain maternal physiological influences can have an impact on later personality. Pavlovian conditioning can take place in the fetus. Disorders such as maternal rubella, placenta previa, and toxemia of pregnancy are associated with an increased incidence of cerebral palsy, epilepsy, mental retardation, and childhood behavior disorders. Prematurity or perinatal cyanosis, anoxia, or high neonatal serum bilirubin levels from any cause are also associated with these conditions.

Personality development can best be thought of as a series of life's stages (Table 3), in each of which specific adaptive changes usually occur. During the initial 3 to 6 weeks of life infants vary considerably in arousal level and sleepiness, in intensity of

Table 3. Stages of personality development—cont'd

Age	Stage	Developmental issues
4-7 yr.	Oedipal	Learning to read; family role definition; basis of comfortable sex identification or castration anxiety and penis envy
7-9 yr.	Latency	Industry and work habits, attainment of concrete logical thinking, role in school and neighborhood, friendships; basis for self-esteem or sense of inferiority
9-12 yr.	Preadolescence	Discipline of memory, attainment of abstract logic, gang and clique formation, homoerotic exploration
12-16 yr.	Early adolescence	Puberty, disillusionment with family myths, intellectual autonomy, and availability of complex or intuitive judgment
16-20 yr.	Late adolescence	Identity formation, career choice, esthetic and religious preference, heterosexual relationships
20-30 yr.	Early adulthood	Intimacy, commitment to parenthood, worldly competition
30-65 yr.	Maturity	Social responsibility, generativity, leadership
Over 65 yr.	Old age	Integrity or despair

hunger, in social responsiveness, in their sensitivity to contact, taste, smell, postural change, sights, and sounds. The principal developmental change here is the *stabilization of vital functions* of eating, sleeping, and tension management through rocking, stroking, bathing, and comforting sounds. If a reasonably stable relationship occurs between a comfortable, intelligent, and observant mother and an infant who has no unusual sensitivities or tendencies to tension buildup and overreactivity, a sound basis for later development is provided. In a similar fashion each later developmental stage has primary change processes. An infant or child may begin early to show his characteristic mode of dealing with new situations, a mode that may become a lifelong style of personality. Kagan and Moss, for example, show that passive, inhibited infants predict dependent unassertive young adults. Studies now have demonstrated that immediately after birth males and females have a different repertoire of response styles. With the maturation of new abilities, however, or with the occurrence of serious conflict at a later developmental stage, the style of personality may be altered considerably.

Careful observation of newborn infants has identified the presence of expressive behavior patterns, including smiling, although the social smile is first seen in most infants between 3 and 7 weeks of age. By 3 to 4 months considerable perceptual competence has developed and sensorimotor coordination of the fingers, hands, eyes, mouth, and head is seen. About this time the infant can begin to notice the difference between the familiar and the unfamiliar. A strange object appearing before him may lead to an anxious sobering. By 5 or 8 months of age "stranger anxiety proper" develops in some infants, presumably indicating that the infant now can perceive clearly the difference between his family and strange persons. It is assumed that during the second 6 months of life the infant clarifies the difference between the inside and outside of his body and between himself and other persons. This comes about as the infant attaches himself more and more specifically to his mother. He may begin in the third 6 months of life to experience increasing separation anxiety when she is away from his presence.

Between 9 and 14 months of age the child stands and shortly thereafter begins to walk. In the subsequent developmental period of 12 to 15 months the child for the first time is prevented from carrying out his goals (stopped from knocking over things) and begins to hear "No." This development facilitates his capacity not only to differentiate perceptually between himself and others (a capacity presumed to have appeared at about 2 to 3 months of age) but also to deal with himself as a separate person and to treat his own impulses with some beginning objectivity. From 18 to 36 months, cognitive capacities and early interpersonal patterns emerge, particularly focused about control of bowel and locomotor functions and about the pleasure in manipulating and sensing the diversity of the physical world. Language capacity matures and the use of fantasy play becomes a major mode for self-expression and for internalization of new learnings about family life. From 4 to 7 years of age the child experiences with intense affect the forces of love and anger and the habitual family defenses against anxiety, and he may attempt to exert his or her own powers to intervene in sibling or parental transactions. A phase of overestimation of his own power to seduce or to overwhelm other family members gives way to a more realistic self-appraisal, except in the instance of an emotionally disturbed youngster. This facilitates movement of the child into the community, via school, and the gradual attenuation through the next few years of the intense family bonds set up in the earliest period of life.

In recent years developmental psychologists have noted that the child develops in a healthy manner when the home and social environment do not contain too many contradictions and when the environment supports the development of new capacities in the child that are appropriate to his age. Certain environmental requirements may be stated for each developmental stage. For example, 3- to 4-year-old children are generally more responsive to and rewarded by women than by men; 6- or 7-year-old children tend to be rewarded more by the opposite sex parent, and at least for a larger group of children, as they grow older, the same sex parent tends to function as the model and as the person who shapes behavior. Social class and subcultural differences are important here. In middle-class families in industrial countries the child's aggression tends to be disciplined by the same sex parent, whereas in families in which the father is unskilled the mother expects him to be the disciplinarian for all the children and expects herself to be the nurturant support.

In *Three Contributions to the Theory of Sex,* Freud schematized these complex developments by the concepts of *oral, anal,* and *phallic* phases of *pregenital development.* The classic Freudian position has been that during each phase a primary instinctual impulse strives for discharge. Each impulse has a specific *aim* (the act, such as sucking, which would provide a mode of discharge and pleasurable reduction of tension), a specific *object* (the breast), and a specific *source* (the erogenous zone—in the oral phase, the mouth of the infant). On the basis of Freudian theory, you would assume that character traits referable to trust, self-confidence, narcissism, and autoeroticism have been dealt with in the oral phase (age 0 to 18 months); that traits of ambivalence, orderliness or sloppiness, punctuality, definance, submission, and impulse control have been dealt with in the anal phase (age 18 months to 3 years); and that in the phallic phase (age 3 to 5 years), in which the child is preoccupied with the significance of having or not having a penis (the *castration complex*), traits of sexual identity or fears, self-esteem, sex role definition, and social facility would begin to be salient. On the basis of the form these early pregenital experiences take and, in particular, upon the manner in which the child resolves them for himself during the *oedipal period* (age 4 to 7 years), the superego is said to be formed. This intrapsychic agency, contained within the ego, represents those aspects of the parental images which the child takes as his own lifelong automatic guideposts to moral and social values.

During *preadolescence* the individual becomes more effective as a worker and strives for the first time to achieve some individuality and intimacy outside the family with his peers. It is usual at this period for the child to find a confidant of the same sex with whom he explores and tests many questions about life. Homosexual experiences are normal here.

With the advent of *adolescence,* an internal upheaval is brought about by the biological pressure of sexual maturation and the social pressure to become emancipated from the family. The ensuing struggle to find a new psychological equilibrium tests the strength of earlier ego development and normally produces, to some degree, symptoms which in the adult would be judged neurotic.

The young family man or woman faces genuine testing of abilities to take economic and emotional responsibilities for others. Here a degree of self-centeredness or self-love *(narcissism),* which may have been consistent with outward mental health in earlier years, can lead to trouble. Or, if chronic tendencies to misperceive reality or to mistrust oneself or others remain, the increasingly intimate and complex relationships at home and at work will be stressful and lead to symptoms.

Finally, as the mature individual grows older, sufficient self-respect and autonomy must have developed to permit the natural social and biological changes of approaching senescence to be accepted with calm (as in serene old age) rather than alarm (as in involutional melancholia).

At any stage of life, disorganizing symptoms may appear for the first time. But the clinician, upon sensitive and careful inquiry into the patient's past, will note lifelong trends in reacting to certain types of events as though they were threatening; he will see that the patient—instead of solving certain types of problems—finds it necessary to bring into play some pathological defense mechanisms. Thus, though symptoms may have been absent, the overuse of certain defense mechanisms has heralded potential mental illness for years.

Prominent characteristics in the developmental pattern are summarized in Table 3.

MECHANISMS OF DEFENSE

A well-adjusted individual frequently reaches conclusions and resolves conflictual situations through a rational consideration and weighing of the facts before making his decision. The person who is emotionally disabled and finds conflicts very anxiety-provoking seeks to escape from the dilemma through one or a variety of behavioral gambits that have been termed "mechanisms of defense." While such mechanisms are clearly seen in psychoneurotics and psychotics, they also exist to some degree in everyone. Such patterns of action, if commonly used, may "character-ize" the individual who comes to rely upon them more or less automatically for handling his anxieties and in resolving interpersonal problems. For such reasons it is useful to have knowledge of these psychological mechanisms that are called upon for the self-defense of the person in times of conflict.

compensation Mechanism in which an approved or admirable character trait is developed to conceal either the absence of some other or the presence of an opposite one. The latter may exist only in the uncon-

scious. A person who has no capacity as an athlete may compensate in
scholarship.

complex formation Interassociation of a number of related or even unrelated ideas in the unconscious, in such a way that any threat to one
brings out the emotional tone and defense of the whole.

condensation Expression of a whole group of ideas with a single word,
phrase, or thought.

conversion Attempt to keep a disturbing wish from realization through
inhibition of motor and/or sensory activities—either partial (blindness, paralysis) or complete (generalized paralysis or refusal to
move).

denial No acknowledgement of a disturbing reality situation or intense
inner affect. Mutually incompatible thoughts can exist side by side in
logic-tight compartments or be completely *isolated* as in circumscribed amnesia.

displacement Substitution of a different object upon whom affect is then
centered or released. The emotional investment (cathexis) is transferred from the unacceptable ideas to other, associated ideas that can
appear in consciousness without causing anxiety.

dissociation Separation in which one idea or several groups of ideas become split off from the main body of thought. Dissociated ideas are not
accessible to consciousness.

dreaming Represssed material appears and conflicts are "worked through"
or solved in one's dreams.

fantasy identification One adapts or patterns behavior after that of an image
or ego ideal whose behavior one admires.

inhibition In an inhibition the aim or goal of an instinctual drive is modified but the original drive is satisfied to some extent. Thus a desire in
the child for sexual relations with a parent may change to an attitude of
love or respect in which there is no overt sexuality.

introjection The object is, as it were, ingested by the mind so that the
psychic energies of the ego appear to be organized as if they were
under the control of the introject. The experience of a feared or a desired person being inside the self.

introversion Introversion occurs when a person withdraws from environmental context and indulges in excessive fantasy. This is usually followed by marked regression.

isolation The impulse to action, the thought, or the act is isolated from the
associated affect and the wider associations connected with it. The
thought, for example, is conscious but minus the distressing associations or affect. This defense is found in obsessional neurosis.

projection. Displacement of one's wishes, fears, or desires upon another
person.

reaction formation Transformation of one drive into seemingly the exact

opposite, as in expressing extreme consideration toward one for whom
hostile feelings are held.

regression Abandonment of mature behavior patterns for increasingly immature or infantile ones. Extreme retreat into fantasy life *(autism)* can
lead to escape from upsetting realities through *delusion formation.*

repression Total exclusion of the idea from consciousness.

somatization Conflict is repressed and becomes represented by physical
symptoms involving parts of the body innervated by the autonomic
nervous system.

sublimation Substitution of a more socially acceptable activity for one that
is unacceptable.

symbolization An object or an act represents a complex group of objects or
acts.

undoing The disturbing thought or action is allowed to occur and is then
followed by the opposite throught or act, which cancels the effect of the
first thought or act in a magical way. This mechanism is especially seen
in obsessions and compulsions.

ROLE OF DEFENSES IN SYMPTOM FORMATION

Defense mechanisms are utilized to some extent by all persons
in their day-to-day living but are seen in extreme form in mental
disorder, where frequently one type of mechanism, used predominantly, fosters a symptom picture characteristic for that disorder.

In many adult patients it appears that the current life situation
has evoked long-forgotten, unresolved anxieties from an earlier
period, which in turn foster inappropriate defenses and symptom
formation. Thus, for example, the complex emotional attachment
to the first object of one's affection, mother, with its attendant fluctuating, mixed (ambivalent) feelings toward father, who threatens
or at least partly usurps that mother love, is often never fully understood or solved by the child. If this occurs, the unacceptable (to
society and the superego) feelings of love and hostility (Oedipus
complex) are repressed instead of accepted. At a later time, under
the pressure of similar affectionate feelings toward an adult lover
or similar competitive feelings toward a business rival, anxiety
may be experienced; in psychoanalytic theory this is considered to
stem from the fact that in the early family situation these similar
feelings, instead of being accepted and mastered, were repressed.

When such anxiety related to repressed complexes occurs,
symptoms or behaviors appear which are determined in part by

the defense employed. For example, with *reaction formation* the individual may feel a need to be excessively considerate of and polite to his rival; or the offending feelings might be *displaced* and experienced openly in relation to political figures or chance or distant acquaintances rather than in relation to their real human object. If the anxiety were to be dealt with still more pathologically, perhaps compulsive acts, obsessive thoughts, or delusions might become related in the patient's mind to the rival or lover.

SUGGESTED READINGS

Blos, P.: On adolescence, New York, 1962, The Free Press of Glencoe, Inc.

Bowlby, J.: Nature of the child's tie to his mother, Int. J. Psychoanal. **39:**350, 1958.

Erikson, E. H.: Childhood and society, ed. 2, New York, 1963, W. W. Norton & Co., Inc.

Fenichel, O.: Outlines of clinical psychoanalysis, New York, 1934, W. W. Norton & Co., Inc.

Freud, A.: The ego and the mechanisms of defense, London, 1937, The Hofarth Press.

Freud, A.: Concept of developmental lines, psychoanalytic study of the child, New York, 1963, International Universities Press, Inc.

Hartmann, H.: Ego psychology and the problem of adaptation, New York, 1958, International Universities Press, Inc.

Kagan, J., and Moss, H.: Birth to maturity, New York, 1962, John Wiley & Sons, Inc.

Kessen, W., and Kuhlman, C.: Thought in the young child, Monogr. Soc. Res. Child Develop. **27**(2):3, 1962.

Piaget, J.: Play, dreams and imitation in childhood, New York, 1962, W. W. Norton & Co., Inc.

Rapaport, D.: Structure of psychoanalytic theory, Psychol. Issues **2:**1, 1960.

Vaillant, G. E.: Natural history of male psychosocial health, Arch. Gen. Psychiatry **33:**535, 1976.

Vaillant, G. E.: Theoretical hierarchy of adaptive ego mechanisms, Arch. Gen. Psychiatry **24:**107, 1971.

9

Symptoms of psychiatric disorders

Behavior, both normal and pathological, derives from sources which include instinctual and hereditary drives, as well as environmentally and socially determined forces. *Instincts* have been defined as inherited neuronal (probably diencephalic) patterns of behavior, which are present at birth and which alter with growth, cerebral myelinization, hormonal development, and the modifying impact of intellect and acquired social patterns. *Emotion* accompanies and colors behavior as a result of the facilitation and impeding of instinctual drives. *Conation* is the inherent urge to all activity, mental as well as physical; its level varies widely from sluggish to hypomanic but is characteristic for any individual throughout his life.

Consciousness can be defined as the organism's capacity to react to stimuli and is displayed in degrees of awareness or *attention* to the surrounding environment. The five senses serve as means for *perception* of all sensory stimuli, which are *recognized* or identified in terms of previous experiences. Such recognized sensations are organized into *concepts* which, subject to intelligence, judgment, and wisdom, are put into function through *motor action*. *Will* is the crystallization of cognition and thought that leads to behavior. *Personality* is the resultant picture of all the habitual patterns displayed by the individual, from a fusion of his genetic endowment and the sum of experiential modifications. A wide variety of normal variations and the combination of behavioral symptoms make up identifiable character types and form the basis for clinical syndromes.

Many different terms have been used to describe the infinite variety of symptoms that are the *psychopathology* of mental disorders. Some of these are but adaptational adjustments that may occur to a lesser degree in the coping behavior of normal persons. Others are the florid manifestations of a malfunctioning brain. Although usually described as disturbances of "separate functions of the mind," it is well to remember that because the organism functions as a whole this designation is merely a convenient fiction.

DISORDERS OF PERCEPTION

The avenues of perception include sight, hearing, touch, taste, and smell—of which the disorders are classically *illusions* and *hallucinations*. An *illusion* is a false interpretation or misinterpretation of a real sight, sound, or other sensation. It may express a hoped for or feared event or be simply the result of a delirious, toxic, or febrile state. A *hallucination* is a false perception for which there exists no actual sensory basis. So-called *pseudo hallucinations, hypnagogic* and *hypnopompic hallucinations* occur while persons are falling asleep and awakening, respectively. These lack the vividness and clarity of *true hallucinations.* Most common are hallucinations of hearing. The auditory type may be *elementary hallucinations,* consisting of noise and music, or more complex *hallucinatory voices (phonemes).* Special cases include *"Gedankenlautwerden,"* in which the patient hears his own thoughts spoken aloud, and *functional hallucinations,* with the phonemes occurring only if there is some external source of noise (e.g., running water). *Hallucinations of vision* may be elementary, consisting only of flashes of light, or be more organized (persons and things) in flashback memories, and even *mass hallucinations* of groups of persons in active scenes. In *heautoscopy ("Doppelgänger")* the subject sees and recognizes himself. *Extracampine hallucinations* are ones identified as outside the visual field (e.g., "behind me"). Other visual hallucinatory experiences include *macropsia,* seeing things enlarged, and *micropsia (lilliputian hallucinations)* in which things seem smaller. *Hallucinations of smell* are usually of disagreeable and noxious odors, while *hallucinations of taste* often refer to poisons "and dope in the food." *Hallucinations of touch* are often interpreted as insects crawling over the skin (e.g., cocaine bug) but may involve *sexual hallucinations* of erection, orgasm, etc. *Hallucinations of deep sensation* and of *vestibular sensation* include feelings such as twisting or flying. A special case of hallucinations is that of *phantom limb"* arising from sensations of an amputated stump. So-called *negative hallucinations* in which something present is perceived as being absent occur in hysteria and as a phenomenon readily demonstrated under hypnosis.

SUGGESTED READINGS

Charlton, M. H.: Visual hallucinations, Psychiatr. Q. **37**:487, 1963.

Egdell, H. G., and Kolven, I.: Childhood hallucinations, J. Child Psychol. Psychiatry **13**:279, 1972.

Gallinek, A.: The phantom limb: its origin and its relationship to the hallucinations of psychotic states, Am. J. Psychiatry **96**:413, 1939.

Havens, L. L.: The placement and movement of hallucinations in space: phenomenology and theory, Int. J. Psychoanal. **43**:426, 1962.

McDonald, C.: A clinical study of hypnagogic hallucinations, Br. J. Psychiatry **118**:543, 1971.

Siegal, R. K.: Cocaine hallucinations, Am. J. Psychiatry **135**:309, 1978.

Siegel, R. K., and West, L. J., editors: Hallucinations: behavior, experience and theory, New York, 1975, John Wiley & Sons, Inc.

DISORDERS OF CONSCIOUSNESS, ORIENTATION, AND ATTENTION

These disorders are closely related to those of perception. *Apperception*, for instance, is the comprehension of what is perceived, or perception supplemented by *recognition* and *interpretation*. The ability to perceive and apperceive depends upon the *state of attention* or focusing ability, which may be hyperactive *(startle) distractible*, easily diverted, or tenaciously adherent to some single stimulus. *Confusion* is a state of impairment of the sensorium which can vary all the way from a slight *clouding of consciousness* to a deep *stupor*. The term *coma* refers to a profound degree of unconsciousness from which the patient cannot be aroused and which usually results from some general organic or cerebral condition. *Disturbances of orientation* (time, place, and person) are those in which the patient does not know where he is, what time it is, or how to identify himself and those around him. This most often occurs with states of toxic delirium but can be seen in *dream states* of psychogenic or unknown origin. Sometimes listed under alteration of consciousness are states of *heightened suggestibility* and *negativism;* in the former the subject is influenced with uncritical acceptance, as in hypnosis and some types of "folie à deux," but in the latter any suggestion produces just the opposite reaction.

DISORDERS OF MEMORY

Disorders of memory involve the mechanisms for the reception and registration of ideas, for their retention, and for later recall and reproduction. These mechanisms show three major types of disorders: *hypermnesia, amnesia,* and *paramnesia.* Hypermnesia is an abnormal mnemonic capacity seen in mild manic and paranoid conditions. The term *amnesia* refers to a loss of memory. In *organic amnesia,* as for example in the aging brain, *recent memory* may be lost while memory for remote past events is retained. In *psychogenic amnesia* recall is inhibited for psychological reasons. There may be a *generalized* or a *selective* type of amnesia in which inconvenient events or topics are forgotten. *Anterograde amnesia* is one that continues progressively, parallel with ongoing activity in which the subject appears to act normally but later has no recollection of his behavior. In *retrograde amnesia* the loss of memory extends backward, as for a period preceding trauma to the head. *Paramnesia* refers to a falsification of memory, commonly observed in Korsakoff's syndrome as *confabulation* in which the patient simply fills in the gaps of his memory by fabrications which have no basis in fact. *Retrospective falsification* occurs when the patient unconsciously distorts or "embroiders" his memories of past life experiences in response to some emotional needs. The illusion of memory known as "déjà vu" refers to a false feeling of familiarity for some new scene; "jamais vu" is the term for a false feeling of unfamiliarity.

SUGGESTED READING

Arlow, J. A.: The structure of the déjà vu experience, J. Am. Psychoanal. Assoc. 7:611, 1959.

DISORDERS OF THINKING

The production of *rational thinking* is complicated business and depends upon the smooth coordinated functioning of very complicated brain mechanisms. Even at best, "normal humans" show frequent lapses from logic *(parapraxis);* and as Freud pointed out in his *Psychopathology of Everyday Life,* emotion is commonly betrayed *(lapsus linguae)* and can interfere with intellectual functioning. When thinking is obviously guided by processes byond awareness and finds its origin in complexes, wishes, and other motivations not under conscious recognition, it is called *autistic* or *dereistic thought.* Disturbances in *progression* of thought *(stream of thought)* include *flight of ideas,* in which one thought follows another in quick succession but with little progress toward a single goal idea. This may be associated with an inner-push *distractibility* and often involves words having a similar sound *(clang associations).* In the opposite vein, speech and thinking may be *retarded* or manifest *blocking* with sudden obstructions, which may be removed as suddenly as they appeared. In schizophrenics there may be *fragmentation* or *scattering* of speech to the point of incoherence; thoughts may be so *tangential* as to be barely related to each other, or entirely new and unusual words *(neologisms, word salad)* may be produced. *Perseveration* occurs when an idea is abnormally repeated and continued, particularly in the retarded, epileptic, or senile. *Circumstantiality* occurs when a person's sequence of spoken words unnecessarily elaborates trivial details. In persons less disabled one finds evidence of extreme *volubility (logorrhea)* and in some a tendency to brood over abstract matters or take refuge in scientific terms *(intellectualization).* Belief that specific thoughts can lead to the fulfillment of wishes or can ward off evil *(magical* or *superstitious thinking)* is found commonly in children and in less sophisticated cultures. Disturbances in the content of thought include preoccupation *(trends)* and overdetermined ideas resulting more from affective factors than from logical reasoning. Ideas that persistently thrust themselves into consciousness are termed *obsessions.* Allied to these are *phobias, fears, doubts,* and *indecisions. Fantasy* occurs in the form of ideas that are hoped for but recognized as unreal. *Pseudologia fantastica* is different from normal *daydreams* in that the patient *(impostor* and *pathological liar)* believes his ideas sufficiently to act upon them. A *delusion* is a false belief not founded upon logical inference and one which cannot be corrected by adequate proof of its falsity. Most common are *delusions of persecution* in which the patient believes that various persons or forces are attempting to harm or manipulate him with hostile intent. Such beliefs may be vague and poorly organized *(unsystematized delusions)* or may be in the form of an elaborate fixed or systematized delusion. Closely related to these are *ideas of reference,* in which the patient falsely interprets remarks and actions of people around him as ridiculing or depreciatory of him. *Litigious behavior* may occur, with the involvement of lawyers and courts. A commonly related everyday phenomenon is *pathological jealousy.* Patients who feel they have great powers, religious significance, or special identity demonstrate *delusions of grandeur.* Patients heavily burdened with feelings of unworthiness develop delusions of *self-accusation,* ideas of guilt, sin, poverty, and the like. *Delusions of disease* arise from extreme hypochondriasis.

DISORDERS OF AFFECT

Disorders of *affect* constitute a large segment of mental illness with changes in emotion or *feeling tone.* (The term *mood* is used for sustained affect). *Depression* is a state of melancholy in which the patient views the world around him with sadness and pessimism. Depression as a symptom occurs in all degrees and with many types of psychiatric illness. *Anaclitic depression* refers to depression in infants who have been deprived of a suitable mother figure. The exact opposite of depression are states of *pleasurable affect, elation, euphoria, hypomania,* and *mania. Exaltation* merges into *ecstasy* as the peak of rapture and is seen in acute schizophrenia with states of religious mysticism. *Ambivalence* refers to the simultaneous coexistence of antithetical emotions, ideas, or wishes toward, and at the same time away from, a given object or situation. Particularly in schizophrenia, affect may appear to be *flat* (absence of feeling tone) or it may be *inappropriate* to the situation (e.g., giggles without reason). *Depersonalization* occurs when the patient has a feeling that things around him seem "unreal" or that the world has undergone a profound change. *Anxiety* is a feeling of apprehension and uneasiness. If it cannot be attributed to any particular idea or object it is labeled "*free-floating anxiety.*" *Tension* is prolonged anxiety. *Panic* is severe overwhelming anxiety which can lead to terror and utter disorganization.

DISORDERS OF THE MOTOR ASPECT OF BEHAVIOR

Behavior disorders may show themselves as disturbances of *conation* or *volition* and *will, attitudes,* and *disposition* toward carrying out some behavior; as *ambivalence* in making decisions; and in aggressive displays of hostility from frustration and "pent-up" emotions. *Motor behavior* may be increased *(drivenness)* or decreased *psychomotor retardation, painful effort).* Repetitious activities include *stereotypy* (persistent repetition) and *automatic obedience (echopraxia*—imitation of the movement of others—or *echolalia*—repetition of the phases of others). *Cerea flexibilitas* describes a high degree of susceptibility in which the subject's limbs may be molded like wax into any position. *Grimaces, tics, peculiarities of gait,* and *other types of mannerisms* occur. *Compulsions* are morbid and often irresistible urges to perform certain acts. *Negativism* refers to a refusal to do what is asked or even a performance of the exact opposite. The term *aversion* refers not simply to passive unwillingness but rather to self-assertive negative reaction characterized by sullen uncooperativeness.

In addition to all the above there may be seen disturbances in appearance, decoration, dress, demeanor, and, indeed, the total life pattern, including the patient's relationship to family, work, and society and his attitudes toward many aspects of the community in which he lives. From these symptoms are derived patterns of behavior, the syndromes of specific diagnosable mental illnesses.

SUGGESTED READINGS

Climent, E. C., Plutchik, R., Estrada, H., Gavina, L., and Arevalo, W.: A comparison of traditional and symptom-checklist based histories, Am. J. Psychiatry **132**:450, 1975.

Kolb, L. C.: Modern clinical psychiatry, ed. 9, Philadelphia, 1977, W. B. Saunders Co.

Nicholi, A. M.: History and mental status. In Nicholi, A. M., editor: The Harvard guide to modern clinical psychiatry, Cambridge, 1978, Belknap Press of Harvard University Press.

Spitzer, R. L., Fleiss, J. L., Burdock, E. I., and Hardesty, A. S.: The mental status schedule—rationale, reliability, and validity, Compr. Psychiatry **5**:384, 1964.

Stevenson, I.: The psychiatric examination, Boston, 1968, Little, Brown and Co.

II

CLINICAL SYNDROMES

10

Problem of classification

The classification of mental disorders is based upon a description of behavioral symptoms and varies over the years with changes in psychological theory. The terms "psychosis" and "neurosis" have been used to dichotomize serious and "major" from less serious or "minor" psychiatric disorders, respectively. Such dichotomy is misleading, as many chronic neurotic disorders are more crippling than some transient psychotic states. The concept of psychosis, traditionally similar to the legal term "insanity," usually implies an emotional (mental) illness whose seriousness is measured by behavior so unacceptable as to necessitate the withdrawal of social privileges. The concept, however, applies not only to the popularly conceived, chronic hallucinatory, delusional, and withdrawn states but also to fleeting states of mental incompetence such as the deliria which accompany various infectious, metabolic, and toxic ills.

A group of behavioral disturbances which interfere to no catastrophic extent with social functions are called *psychoneuroses*. In these disorders the symptoms may include anxiety, depression, obsessions, or fears, as well as a host of autonomic disturbances. Where the symptomatology is primarily visceral in nature, the terms "organ neurosis" and "psychophysiological disorder" have been applied.

The category *psychopath* was once used as the wastebasket of psychiatry. Cases of dubious diagnosis not clearly psychotic or psychoneurotic were often classified under this heading. More frequently, now, the term "psychopath" is used to refer only to asocial or antisocial behavior disorders classed under the term "sociopathic" personality disorder. The concept *personality disorder* is now used for a category within which the classic psychopath is but one type.

Each patient's mental disorder is a highly individual affair. Often exact categorization of an individual case is so fraught with difficulty as to appear impossible. If followed over a period of time, the patient may seem to pass from one diagnostic category into another. With some reservations, however, categorization of mental disorder proves useful in estimating the type of risk and problems likely to be encountered in planning therapy and in judging prognosis.

It should be borne in mind that a single dramatic symptom taken by itself can lead to erroneous diagnosis. Depression and anxiety can occur to some extent in many mental disorders, and the occurrence of paranoid symptomatology does not always mean schizophrenia, as paranoid delusions may occur also in general paresis, involutional or senile psychosis, acute alcoholic hallucinosis, and other conditions.

In understanding the production of behavioral abnormalities, the roles of genetic predisposition, organ dysfunctions, and the exogenous and endogenous toxins must be emphasized, as well as social tensions, defects in family social structure or environmental attitudes, and traumatic childhood experiences. The complex interplay of these factors must be grasped by the psychiatrist; who therefore finds it impossible to settle upon a single etiological factor to explain any behavior disorder.

The standard nomenclature of mental disorders is revised approximately every 10 years. The terms used in the third edition of the *Diagnostic and Statistical Manual* as prepared by the American Psychiatric Association (DSM III) differ considerably from those of DSM II which have been in general use. To assist with the transition in terminology, we have reproduced both classifications in Chapter 11.

SUGGESTED READINGS

Blashfield, R. K., and Draguns, J. G.: Toward a taxonomy of psychopathology: the purpose of psychiatric classification, Br. J. Psychiatry **129:**574, 1976.

Cooper, J. E., Kendell, R. E., Gurland, B. J., Sartorious, N., and Farkas, T.: Cross-national study of diagnosis of mental disorders: some results in the first comparative investigation, A. J. Psychiatry **125:**21, 1969.

Diagnostic and statistical manual of mental disorders, ed. 2, Washington, D. C., 1968, American Psychiatric Association.

Diagnostic and statistical manual of mental disorders, ed. 3, Washington, D.C., 1979, American Psychiatric Association.

Falek, A., and Moser, H. M.: Classification in schizophrenia, Arch. Gen. Psychiatry **32**(1):59, January 1975.

Feighner, J. P., Robins, E., Guze, S. B., and others: Diagnostic criteria for use in psychiatric research, Arch. Gen. Psychiatry **26:**57, 1972.

Fish, F.: A guide to the Leonhard classification of chronic schizophrenia, Psychiatr. Q. **38:**438, 1964.

Helzer, J. E., Clayton, P. J., Pambakian, R., and others: Reliability of psychiatric diagnosis. II. The test/retest reliability of diagnostic classification, Arch. Gen. Psychiatry **34:**136, 1977.

Katz, M. M., Cole, J. O., and Lowery, H. A.: Studies of the diagnostic process, Am. J. Psychiatry **125:**937, 1969.

Kendell, R. E.: The classification of depressions: a review of contemporary confusion, Br. J. Psychiatry **129:**15, 1976.

Koehler, K., and Steigerwald, F.: Consistency of Kurt Schneider-oriented diagnosis over 40 years, Arch. Gen. Psychiatry **34:**51, 1977.

Kuriansky, J. B., Gurland, B. J., and Spitzer, R. L.: Trends in the frequency of schizophrenia by different diagnostic criteria, Am. J. Psychiatry **134:**631, 1977.

Spitzer, R. L.: More on pseudoscience in science and the case for psychiatric diagnosis, Arch. Gen. Psychiatry **33:**459, 1976.

Spitzer, R. L., Endicott, J., and Robins, E.: Research diagnostic criteria (RDC), New York, 1974, State Department of Mental Hygiene.

Tseng, W. S., Arensdorf, A. M., McDermott, J. F., Jr., and others: Family diagnosis and classification, J. Am. Acad. Child Psychiatry **15**(1):15, Winter 1976.

Woodruff, R. A., Goodwin, D. W. and Guze, S. B.: Psychiatric diagnosis, New York, 1974, Oxford University Press.

11

Standard nomenclature of mental disorders

CLASSIFICATION OF DSM II

The following is the classification of DSM II, adapted from *Diagnostic and Statistical Manual of Mental Disorders*, ed. 2, Washington, D.C., 1968, American Psychiatric Association.

I. ORGANIC BRAIN SYNDROMES (O.B.S.)
A. PSYCHOSES

Senile and presenile dementia

290.0	Senile dementia
290.1	Presenile dementia

Alcoholic psychosis

291.0	Delirium tremens
291.1	Korsakoff's psychosis
291.2	Other alcoholic hallucinosis
291.3	Alcoholic paranoid state
291.4	Acute alcoholic intoxication
291.5	Alcoholic deterioration
291.6	Pathological intoxication
291.9	Other alcoholic psychosis

Psychosis associated with intracranial infection

292.0	General paralysis
292.1	Syphilis of central nervous system
292.2	Epidemic encephalitis
292.3	Other and unspecified encephalitis
292.9	Other intracranial infection

Psychosis associated with other cerebral condition

293.0	Cerebral arteriosclerosis
293.1	Other cerebravascular disturbance
293.2	Epilepsy
293.3	Intracranial neoplasm
293.4	Degenerative disease of the C.N.S.
293.5	Brain trauma
293.9	Other cerebral condition

Psychosis associated with other physical condition

294.0	Endocrine disorder
294.1	Metabolic and nutritional disorder
294.2	Systemic infection
294.3	Drug or poison intoxication (other than alcohol)
294.4	Childbirth
294.8	Other and unspecified physical condition

B. NONPSYCHOTIC O.B.S.

309.0	Intracranial infection
309.13	Alcohol (simple drunkenness)
309.14	Other drug, poison, or systemic intoxication
309.2	Brain trauma
309.3	Circulatory disturbance
309.4	Epilepsy
309.5	Disturbance of metabolism, growth, or nutrition
309.6	Senile or presenile brain disease
309.7	Intracranial neoplasm
309.8	Degenerative diseases of the C.N.S.
309.9	Other physical condition

II. PSYCHOSES NOT ATTRIBUTED TO PHYSICAL CONDITIONS LISTED PREVIOUSLY

Major affective disorders

296.0	Involutional melancholia
296.1	Manic-depressive illness, manic
296.2	Manic-depressive illness, depressed
296.3	Manic-depressive illness, circular
296.33	Manic-depressive, circular, manic
296.34	Manic-depressive, circular, depressed
296.8	Other major affective disorder

Schizophrenia

295.0	Simple
295.1	Hebephrenic
295.2	Catatonic
295.23	Catatonic type, excited

Schizophrenia—cont'd

295.24	Catatonic type, withdrawn
295.3	Paranoid
295.4	Acute schizophrenic episode
295.5	Latent
295.6	Residual
295.7	Schizoaffective
295.73	Schizoaffective, excited
295.74	Schizoaffective, depressed
295.8	Childhood
295.90	Chronic undifferentiated
295.99	Other schizophrenia

Paranoid states

297.0	Paranoia
297.1	Involutional paranoid state
297.9	Other paranoid state

Other psychoses

298.0	Psychotic depressive reaction

III. NEUROSES

300.0	Anxiety
300.1	Hysterical
300.13	Hysterical, conversion type
300.14	Hysterical, dissociative type
300.2	Phobic
300.3	Obsessive compulsive
300.4	Depressive
300.5	Neurasthenic
300.6	Depersonalization
300.7	Hypochondriacal
300.8	Other neurosis

IV. PERSONALITY DISORDERS AND CERTAIN OTHER NONPSYCHOTIC MENTAL DISORDERS

Personality disorders

301.0	Paranoid
301.1	Cyclothymic
301.2	Schizoid
301.3	Explosive
301.4	Obsessive compulsive
301.5	Hysterical
301.6	Asthenic
301.7	Antisocial
301.81	Passive-aggressive

| 301.82 | Inadequate |
| 301.89 | Other specified types |

Sexual deviation

302.0	Homosexuality
302.1	Fetishism
302.2	Pedophilia
302.3	Transvestitism
302.4	Exhibitionism
302.5	Voyeurism
302.6	Sadism
302.7	Masochism
302.8	Other sexual deviation

Alcoholism

303.0	Episodic excessive drinking
303.1	Habitual excessive drinking
303.2	Alcohol addiction
303.9	Other alcoholism

Drug dependence

304.0	Opium, opium alkaloids, and their derivatives
304.1	Synthetic analgesics with morphinelike effects
304.2	Barbiturates
304.3	Other hypnotics and sedatives or tranquilizers
304.4	Cocaine
304.5	Cannabis sativa (hashish, marihuana)
304.6	Other psychostimulants
304.7	Hallucinogens
304.8	Other drug dependence

V. PSYCHOPHYSIOLOGICAL DISORDERS

305.0	Skin
305.1	Musculoskeletal
305.2	Respiratory
305.3	Cardiovascular
305.4	Hemic and lymphatic
305.5	Gastrointestinal
305.6	Genitourinary
305.7	Endocrine
305.8	Organ of special sense
305.9	Other type

VI. SPECIAL SYMPTOMS

306.0	Speech disturbance
306.1	Specific learning disturbance
306.2	Tic

VI. SPECIAL SYMPTOMS—cont'd

306.3	Other psychomotor disorder
306.4	Disorders of sleep
306.5	Feeding disturbance
306.6	Enuresis
306.7	Encopresis
306.8	Cephalalgia
306.9	Other special symptom

VII. TRANSIENT SITUATIONAL DISTURBANCES

307.0	Adjustment reaction of infancy
307.1	Adjustment reaction of childhood
307.2	Adjustment reaction of adolescence
307.3	Adjustment reaction of adult life
307.4	Adjustment reaction of late life

VIII. BEHAVIOR DISORDERS OF CHILDHOOD AND ADOLESCENCE

308.0	Hyperkinetic reaction
308.1	Withdrawing reaction
308.2	Overanxious reaction
308.3	Runaway reaction
308.4	Unsocialized aggressive reaction
308.5	Group delinquent reaction
308.9	Other reaction

IX. MENTAL RETARDATION

310	Borderline
311	Mild
312	Moderate
313	Severe
314	Profound
315	Unspecified

With each: following or associated with

.0	Infection or intoxication
.1	Trauma or physical agent
.2	Disorders of metabolism, growth or nutrition
.3	Gross brain disease (postnatal)
.4	Unknown prenatal influence
.5	Chromosomal abnormality
.6	Prematurity
.7	Major psychiatric disorder
.8	Psychosocial (environmental) deprivation
.9	Other condition

X. CONDITIONS WITHOUT MANIFEST PSYCHIATRIC DISORDER AND NONSPECIFIC CONDITIONS

Social maladjustment without manifest psychiatric disorder
- 316.0   Marital maladjustment
- 316.1   Social maladjustment
- 316.2   Occupational maladjustment
- 316.3   Dyssocial behavior
- 316.9   Other social maladjustment

Nonspecific conditions
- 317   Nonspecific conditions

No mental disorder
- 318   No mental disorder

XI. NONDIAGNOSTIC TERMS FOR ADMINISTRATIVE USE

- 319.0   Diagnosis deferred
- 319.1   Boarder
- 319.2   Experiment only
- 319.3   Other

Fifth digit qualifying phrases

Section I	.x1	Acute
	.x2	Chronic
Section II	.x6	Not psychotic now
Sections III-VIII	.x6	Mild
	.x7	Moderate
	.x8	Severe
All disorders	.x5	In remission

CLASSIFICATION OF DSM III

The following is the classification of DSM III, a draft of axes I and II of *Diagnostic and Statistical Manual of Mental Disorders*, ed. 3, January 16, 1977, American Psychiatric Association.

ORGANIC MENTAL DISORDERS

Section 1. *Organic mental disorders in which the etiology or pathogenesis is listed below (taken from the mental disorders section of ICD-9-CM).*

SENILE AND PRE-SENILE DEMENTIAS

Code phenomenology in fifth digit as 0 = (uncomplicated), 1 = with delirium, 2 = with delusional features, 3 = with depressive features.
- 290.0x   Progressive idiopathic dementia, senile onset
- 290.1x   Progressive idiopathic dementia, presenile onset
- 290.4x   Multi-infarct dementia

SUBSTANCE INDUCED

Alcohol

303.00	Intoxication
291.40	Idiosyncratic intoxication (pathological intoxication)
291.80	Withdrawal
291.00	Withdrawal delirium (Delirium tremens)
291.30	Hallucinosis
291.10	Amnestic syndrome (Korsakoff syndrome)

Indicate severity of dementia as 1 = mild, 2 = moderate, 3 = severe, 0 = unspecified.

291.2x	Dementia associated with alcoholism

Barbiturate or similarly acting sedative or hypnotic

292.71	Intoxication
292.81	Withdrawal
292.01	Withdrawal delirium
292.21	Amnestic syndrome

Opioid

292.72	Intoxication
292.82	Withdrawal

Cocaine

292.73	Intoxication

Amphetamine or similarly acting sympathomimetic

292.74	Intoxication
292.04	Delirium
292.34	Delusional syndrome
292.84	Withdrawal

Hallucinogen

292.45	Hallucinosis
292.35	Delusional syndrome
292.55	Affective syndrome

Cannabis

292.76	Intoxication
292.36	Delusional syndrome

Tobacco

292.87	Withdrawal

Caffeine

292.78	Intoxication (Caffeinism)

Other or unspecified substance

292.09	Delirium
292.19	Dementia
292.29	Amnestic syndrome
292.39	Delusional syndrome

292.49   Hallucinosis
292.59   Affective syndrome
292.69   Personality syndrome
292.89   Withdrawal
292.79   Intoxication
292.99   Other or mixed organic brain syndrome

Section 2. *Organic mental disorders in which the etiology or pathogenesis is either noted as an additional diagnosis from outside of the mental disorders section of ICD-9-CM or is unknown.*

293.00   Delirium
294.10   Dementia
294.00   Amnestic syndrome
293.81   Organic delusional syndrome
293.82   Organic hallucinosis
293.83   Organic affective syndrome
310.10   Organic personality syndrome
294.80   Other or mixed organic brain syndrome

SUBSTANCE USE DISORDERS

Code course of illness in fifth digit as 1 = continuous, 2 = episodic, 3 = in remission, 0 = unspecified.

305.0x   Alcohol abuse
303.9x   Alcohol dependence (alcoholism)
305.4x   Barbiturate or similarly acting sedative or hypnotic abuse
304.1x   Barbiturate or similarly acting sedative or hypnotic dependence
305.5x   Opioid abuse
304.0x   Opioid dependence
305.6x   Cocaine abuse
304.2x   Cocaine dependence
305.7x   Amphetamine or similarly acting sympathomimetic abuse
304.4x   Amphetamine or similarly acting sympathomimetic dependence
305.3x   Hallucinogen abuse
305.2x   Cannabis abuse
304.3x   Cannabis dependence
305.1x   Tobacco use disorder
305.9x   Other or unspecified substance abuse
304.6x   Other specified substance dependence
304.9x   Unspecified substance dependence

SCHIZOPHRENIC DISORDERS

Code course of illness in fifth digit as 1 = subchronic, 2 = chronic, 3 = sub-chronic with acute exacerbation, 4 = chronic with acute exacerbation, 5 = in remission, 0 = unspecified.

295.1x	Disorganized (Hebephrenic)
295.2x	Catatonic
295.3x	Paranoid
295.9x	Undifferentiated
295.6x	Residual

PARANOID DISORDERS

297.10	Paranoia
297.30	Shared paranoid disorder (Folie à deux)
297.90	Paranoid state

SCHIZOAFFECTIVE DISORDERS

295.7x	Schizoaffective disorder

Code phenomenology and course in fifth digit as:

1 = Manic, episodic
2 = Manic, chronic
3 = Manic, in remission
4 = Depressed, episodic
5 = Depressed, chronic
6 = Depressed, in remission
7 = Mixed, episodic
8 = Mixed, chronic
9 = Mixed, in remission

AFFECTIVE DISORDERS
EPISODIC AFFECTIVE DISORDERS

Code severity of episode in fifth digit as 1 = moderate, 2 = marked, 3 = severe but not psychotic, 4 = psychotic, 5 = in partial remission, 6 = in full remission, 0 = unspecified.

Manic disorder

296.0x	Single episode
296.1x	Recurrent

Major depressive disorder

296.2x	Single episode
296.3x	Recurrent

Bipolar affective disorder

296.4x	Manic
296.5x	Depressed
296.6x	Mixed

CHRONIC AFFECTIVE DISORDERS

301.11   Chronic hypomanic disorder (Hypomanic personality)
301.12   Chronic depressive disorder (Depressive personality)
301.13   Cyclothymic disorder (Cyclothymic personality)

ATYPICAL AFFECTIVE DISORDERS

296.81   Atypical manic disorder
296.82   Atypical depressive disorder
296.70   Atypical bipolar disorder

PSYCHOSES NOT ELSEWHERE CLASSIFIED

295.40   Schizophreniform disorder
298.80   Brief reactive psychosis
298.90   Atypical psychosis

ANXIETY DISORDERS

Phobic disorders
300.21   Agoraphobia with panic attacks
300.22   Agoraphobia without panic attacks
300.23   Social phobia
300.29   Simple phobia
300.01   Panic disorder
300.30   Obsessive compulsive disorder
300.02   Generalized anxiety disorder
300.00   Atypical anxiety disorder

FACTITIOUS DISORDERS

300.16   Factitious illness with psychological symptoms
301.51   Chronic factitious illness with physical symptoms (Mun-
          chausen syndrome)
300.18   Other factitious illness with physical symptoms

SOMATOFORM DISORDERS

300.81   Somatization disorder (Briquet's syndrome)
300.11   Conversion disorder
307.80   Psychalgia
300.70   Atypical somatoform disorder

DISSOCIATIVE DISORDERS

300.12   Psychogenic amnesia
300.13   Psychogenic fugue
300.14   Multiple personality

DISSOCIATIVE DISORDERS—cont'd

300.60	Depersonalization disorder
300.15	Other

PERSONALITY DISORDERS

Note: These are coded on Axis II.

301.00	Paranoid
301.21	Introverted
302.22	Schizotypal
301.50	Histrionic
301.81	Narcissistic
301.70	Antisocial
301.83	Borderline
301.82	Avoidant
301.60	Dependent
301.40	Compulsive
301.84	Passive - aggressive
301.89	Other or mixed

PSYCHOSEXUAL DISORDERS

Gender identity disorders

Indicate sexual history in the fifth digit of Transsexualism code as 1 = asexual, 2 = homosexual, 3 = heterosexual, 4 = mixed, 0 = unspecified.

302.5x	Transsexualism
302.60	Gender identity disorder of childhood
302.85	Other gender identity disorder of adolescence or adult life

Paraphilias

302.81	Fetishism
302.30	Transvestism
302.10	Zoophila
302.20	Pedophilia
302.40	Exhibitionism
302.82	Voyeurism
302.83	Sexual masochism
302.84	Sexual sadism
302.89	Other

Psychosexual dysfunctions

302.71	With inhibited sexual desire
302.72	With inhibited sexual excitement (frigidity, impotence)
302.73	With inhibited female orgasm
302.74	With inhibited male orgasm
302.75	With premature ejaculation
302.76	With functional dyspareunia

306.51   With functional vaginismus
302.79   Other

Other psychosexual disorders

302.01   Ego-dystonic homosexuality
302.90   Psychosexual disorder not elsewhere classified

DISORDERS USUALLY ARISING IN CHILDHOOD OR ADOLESCENCE

This section lists conditions that usually first manifest themselves in childhood or adolescence. Any appropriate adult diagnosis can be used for diagnosing a child.

Mental retardation

Code a 1 in the fifth digit to indicate association with a known biological factor which must be coded on Axis III. Otherwise code 0.

317.0x   Mild mental retardation
318.0x   Moderate mental retardation
318.1x   Severe mental retardation
318.2x   Profound mental retardation
319.0x   Unspecified mental retardation

Pervasive developmental disorders

Code in fifth digit, 0 = full syndrome present, 1 = residual state.

299.0x   Infantile autism
299.8x   Atypical childhood psychosis

Specific developmental disorders

Note: *These are coded on Axis II.*

315.60   Specific reading disorder
315.10   Specific arithmetical disorder
315.32   Developmental language disorder
315.39   Developmental articulation disorder

Indicate course in the fifth digit as 1 = primary, 2 = secondary, 0 = unspecified.

307.6x   Enuresis
307.7x   Encopresis
315.50   Mixed
315.80   Other

Attention deficit disorders

Code severity in fifth digit as 1 = mild, 2 = moderate, 3 = severe, 0 = unspecified.

314.0x   With hyperactivity
314.1x   Without hyperactivity

Conduct disorders

Code severity in fifth digit as 1 = mild, 2 = moderate, 3 = severe, 0 = unspecified.

Conduct disorders—cont'd
312.0x   Undersocialized conduct disorder, aggressive type
312.1x   Undersocialized conduct disorder, unaggressive type
312.2x   Socialized conduct disorder

Anxiety disorders of childhood or adolescence
309.21   Separation anxiety disorder
313.21   Shyness disorder
313.00   Overanxious disorder

Other disorders of childhood or adolescence
313.22   Introverted disorder of childhood
313.81   Oppositional disorder
313.23   Elective mutism
313.83   Academic underachievement disorder

Disorders characteristic of late adolescence
309.22   Emancipation disorder of adolescence or early adult life
313.82   Identity disorder
309.23   Specific academic or work inhibition

Eating disorders
307.10   Anorexia nervosa
307.51   Bulimia
307.52   Pica
307.53   Rumination
307.59   Atypical

Speech disorders
307.00   Stuttering

Stereotyped movement disorders
307.21   Transient tic disorder
307.22   Chronic motor tic disorder
307.23   Tourette's disorder
307.20   Atypical tic disorder
307.30   Other

REACTIVE DISORDERS NOT ELSEWHERE CLASSIFIED

Posttraumatic stress disorder
308.30   Acute
309.81   Chronic

Adjustment disorders
309.00   With depressed mood
309.24   With anxious mood
309.28   With mixed emotional features
309.82   With physical symptoms
309.30   With disturbance of conduct
309.40   With mixed disturbance of emotions and conduct

309.83   With withdrawal
309.89   Other

DISORDERS OF IMPULSE CONTROL NOT ELSEWHERE CLASSIFIED

312.31   Pathological gambling
312.32   Kleptomania
312.33   Pyromania
312.34   Intermittent explosive disorder
312.35   Isolated explosive disorder
312.39   Other impulse control disorder

SLEEP DISORDERS (to be revised)
Nonorganic
307.41   Temporary insomnia
307.42   Persistent insomnia
307.43   Temporary hypersomnia
307.44   Persistent hypersomnia
307.45   Non-organic sleep-wake cycle disturbance
307.46   Somnambulism
307.47   Night terrors
307.48   Other nonorganic dyssomnias
307.49   Unspecified nonorganic sleep disorder
Organic
780.51   Insomnia associated with diseases elsewhere classified
780.52   Insomnia with central sleep-apnea
780.53   Other organic insomnia
780.54   Hypersomnia associated with diseases elsewhere classified
780.55   Hypersomnia associated with obstructive or mixed sleep-apnea
780.56   Other organic hypersomnia
780.57   Organic sleep-wake cycle disturbance
780.58   Organic dyssomnias
780.59   Unspecified organic sleep disorder

OTHER DISORDERS

Unspecified mental disorder (nonpsychotic)
V40.90   Unspecified mental disorder (nonpsychotic)
Psychological factors affecting physical disorder
Specify physical disorder on Axis III.
316.10   Psychological factor probably affecting physical disorder
316.20   Psychological factor definitely affecting physical disorder
No mental disorder
V71.00   No mental disorder

CONDITIONS NOT ATTRIBUTABLE TO A MENTAL DISORDER

V65.20	Malingering
V71.01	Adult antisocial behavior
V71.02	Childhood or adolescent antisocial behavior
V61.10	Marital problem
V61.20	Parent-child problem
V61.21	Child abuse
V62.81	Other interpersonal problem
V62.20	Occupational problem
V62.82	Uncomplicated bereavement
V15.81	Noncompliance with medical treatment
V62.88	Other life circumstance problem

ADMINISTRATIVE CATEGORIES

799.90	Diagnosis deferred
V70.70	Research subject
V63.20	Boarder
V68.30	Referral without need for evaluation

12

Organic brain syndromes (O.B.S.)

This classification of mental disorders includes a broad group of illnesses of both known and unknown etiology. Some, such as *general paralysis*, are the direct result of a known brain infection; others result from organic brain changes due to head trauma, growth of neoplasms, toxic agents, or (like *presenile dementia*) from some other as yet poorly defined or unknown cerebral condition. Under this heading too are disorders of the brain that result from general physical conditions such as systemic infection, metabolic change, or endocrine disorder. The number of such conditions is very large; examples of only the more important will be given here.

In this section we will discuss both acute and chronic brain disorders. We would here stress the similarities among the toxic and organic psychoses and point out that, although some rather characteristic differences can occur with a specific agent or anatomical predilection of lesion, yet perhaps more striking are the similarities which produce a basic syndrome consisting of (1) impairment of orientation; (2) impairment of intellectual functions, including comprehension, calculation, knowledge, learning, judgment, and recent memory (remote memory being at times preserved); and (3) lability and shallowness of affect.

Differences in the clinical picture may occur. Presumably differences in personality structure account for the appearance of such types as paranoid, depressed, manic, etc., listed under individually described psychoses due to widely different agents.

The term "acute brain disorder" has been used for organic brain syndromes from which the patient recovers. They are the result of temporary, reversible, diffuse impairment of brain tissue function such as is present in acute alcoholic intoxication or acute delirium. The basic disturbance of the sensorium may release other disturbances, such as hallucinations, poorly organized transient delusions, and behavior disturbances of varying degree.

These disorders are subclassified according to the cause of the impairment of brain tissue function. Some of the more commonly seen acute brain disorders are discussed in this section. They may be associated with such conditions as intracranial infections, systemic infections, trauma, circulatory disturbances, metabolic disorders, etc. These typically reversible, toxic psychoses may also, on occasion, when the brain damage is severe, progress to an irreversible organic syndrome.

Organic brain disorders are considered *chronic* when they result from relatively permanent and usually diffuse impairment of function of cerebral tissue. While the underlying pathological process may subside or respond to specific treatment, as in syphilis, there remains always a certain irreducible minimum of brain tissue destruction which cannot be reversed, even though the loss of function may be almost imperceptible clinically. As time passes, the chronic brain syndrome may become milder, vary in degree, or progress; but some disturbance of memory, judgment, orientation, comprehension, and affect persists permanently.

These disorders are classified according to the cause of the impairment of brain function. Some of the diagnostic categories are identical with those of the acute brain syndromes; the differentiation is based on the permanent impairment of brain function in the chronic group.

Finally, there is a group of conditions with organic brain change and behavior disorder but in which the behavioral symptoms are not of a degree to warrant the term "psychosis." For such, the term "nonpsychotic organic brain syndrome" is used. Such a diagnosis may often be appropriately applied in the case of children where mild brain damage may result in hyperactivity, short attention span, easy distractibility, and impulsiveness. Other children with this diagnosis may be withdrawn, listless, apathetic, or unresponsive.

SUGGESTED READINGS

Benson, D. F., Lemay, M., Patten, D. H., and others: Diagnosis of normal pressure hydrocephalus, N. Engl. J. Med. **83**:609, 1970.

Ehrentheil, O. F.: Differential diagnosis of organic dementias and affective disorders in aged patients, Geriatrics **12**:426, 1957.

Freemon, F. R.: Evaluation of patients with progressive intellectual deterioration, Arch. Neurol. **33**:658, 1976.

Seltzer, B., and Sherwin, I.: Organic brain syndromes: an empirical study and critical review, Am. J. Psychiatry **135**:13, 1978.

Terry, R. D.: Dementia. A brief and selected review, Arch. Neurol. **33**:1, 1976.

Waggoner, R. W., and Bagchi, B. K.: Initial masking of organic brain changes by psychiatric symptoms. Am. J. Psychiatry **110**:904, 1954.

Wells, C.: Chronic brain disease: an overview, Am. J. Psychiatry **135**:1, 1978.

GENERAL MANAGEMENT OF ORGANIC BRAIN DISTURBANCES

The management of organic brain disturbances is a problem often faced by both the psychiatrist and the general practitioner. The term "delirium" is commonly used for acute brain disorders which, although classed as psychoses, are more or less temporary conditions characterized by disorientation and accompanied by illusions and hallucinations and a predominant affect of fear. Disturbances in brain metabolism may be of infectious, toxic, vascular, nutritional, or traumatic origin and are usually reversible, so that complete recovery may occur.

The symptoms of delirium seem to *depend* on underlying personality and life experiences of the subject. For example, paranoid misinterpretations are not uncommon in persons known to have been of suspicious nature.

The *chief complaint* is usually indicated in a referral by private physician or by family, stating that the patient is becoming restless and uneasy and shows increasing tendency to emotional instability and sensitivity to light and sound. *History* may reveal evidence of some underlying infectious, metabolic, or nutritional illness, a head injury, or chronic drug ingestion. One suspects delirium in a patient over 40 years of age, when hospitalized for cardiac decompensation, kidney or liver disease, hypertension, or metabolic disorder, or following surgical procedures, particularly those involving the eyes or ears. The administration of barbiturate sedation may be the final insult in those patients whose sluggish circulation is laden with other medication.

From the *behavioral* standpoint there is outstanding disturbance in intellectual functions, with disorientation as to time, place, and person, poor recent and remote memory, defects in fund of general information, and defects in ability to calculate and in judgment. Illusions and hallucinations (predominantly visual, sometimes tactile) may be present. Unsystematized paranoid ideas are not infrequent. The mood is usually fearful although elation and depression can occur. A patient may jump out of the window to his death in a sudden attempt to escape envisioned attackers. Speech may be indistinct. The patient may be restless and irritable, with insomnia and a tendency to emotional instability if seen early, but later he may be semicomatose or in coma. On *physical* examination tremors, incoordination, urinary incontinence, dehydration, malnutrition, signs of vitamin deficiency, and elevated temperature are found. *Laboratory* reports indicate leukocytosis, albuminuria, and glycosuria. The EEG often shows slowing of basic rhythms.

PROGNOSIS. Prognosis is good with active treatment, but the ultimate course depends upon the underlying disease and the extent of arteriosclerotic and senile change.

TREATMENT. Precautions against suicide are essential.

Stop sedatives and all other nonvital drugs.

Promote rest and sleep. Do not disturb when asleep. Hydrotherapy, 95° to 96° F., may be useful.

Avoid wet packs if circulatory difficulties exist; use no mechanical restraints.

Give parenteral fluids if patient is dehydrated—and as long as urine output can increase (1000 ml. 10% glucose in H_2O, I. V.).

Get patient up as soon as medical condition permits. Provide constant companionship and a light in the room while the patient is awake.

Do not joke about hallucinations. Urge the patient to accept them as bad dreams (note content, as it may give clues for later psychotherapy).

Sedate with 5 to 10 mg. haloperidol given orally or intravenously. Do not use barbituates as they may increase confusion in the elderly. Chloropromazine is helpful for insomnia and aggressive-destructive behavior. Begin with 10 mg. orally three times a day and gradually raise dose if hypotension does not develop.

This condition fluctuates: The patient may be clear in the morning but confused as the evening shadows fall. The harm that comes to the patient from yelling is little when compared to the possible toxic effects of medication that not only may fail to make him quiet but actually may also make him worse.

SUGGESTED READINGS

Anderson, W. H., Kuehnle, J. C., and Catanzara, D. M.: Rapid treatment of acute psychosis, Am. J. Psychiatry **133**:1076, 1976.

Carter, R. G.: Psychotolysis with haloperidol: rapid control of the acutely disturbed psychotic patient, Dis. Nerv. Syst. **38**:237, 1977.

Cohen, M. D.: The management of disturbed cardiac patients, Mod. Concepts Cardiovasc. Dis. **22**:182, 186, 1953.

Cohen, S.: The toxic psychoses and allied states, Am. J. Med. **15**:813, 1953.

Engel, G. L., and Romano, J.: Delirium, a syndrome of cerebral insufficiency. J. Chron. Dis. **9**:260, 1959.

Fantus, B., and Kraines, S. H.: The therapy of acute delirium, J.A.M.A. **115**:929, 1940.

Lipowski, Z. J.: Delirium, clouding of consciousness and confusion, J. Nerv. Ment. Dis. **145**:227, 1967.

Moore, D. P.: Rapid treatment of delirium in critically ill patients, Am. J. Psychiatry **134**:1431, 1977.

Shear, M. K., and Michael, H. S.: Digitalis delirium: report of two cases, Am. J. Psychiatry **135**:109, 1978.

Siegel, R. K., and West, L. J., editors: Hallucinations, London, 1975, John Wiley & Sons, Inc.

PSYCHOSES ASSOCIATED WITH ORGANIC BRAIN SYNDROMES
Senile and presenile dementia
Senile dementia (and psychoses with cerebral arteriosclerosis; multi-infarct dementia)

Although the processes of both arteriosclerosis and senile degeneration not infrequently affect the same brain, it is usual for one to predominate over the other. The two disorders are to some degree clinically distinguishable, they represent separate pathological entities, and each may exist without the other. Relative to the size of the population from which mental disturbances are drawn, the senile and arteriosclerotic psychoses are by far the most frequent of all psychoses. Senile psychosis is twice as common in women and psychosis with cerebral arteriosclerosis three times as common in men.

ANAMNESIS. The *chief complaint* is given by the family, who may state that the patient's behavior (confusion, delusions, weakness, incontinence, etc.) is no longer manageable. The *history* in both disorders reveals gradual onset over previous months or years—of forgetfulness, failure of efficiency, exaggeration of previous personality weaknesses, deterioration of judgment and personal habits, loss of emotional control, and physical weakness. Social changes may precipitate a worsening of symptoms. A history of headache, dizziness, explosive emotional outbursts, syncopal attacks, or cardiac disturbance strongly suggests arteriosclerotic psychosis, whereas predominance of personality disturbance favors a diagnosis of senile psychosis.

EXAMINATION. Examination reveals one of a great variety of clinical pictures appearing in the sixth to ninth decade which have in common progressive signs of organic mental deficit, an exaggeration of the aging process. In the *behavioral* patterns we find untidiness of dress, easy emotionality with fluctuation, restlessness and confusion at night, and defects in recent memory appearing early. During initial stages the failure of memory for recent events causes excessive reminiscence of past life, which may lead the family to think the patient has a keen mind. Fabrication, disorientation, and rambling incoherent speech develop later. Patients show poor judgment and tend to hoard objects of little worth. Prolonged depression, periods of confusion which remit, dizziness, aphasias, apraxias, fainting spells, and convulsive seizures are useful diagnostic signs, since they are rare in senile cases but not uncommon with cerebral arteriosclerosis. The picture of gradual, progressive deterioration of intellectual functions (rather than a sudden exacerbation of symptions) usually indicates a senile psychosis. The illness may release traits that caricature the prepsychotic personality. Neurotic trends with hypochondriasis are common. Results from *physical* tests indicating hypertension and peripheral arteriosclerosis do *not* favor either diagnosis. In the end there results a completely bedridden organism, responding with primitive reflexes and suffering malnutrition, generalized weakness, incontinence, fractures, and decubitus ulcers. Early loss of abstract thinking and inability to organize and retain new observations are revealed by *psychological* tests.

Pathological examination frequently reveals no correlation between the degree of brain damage and symptomatology. Senile psychosis presents a diffuse atrophy of cortical convolutions and individual nerve cells with preservation of cortical architecture. Senile plaques which stain with silver are found in great number throughout the cortex. The Alzheimer type of neurofibril change is sometimes seen. Cerebral arteriosclerosis presents a great variety of focal lesions accompanied by atherosclerosis (large vessels are rarely spared), arteriolosclerosis, and capillary fibrosis. Anemic or hemorrhagic areas of softening occurring in any part of the brain are usual. The term "multi-infarct dementia" has replaced the older term "cerebral arteriosclerosis." There is no correlation between arteriosclerosis of the brain and of other body areas.

PROGNOSIS. In senile cases the total course of illness may be from 1 to 10 years; death occurs from infection (pneumonia, bacteremia from decubitus ulcers, etc.). In arteriosclerotic cases the course is extremely variable and depends on the state of vessels in vital organs.

TREATMENT. In very early stages the family should prepare for the resulting failing judgment with tactful suggestions of retirement. Limit work routine within the tolerance of the patient.

Provision of a protected physical and social environment with proper diet, simple activities, and quiet companionship pays dividends. Regularity and hobbies should be encouraged.

A high-nitrogen diet (including powdered milk and egg) has been advocated to overcome the negative nitrogen balance that occurs in the aged. Hydergine (dehydrated ergot, 1 mg.) tablets have been given 6 to 8 per day with reported good results. Metrazol alone, 0.1 Gm. orally, 1 to 2 tablets t.i.d., and in combination with nicotinamide, 400 mg. daily, has been reported to aid in relieving the confusion seen in these patients.

Angiolytics and hypnotics relieve restlessness and insomnia. Avoid daytime catnaps.

Immobilization in bed—even in case of fractures—is to be avoided, as it hastens confusion and physical deterioration.

Occupational therapy and group psychotherapy have been found useful even in fairly advanced states of deterioration. Often the earliest action to be taken is the removal of major occupational, financial, and family responsibilities. Frequently the failure of judgment requires the appointment of a guardian.

Beware of risking injuries through falling.

Avoid sexual stimulation, which may lead to difficulties with children of opposite sex. These patients recognize a child's sex but ignore age.

The alert physician who detects the onset of senility may save the family shame and disgrace by advising for trust funds and competent legal guardianship before the onset of poor business and social judgment. Remember these conditions are characterized by fluctuation both in intellectual function and in mood. The diagnosis is best made in the evening hours, when the patient is fatigued and shadows fall.

SUGGESTED READINGS

Blessed, G., Tomlinson, B. E., and Roth, M.: The association between quantitative measures of dementia and of senile change in the cerebral grey matter of elderly subjects, Br. J. Psychiatry **114**:797, 1968.

Busse, E. W., and Pfeiffer, E., editors: Mental illness in later life, Baltimore, 1973, American Psychiatric Association Publishing Division, Garamond/Pridemark Press.

Fox, J. H., Topel, J. L., and Huckman, M. S.: Use of computerized tomography in senile dementia, J. Neurol. Neurosurg. Psychiatry **38**:948, 1975.

Hachinski, V. C., Lassen, N. A., and Marshall, J.: Multi-infarct dementia: a cause of mental deterioration in the elderly, Lancet **2**:207, 1974.

Kiloh, L. G.: Pseudodementia, Acta Psychiat. Scand. **37**:336, 1961.

Roth, M.: The natural history of mental disorders in old age, J. Ment. Sci. **101**:281, 1955.

Tomlinson, B. E., Blessed, G., and Roth, M.: Observations on the brains of demented old people, J. Neurol. Sci. **11**:205, 1970.

Presenile dementia

Abnormalities of behavior which occur in middle life as a result of permanent loss of brain substance include two generally recognized clinical entities: *Alzheimer's disease* and *Pick's disease*. Although there apparently are clinical differences, the differential diagnosis between the two can be made definitely only at autopsy, where the distinguishing characteristics are seen on microscopic examination of the brain. Pick's disease is rare and is now felt to be a specific heredodegenerative process caused by a mendelian dominant trait. On the basis of pathological data, a close relationship between Alzheimer's disease and senile psychosis has been postulated.

ANAMNESIS. The *chief complaint* made by those around the patient is that he has been showing a poorly defined personality change over the previous 1 to 10 years. Forgetfulness, carelessness in dress or work habits, apathy, antisocial or unethical acts (usually of minor importance, such as increased use of profanity, pilfering, etc.), and a tendency to repeat ideas or statements have appeared gradually. Occasionally the initial *history* may, instead, present the picture of a sudden onset of confusion or apathy following severe emotional or physical trauma. But careful inquiry in these cases will reveal preceding changes of the type noted above. In a small percentage of cases *family history* reveals other cases of organic brain damage appearing before senescence. Onset occurs in the third to the sixth decade of life and both syndromes occur more frequently in females than in males.

During the first years of the illness, only careful history and observation will prevent mistaken diagnosis of psychogenic disturbance.

EXAMINATION. In the early stages, the patient's *behavioral* pattern tends to show affability, periods of mild euphoria and depression, defects in recent memory, with perseverative ideas and behavior. Frequently a complete denial of these symptoms may necessitate relying on careful observation for diagnosis. In later stages, confusion, inertia, protracted states of panic, or psychotic symptoms develop. Making a differential diagnosis on the basis of clinical observations is fraught with difficulty. There is a tendency in Alzheimer's disease to show a greater loss of memory and a greater confusion at the onset of the illness. After the syndrome is well developed, the presence of confabulation, motor restlessness, tremors, and epilepsy also favors the diagnosis of Alzheimer's disease. In the early stages, patients with Pick's disease may show only slight defects in recent memory with the predominating defects being loss of initiative, difficulty in attention, and stereotypy of behavior. In advanced stages, patients with Pick's disease tend toward marked inertia. Confabulation is rare, and even in advanced cases memory is likely to be less affected. No abnormalities appear on *physical* examination in early cases. Weight loss, aphasia, gait disturbances, changes in muscle tonus, and other focal neurological signs occur in advanced cases. Pneumo-encephalograms as *diagnostic* tests are valuable principally to demonstrate cortical atrophy, not to differentiate the type. Local-ized atrophy over frontal or temporal lobes suggests Pick's rather than Alzheimer's disease. In Alzheimer's disease *pathological* findings are as follows: There is a generalized marked atrophy of the cortex with approximately one-third of the cells showing fibrillary degeneration (of Alzheimer). Microscopically these cells and the characteristic miliary plaques accompanied by hyaline degeneration of small blood vessels present the diagnostic fea-tures of Alzheimer's disease. In Pick's disease the gross pathology shows visible atrophic areas circumscribed to a single convolution or a lobe, with the lesion often occurring symmetrically. Micro-scopically, all that is seen is cell degeneration, which may be localized over the frontal and temporal lobes and usually involves the first three layers of cortical ganglia.

PROGNOSIS. Two to twenty years' total duration of illness.

TREATMENT. No specific treatment. Eventual hospitaliza-tion is inevitable. At that time helping the family to accept the situation aids in the patient's hospital adjustment.

SUGGESTED READINGS

Alpers, B. J., editor: The pre-senile dementias—symposium, Trans. Amer. Neurol. Assoc. **89**:9, 1964.

Bellak, L., Karasu, T. B., and Birenbaum, C., editors: Geriatric psychiatry: a handbook for psychiatrists and primary care physicians, New York, 1976, Grune & Stratton, Inc.

Liston, E. H., Jr.: Occult presenile dementia, J. Nerve. Ment. Dis. **164**:263, 1977.

Newton, R. D.: Identity of Alzheimer's disease and senile dementia and their relationship to senility, J. Ment. Sci. **94**:225, 1948.

Williams, G. R. Genetics of the pre-senile dementias, Trans. Amer. Neurol. Assoc. **89**:9, 1964.

Ziegler, D.: Cerebral atrophy in psychiatric patients, Am. J. Psychiatry **111**:454, 1954.

Alcoholic psychoses

The personality difficulties that lead to alcohol addiction may include various types of emotional and behavioral disorders. Of these conditions, immoderate drinking is but a symptom. The present section will be concerned, however, not with addiction to alcohol but rather with the psychotic disturbances that result from states of alcoholic intoxication which have been prolonged or repeated and often associated with dietary deficiencies.

DELIRIUM TREMENS (withdrawal dementia). This is a type of delirium occurring in about 5% of chronic alcoholics, characteristically with sudden onset at night associated with a period of heavy drinking. Symptoms occur characteristically with the withdrawal of alcohol. Hallucinations and illusions are predominantly visual, typically moving, colored, and with large numbers of the same objects or small animals. Patients are usually disoriented, although they may sense the unreality of their illusions. There is a hypersensitivity of sensory perception and a predominant mood of fear. They are restless and hyperactive and have insomnia. There is a coarse arrhythmic tremor of the tongue, face, fingers, legs, eyes, and even trunk. These may early be felt more readily than seen. Convulsions occur in 9% of cases. Nausea, vomiting, and dehydration may occur. There is fever in 90% of cases and albuminuria at the height of the delirium. This condition can, in itself, be fatal and is often complicated by head injuries, unrecognized fractures, pneumonia, and cardiac decompensation.

KORSAKOFF'S PSYCHOSIS (amnestic syndrome). This amnestic polyneuritic syndrome can be caused by other toxins but occurs in about 1 per 100 chronic alcoholics, in women more frequently than in men, and with mean age of onset at 51 years. The condition begins insidiously, and it may be difficult to detect the intellectual impairment. Anterograde amnesia is typical, but remote memory and learning ability may also be impaired. There may be disorientation for time and place with attempt to cover defects by confabulation. Aphasia, agraphia, and stereotyped speech occur; mood is indifferent or may be euphoric. Polyneuritis occurs, usually symmetrical, involving both upper and lower extremities and with sensory and motor deficit. Mortality is high.

ALCOHOLIC HALLUCINOSIS (withdrawal hallucinosis). Only one fifth as common as delirium tremens, this occurs after a shorter period of drinking, typically in younger persons with family or personal history of psychopathology. There is a prodromal period of anxiety, headache, insomnia, and increased sensitivity to sounds. Patients are well oriented. There are occasional cutaneous sensations but more typical are auditory hallucinations in which voices talk about the patient in the third person. Such hallucinations may be delusionally rationalized by the patient. Fear is the predominant mood and suicidal attempts are common. Prognosis is good for the individual attack, but symptoms may last several months or the condition may become chronic.

ALCOHOLIC PARANOID STATE. This term is used to describe the occurrence of paranoid ideas but without other changes due to chronic drinking.

ACUTE ALCOHOLIC INTOXICATION. Uncomplicated intoxication with or without delirium, mood change, or tremor is often seen as one of many acute episodes in the course of chronic alcoholism.

ALCOHOLIC DETERIORATION. The continued excessive use of alcohol over a period of time may result in deterioration, with brutality, ethical dulling, labile affect, impaired memory, diminished will power, dilated facial vessels, tremor, and "rum fits." *Alcoholic encephalopathy,* or *Wernicke's syndrome,* shows clouding of consciousness, opthalmoplegia, and ataxia. Pathologically lesions are in the periventricular nuclei. Beginning with delirium, the condition may end fatally or with a residual Korsakoff's syndrome.

PATHOLOGICAL INTOXICATION (idiosyncratic intoxication). This is seen in 1% of alcoholic hospital admissions as a reaction of blind rage and confusion or paranoid feelings with acts of violence or occasionally an ecstatic state of a few minutes' to a few hours' duration with later amnesia for the attack. Symptoms of intoxication may be transitory or absent and the condition is independent of the amount taken. It occurs most frequently in persons with psychopathic character traits.

OTHER ALCOHOLIC PSYCHOSIS. *Marchiafava's disease* is a rare, progressive mental decadence which may end in confusion, dementia, and epileptiform seizures. Neurological signs include aphasia, agnosia, apraxia, hemiparesis, and cerebellar ataxia. Mental changes include mania, depression, and paranoid states. It occurs in middle or later years, typically in persons of Italian extraction and following the consumption of large quantities of red wine. There is degeneration of the corpus callosum and multiple cortical and subcortical areas of encephalomalacia. Death occurs within a few years.

SUGGESTED READINGS

Hanson, J. W., Jones, K. L., and Smith, D. W.: Fetal alcohol syndrome; experience with 41 patients, J.A.M.A. **235:**1458, 1976.

Leventhal, C. M., Baringer, J. R., Arnason, B. G., and Fisher, C. M.: A case of Marchiafava-Bignami disease with clinical recovery, Trans. Amer. Neurol. Assoc. **90:**87, 1965.

Lynch, M. J. H.: Brain lesions in chronic alcoholism, Arch. Pathology **69:**342, 1960.

Maletzky, B. M.: The diagnosis of pathological intoxication, J. Stud. Alcohol **37:**1215, 1976.

Seixas, F. A., editor: Currents in alcoholism, New York, 1977, Grune & Stratton, Inc.

Victor, M.: Alcoholism. In Baker, A. B., and Baker, L. H., editors: Clinical neurology, New York, 1975, Harper and Row, Publishers.

Psychosis associated with intracranial infection
General paresis

General paresis is a chronic spirochetal meningoencephalitis which severely disturbs the function of the cerebral cortex, thereby producing clinical neurological signs, including marked changes in personality and mental abilities, often a psychosis characterized by depression, expansiveness, or agitation, and terminally a dissolution of mental and physical capacities.

TYPES. The following distribution has been observed: (1) simple deteriorating (40%), (2) depressed (25%), (3) expansive (15% to 20%), (4) manic (10% to 15%), and (5) paranoid (less than 10%).

ANAMNESIS. Occasionally the onset may be sudden with a person apparently in the best of health developing a classic paretic syndrome or with sudden onset of a cerebral accident, aphasia, hemiplegia, convulsion, or psychotic episode which may be of but a few hours' or days' duration and precede the classic psychiatric mental picture by months or years. More often the onset is insidious, with the development of forgetfulness, discourtesy, carelessness of personal appearance, unsound judgment, periods of depression, undue optimism, and overactivity. The consequences of these symptoms for the individual have led this period of onset to be termed the "medicolegal period."

In fully developed paresis the psychotic symptoms occur, and although the syndromes produced are multiform in variety, the types listed above have been classically delimited on the basis of the most conspicuous symptoms. The age of onset is usually between 30 and 50 years, and a period of 5 to 15 years often elapses between the initial syphilitic infection and the development of paresis.

EXAMINATION. The essence of paretic neurosyphilis, *behaviorally,* is mental deterioration with confusion, memory defect, impaired judgment, and lability of mood occurring in all forms; but these may be masked by more dramatic symptoms. The classic expansive paretic syndrome (less common than popularly believed) is characterized by delusions of grandeur in which the patient brags of great riches or power, with an accompanying euphoria. The patient is often hypersuggestible and can be persuaded to do almost anything that is asked of him. Depressed and manic forms may both show agitation and are often like similar states of other etiology. A paranoid type is occasionally seen, with systematized delusions and with good retention of most intellectual faculties.

On *physical* examination, neurological abnormalities are not essential for the diagnosis of early paretic neurosyphilis. Pupillary disorders are common. Advancing infirmity of the body is manifested by slouching carriage, hypotonia, and flattening and smoothing out of the facial lines (paretic facies). Tremors of the facial muscles, extended tongue, and outstretched fingers occur early. Highly typical of paresis is the speech disorder characterized by faulty enunciation, slurring of consonants with rapid speech, poor articulation with elision, and mispronunciation. Handwriting typically shows defects, with evidence of tremor, poor spacing and spelling, and transposition and omission of letters. The tendon reflexes may be normal, increased, decreased, or absent at any stage of the disease.

By *laboratory* tests, blood serology is usually positive. Cerebrospinal fluid is clear under normal or slightly increased pressure and shows pleocytosis (25 to 75 cells/c.mm.); globulin test is positive, and protein is increased 50 to 100 mg./100 ml.; the colloidal gold reaction is markedly abnormal with a first-zone curve (i.e., 5555443211); there is usually a strongly positive Wassermann reaction (over 95% of cases positive if two or more tests used). EEG's show high-voltage slow waves in cases with severe mental impairment, the EEG pattern usually improving with treatment. *Psychometric* examination may demonstrate an organic picture and decrease in I.Q. which usually fails to improve with treatment.

In macroscopic studies of *pathology* are seen thickened and opaque meninges, cerebral atrophy shown by widening of sulci and dilatation of ventricles, and granular ependymitis. Microscopically, there are meningeal and perivascular infiltrates (lymphocytes and plasma cells), loss and degenerative changes in nerve cells, reaction of microglia (rod cells) and astrocytes, and presence of the organism *Treponema pallidum.*

PROGNOSIS. Without treatment the disease is progressive. The grandiosity, mania, depression, agitation, and paranoid ideas recede into the background. The patient is less active and dementia becomes the outstanding characteristic. This period of decline may take a few weeks or 2 or 3 years, and the patient terminally becomes bedridden and paralyzed, with development of emaciation and decubital ulcers, with death from intercurrent infection, or with convulsive seizures. With adequate treatment complete recovery is possible, the best results occurring with early institution of therapy.

DIFFERENTIAL DIAGNOSIS. The mental disturbance of meningovascular syphilis may be indistinguishable from that of the meningoencephalitic form. A differential diagnosis may be possible in those cases in which the history, signs, and symptoms, including serology, suggest a primary and predominating involvement of the meninges and blood vessels rather than of the parenchyma of the nervous system. Suggestive of this type of syphilis, rather than of general paresis, are comparatively early onset after infection, sudden onset of mental disturbance, focal signs, particularly cranial nerve palsy, apoplectiform seizures, very high spinal fluid cell count, positive blood and spinal fluid serology, and prompt response to general systemic and antisyphilitic treatment.

TREATMENT. Administer procaine penicillin G in aqueous suspension, 600,000 units daily for 15 days, or administer benzathine penicillin G (Bicillin), 2.4 million units intramuscularly weekly for 4 doses. If allergic to penicillin, administer doxycycline hydrate, 100 mg. every 12 hours for 30 days. Spinal fluid cells and protein should be decreased at 6 months. Complete fixation test and colloidal gold may not revert for years.

Fever therapy was frequently used until recent years: (1) malaria, *Plasmodium vivax*, 10 to 12 paroxysms (total of 150 hours above 100° F.) or (2) fever cabinet, 10 treatments (total of 5 hours at 106° F.).

SUGGESTED READINGS

Harrison, T. R., and others: Principles of internal medicine, ed. 5, New York, 1966, McGraw-Hill Book Co.

Hurdle, E. S.: Neurosyphilis. In Conn, H. F., editor: Current therapy 1976, Philadelphia, 1976, W. B. Saunders Co.

Acute (Sydenham's) chorea

Acute chorea (St. Vitus' dance) is an infectious encephalitis involving the cerebral cortex and the basal ganglia. An exudative process similar to that in rheumatic fever seems related to the streptococcus. Involuntary jerky movements and grimacing are accompanied by emotional instability (tearfulness and irritability), restlessness, disobedience, impaired concentration, and an inability to remember. Insomnia, night terrors, and sleepwalking may be present. There may be a history of rheumatism, repeated attacks of tonsillitis, fever, or heart disease. This disease must be differentiated from tics, athetoid movements, and hysteria. Both physical and mental rest away from other persons in a hospital is advisable, combined with sodium salicylate and aspirin treatment; a sedative may be needed if restlessness is marked.

SUGGESTED READING

Shaskan, D.: Mental changes in chorea minor, Am. J. Psychiatry **95:**193, 1938.

Psychosis associated with other cerebral conditions
Cerebral arteriosclerosis

See under "Senile dementia."

Other cerebrovascular disturbance

Acute confusional states are seen with infarction of the inferomedial surface of the occiptal lobe and the right middle cerebral artery.

SUGGESTED READINGS

Horenstein, S., Chamberlain, W., and Conomoy, J.: Infarction of the fusiform and calcarine regions: agitated delirium and hemianopia, Trans. Am. Neurol. Assoc. **92:**85, 1967.

Mesulam, M. M., Waxman, S. G., and Geschwind, N.: Acute confusional states with right middle cerebral artery infarctions, J. Neurol. Neurosurg. Psychiatry **39:**84, 1976.

Epilepsy

Psychotic states that are neither seizures nor postictal phenomena may occur in epileptics. They are thought to result from chronic alteration of the brain as a result of severe and repeated seizures. Such conditions occur after several years of seizures and usually after a bout of several convulsions. Overactivity, speech abnormalities, wide variations in mood, visual and auditory hallucinations, delusions, and lack of insight characterize the condition.

Of considerable importance not only in connection with epilepsy but also regarding the pathogenesis of schizophrenia are the schizophrenic-like psychoses of epilepsy. These occur in persons with otherwise normal personalities, save for epileptic personality changes in cases where the seizure disorder was of long duration. The genetic background is of epilepsy rather than schizophrenia. The average age of onset is 30 years. The psychosis is usually of insidious onset after many years (average 14) epilepsy. Onset in some cases can be acute and the symptoms may improve or become chronic; and although the seizure disorder may tend to improve, the psychiatric illness runs toward an end state of general impairment of an organic type. Paranoid features are common, and typical schizophrenic type delusional formation and hallucinary experiences with clear consciousness occur frequently. Flatness of affect, catatonic features, and schizophrenic thought disorders are regularly seen.

SUGGESTED READINGS

Ferguson, S. M., Rayport, M., Gardner, R., Kass, W., Weiner, H., and Reiser, M. F.: Similarities in mental content of psychotic states, spontaneous seizures, dreams, and responses to electrical stimulation in patients with temporal lobe epilepsy, Psychosom. Med. **31:**479, 1970.

Flor, Henry P.: Schizophrenic-like reactions and affective psychoses associated with temporal lobe epilepsy etiological factors, Amer. J. Psychiat. **126**:400, 1969.

Mulder, D. W., Bickford, R. G., and Dodge, H. W., Jr.: Hallucinatory epilepsy complex hallucinations as focal seizures, Amer. J. Psychiat. **113**:1100, 1957.

Slater, E., Beard, A. W., and Glithero, E.: The schizophrenia-like psychoses of epilepsy, I to V, Br. J. Psychiatry **109**:95, 1963.

Solomon, G. E., and Plum, F.: Clinical management of seizures, Philadelphia, 1976, W. B. Saunders Co.

Intracranial neoplasm

Too frequently overlooked in admissions to chronic hospitals and unrecognized until autopsy are those cases whose mental symptoms may occur at any stage of growth of a cerebral neoplasm. Slight behavior alteration, irritability, forgetfulness, and lack of interest are primary symptoms. Disturbance of sensorium may occur with consequent delirium. Affect is labile, with euphoria and facetiousness *(Witzelsucht)*, seen particularly in frontal lobe lesions. Depression and anxiety may occur. Intellectual functioning declines. Simple auditory hallucinations of whistles, bells, etc., or visual hallucinations of flashing or colored lights may be a clue to focal pathology. Uncinate gyrus tumors may give olfactory or déjà vu symptoms.

SUGGESTED READINGS

Bilckiewicz, A., and Gromska, J.: Diagnostic value of mental disorders in temporal lobe tumors, Neurol. Neurochir. Psychiat. Pol. **13**:397, 1963.

Guvener, A., Bagchi, B. K., Kooi, K. A., and Calhoun, H. D.: Mental and seizure manifestations in relation to brain tumors—a statistical study, Epilepsia (Amst.) **5**:166, 1964.

Pool, J. L., and Correll, J. W.: Psychiatric symptoms masking brain tumor, J. Med. Soc. N.J. **55**:4, 1958.

Remington, F. B., and Rubert, S. L.: Why patients with brain tumors come to a psychiatric hospital: a thirty year survey, Am. J. Psychiatry **119**:256, 1962.

Selecki, B. R.: Intracranial space occupying lesions of all patients admitted to a mental hospital, Med. J. Aust. **1**:383, 1965.

Soniat, T. L. L.: Psychiatric symptoms associated with intracranial neoplasm, Am. J. Psychiatry **108**:19, 1951.

Huntington's chorea

A heredofamilial degenerative disease of the nervous system, Huntington's chorea occurs in adult life (35 to 40 years) and is distinguished by persistent and progressive choreiform movements and mental deterioration. The earliest mental symptoms are of emotional lability with irritability and temper, sexual assault, or destructive violence. Psychotic episodes may occur, resembling manic-depressive psychoses or hebephrenic type of schizophrenia. Feelings of unworthiness and self-accusation may lead to suicidal attempts. Memory becomes poor and there is inattention. Suspicion, jealousy, and paranoid trends and later agnosias, apraxia, and disorientation are apparent. The pathological picture includes leptomeningitis, brain atrophy, and dilatation of ventricles.

SUGGESTED READINGS

Enna, S. J., and others: Huntington's chorea. Changes in neurotransmitter receptors in the brain, N. Engl. J. Med. **294:**1305, 1976.

Huntington, G.: On chorea, Med. Surg. Reporter **26:**317, 1872.

James, W. E., Mefferd, R. B., and Kimball, I.: Early signs of Huntington's chorea, Dis. Nerv. Syst. **30:**556, 1969.

McCaughey, W. T. E.: The pathologic spectrum of Huntington's chorea. J. Nerv. Ment. Dis. **133:**91, 1961.

McHugh, P. R., and Folstein, M.: Psychiatric syndromes of Huntington's chorea: a clinical and phenomenologic study. In Benson, D. F., and Blumer, D., editors: Psychiatric aspects of neurological disease, New York, 1975, Grune & Stratton, Inc.

Vessie, P. R.: On transmission of Huntington's chorea for 300 years—Bures family group, J. Nerv. Ment. Dis. **76:**553, 1932.

Whittier, J. R., and Koreny, C.: Effect of oral fluphenazine on Huntington's chorea, Int. J. Neuropsychiatry **4:**1, 1968.

Wilson's disease

Wilson's disease is a familial disease usually with onset in adolescence and fatal in 2 to 7 years, with cirrhosis of the liver and glial proliferation of the globus pallidus (hepatolenticular degeneration). Intention tremor, athetosis, dysarthria, dysphagia, contractures, muscle weakness, progressive dementia, and emaciation are observed. Beginning with facile laughter, the patients may become silly and noisy. Instability of mood, irritability, excitement, hallucinations, and even a picture resembling schizophrenia have been described.

This disease has recently been considered the result of an inborn error of mineral metabolism. The blood and liver of the patients show high copper content. It has been reported that treatment with dimercaprol (BAL) resulted in an increased elimination of copper with a decrease in symptoms and improvement in the EEG.

SUGGESTED READINGS

Evans, G. W., Dubois, R. S., and Hambridge, K. M.: Wilson's disease: Identification of an abnormal protein, Science **181**:1175, 1975.

Wilson, S. A. K.: Neurology, ed. 2, Baltimore, 1955, The Williams & Wilkins Co.

Creutzfeldt-Jakob disease

Creutzfeldt-Jakob disease (cortical-striatal-spinal degeneration) is a rapidly developing secondary dementia presumably caused by a slow virus, which is associated with extrapyramidal disorders and sometimes with lower motor neuron disorders. Ataxia, dysarthrias, spasticity, choreoathetoid movements, tremor, cogwheel rigidity, and muscular wasting occur. Death occurs within 6 months to 2 years of the onset.

SUGGESTED READINGS

Fisher, C. M.: The clinical picture of Creutzfeldt-Jakob disease, Trans. Amer. Neurol. Assoc. **85**:147, 1960.

Gibbs, C. J., and Gajdusek, D. C.: Infection as the etiology of spongiform encephalopathy (Creutzfeldt-Jakob Disease), Science **165**:1023, 1969.

Seidler, H., Gajdusek, D. C., and Zigas, V.: Creutzfeldt-Jakob disease: clinicopathologic report of 15 cases and review of the literature, J. Neuropath. Exper. Neurol. **22**:381, 1963.

Multiple sclerosis

Multiple sclerosis, like any brain disease with scattered degenerative foci, may produce a variety of psychiatric pictures. Paranoid, depressive, hypomanic, and schizophrenic-like states have been described and seem to be related both to the site of the lesion and to the previous personality patterns. In early cases a differentiation from hysteria is sometimes a problem, due to the apparent indifference of the patient to his disease. Thus eutonia sclerotica, or false sense of physical well-being, has been attributed (along with the frequent lability of mood) to the typical subependymal periventricular lesions in the region of the thalamus. Schilder points out, however, that such eutonia is but one manifestation of the attitude not infrequently found in many who are gravely ill.

SUGGESTED READINGS

Baldwin, M.: A clinico-experimental investigation into the psychologic aspects of multiple sclerosis, J. Nerv. Ment. Dis. **115:**299, 1952.

Braceland, F., and Giffin, M.: The mental changes associated with multiple sclerosis, Proc. Assoc. Res. Nerv. Ment. Dis **28:**450, 1950.

Harrower, M.: The results of psychometric and personality tests in multiple sclerosis, Proc. Assoc. Res. Nerv. Ment. Dis. **28:**461, 1950.

Hartstein, J., and Ulett, G.: Galactose treatment of multiple sclerosis (a preliminary report), Dis. Nerv. Syst. **18:**1, 1957.

Langworthy, O., and LeGrand, D.: Personality structure and psychotherapy in multiple sclerosis, Am. J. Med. **12:**586, 1952.

Pratt, R. T. C.: An investigation of the psychiatric aspects of disseminated sclerosis, J. Neurol. Neurosurg. Psychiat. **14:**326, 1951.

Ross, A. T., and Reitan, R. N.: Intellectual and affective functions in multiple sclerosis, Arch. Neurol. Psychiatry **73:**633, 1955.

Swank, R.: The multiple sclerosis diet book, Garden City, N.Y., 1978, Doubleday & Co.

Ulett, G.: Geographic distribution of multiple sclerosis, Dis. Nerv. Syst. **9:**342, 1948.

Brain trauma

We are concerned here with the psychic sequelae of a head injury. In describing the acute injury itself the term "concussion" is properly used only when some amount of amnesia is present. States of impaired consciousness following head injury are described as confusion (mild, moderate, or severe), subcoma, or coma. Following head injuries of varying degrees of severity, there may occur deliria, amnesic states, the "posttraumatic constitution" of Meyer (i.e., easy reaction to alcohol, influenza, etc.), lasting vasomotor neurosis (with headaches, irascibility, and hysterical or even epileptic episodes), traumatic defect conditions such as the aphasias, and even marked progressive cerebral degeneration.

It has been pointed out that in most cases posttraumatic symptoms are substantially receding by 3 months following the injury. In one series approximately 15% of patients had symptoms persisting 1 year or longer. It is felt that patients with pretraumatic psychoneurotic personalities are more likely to develop posttraumatic psychiatric symptoms, but patients with normal pretraumatic personalities are not uncommon. A high correlation has been found between the existence of persistent complicating psychosocial factors—such as continuing compensation, pending litigation, occupational stresses, persistent associated bodily injuries, etc.—and the severity and persistence of psychiatric sequelae.

SUGGESTED READINGS

Allen, A. M., Moore, M., and Daly, B. B.: Subdural hemorrhage in patients with mental disease, N. Engl. J. Med. **223**:324, 1940.

Brock, S., editor: Injuries of the brain and the spinal cord and their coverings, ed. 4, New York, 1960, Springer Publishing Co.

Fras, I., Litin, E. M., and Pearson, J. S.: Comparison of psychotic symptoms in carcinoma of the pancreas and those in some other intra-abdominal neoplasms, Am. J. Psychiatry **123**:1553, 1967.

Garrett, J. F., and Levine, E. F.: Psychological practices with the physically disabled, New York, 1962, Columbia University Press.

Heine, B. E.: Psychiatric aspects of systemic lupus erythematosus, Acta Psychiat. Scand. **45**:307, 1969.

Kamman, G.: Traumatic neurosis, compensation neurosis or attitudinal pathosis? Arch. Neurol. Psychiatry **65**:593, 1951.

Malamud, N., and Saner, G.: Neuropathological findings in lupus erythematosus, Arch. Neurol. Psychiatry **71**:723, 1954.

McKissock, W.: Subdural hematoma; a review of 389 cases, Lancet **1**:367, 1960.

Merskey, H., and Woodforde, J. M.: Psychotic sequelae of minor head injury, Brain **95**:521, 1972.

Rowbotham, G. F.: Acute injuries of the head, ed. 4, Edinburgh, 1964, E. & S. Livingstone, Ltd.

Stuteville, P., and Walsh, K.: Subdural hematoma in the elderly person, J.A.M.A. **168**:1455, 1958.

Ulett, G., and Parsons, E. H.: Psychiatric aspects of carcinoma of the pancreas, J. Missouri Med. Assoc. **45**:490, 1948.

Psychosis associated with other physical conditions
Pernicious anemia

Minor mental symptoms are extremely common in patients with pernicious anemia. Psychotic reactions have been reported in up to 15% of patients from some clinics. Delirium, delusions, hallucinations, depression, agitation, and signs of organic deterioration may all occur. The role of associated vitamin deficiencies may be a factor. The psychiatric symptoms tend to disappear with treatment of the anemia.

SUGGESTED READINGS

Betts, W. C.: The use of electroshock therapy in psychosis associated with pernicious anemia, N. Carolina Med. J. **13**:321, 1952.

Lewin, K. K.: Role of depression in the production of the illness in pernicious anemia, Psychosom. Med. **23**:23, 1959.

Samson, D., Swisher, S., Christian, R., and Engel, G.: Cerebral metabolic disturbance and delirium in pernicious anemia, Arch. Intern. Med. (Chicago) **90**:4, 1952.

Shulman, R.: Psychiatric aspects of pernicious anemia: a prospective study, Br. Med. J. 3:266, 1967.

Paralysis agitans

Paralysis agitans is characterized by degenerative lesions in the globus pallidus and substantia nigra, due to either senile or vascular parenchymatous changes. Similarly the syndrome may occur with virus encephalitis, carbon monoxide poisoning, or following trauma. Progressive muscular rigidity, immobile facies, flexion of neck, trunk, and extremities, a propulsive gait, and slow rhythmic tremor characterize the syndrome. In many patients there are no mental symptoms. Most patients are good natured but some react to their disability with irritability, peevishness, and dissatisfaction. In others senile or vascular changes may produce psychotic symptoms.

SUGGESTED READINGS

Calne, D. B.: Developments in the pharmacology and therapeutics of parkinsonism, Ann. Neurol. **1**:111, 1977.

Goodwin, F. K.: Psychiatric side effects of levodopa in man, J.A.M.A. **218**:1915, 1971.

Parkinson, J.: An essay on the shaking palsy, London, 1817, Neely & Jones.

Robins, A. H.: Depression in patients with parkinsonism, Br. J. Psychiatry **128:**141, 1976.

Sweet, R. D., McDowell, F. H., Feigenson, J. S., Loranger, A. W., and Goodell, H.: Mental symptoms in Parkinson's disease during chronic treatment with levodopa, Neurology **28:**305, 1976.

Pellagra

Pellagra occurs with a polyavitaminosis of the B complex. It tends to appear in communities where dietary standards are low, and it may develop in institutionalized persons who are already psychotic. Neuronal and capillary changes are found throughout the neuraxis, usually most marked in the cerebrum. Stomatitis, glossitis, achlorhydria, and diarrhea are common. In early cases erythema of the skin, especially on the extensor surfaces of the extremities and the inner thighs, is followed by scaling and red-brown pigmentation. The early mental symptoms include irritability, headache, restlessness, lassitude, insomnia, emotional instability, difficulty in concentration, apprehension, and forgetfulness. Later, memory defects, confusion, disorientation, delirium, and finally dementia may occur. Late in the disease severe neurological complications develop with stupor, incontinence, varied sensory disturbances, irregular involuntary movements, convulsions, rigidity, and paralyses. Niacin is the specific therapeutic agent given, 100 mg. t.i.d. in mild cases and in severe cases 1200 to 1500 mg. per day. Brewer's yeast, 40 to 200 Gm., is added to a liberal diet.

SUGGESTED READINGS

Sebrell, W. H., Jr., and Harris, R. S., editors: The vitamins: chemistry, physiology, pathology, New York, 1954, Academic Press, Inc., vol. 1.

Spillane, J. D.: Nutritional disorders of the nervous system, Baltimore, 1947, The Williams & Wilkins Co., especially chaps. 2, 5, 6, and 13.

Porphyria

Acute porphyria is said to occur in families in which psychiatric disorders run rife. Occurring most frequently in women and in the third or fourth decades of life, the attack may be precipitated by sulfonal or barbiturates. Beginning with colicky abdominal pains and the appearance of a urine which darkens to a port-wine color on standing, the condition advances rapidly to the production of convulsions, paralyses, and sensory disturbances whose bizarre character (e.g., transient amaurosis) may be confused with symptoms of conversion hysteria. Transient confusional psychoses are common.

SUGGESTED READINGS

Markowitz, M.: Acute intermittent porphyria. A report of five cases and a review of the literature, Ann. Intern. Med. **41:**1170, 1954.

Roth, N.: The neuropsychiatric aspects of porphyria, Psychosom. Med. **7:**291, 1945.

Sikes, Z. S.: Electroencephalographic abnormalities and psychiatric manifestations in intermittent porphyria, Dis. Nerv. Syst. **21:**226, 1960.

Tschudy, D. P.: In Conn, H. F., editor: Porphyrias—current therapy, Philadelphia, 1965, W. B. Saunders Co.

Psychosis associated with drug or poison intoxication

BROMIDE INTOXICATION. A very common cause of delirium in psychiatric practice is the ingestion of bromide medication, usually as a sedative. With an excessive amount, unsteadiness, confusion, memory loss, and hallucinations occur and in some cases an acneform eruption.

Anamnesis. Among early symptoms, *chief complaints* are fatigue and sleepiness with generalized ataxia which the patient himself may bring to the physician's attention. Later, symptoms of brain dysfunction develop. The *history* is commonly one of underlying personality disorder, with increasing nervousness and ingestion of Bromo Seltzer, B. C., Neurosine, or some "salty liquid preparation." Too often the patient will deny any history of medication. The elderly, arteriosclerotic, chronic alcoholic or patient with cardiorenal disease has a lower tolerance for bromides. In such individuals 2 Gm. per day may produce intoxication in a few weeks. Weight loss, constipation, and insomnia occur.

Examination. In the *behavioral* picture, confusion, memory loss, delusions, and hallucinations occur frequently; the latter are predominantly visual and often of colors, lights, and large animals. There may be excitement, fear, or depression. As *physical* symptoms, ataxia, weakness, and slurred speech may occur. In some cases (10%) acneform eruption is present. This seems dependent more upon a dermatological predisposition than upon amount of drug ingested. Weight loss, cachexia, and even stupor can result. Based on *laboratory* tests, a serum bromide level of 150 mg./100 ml. is cited as the average at which symptoms begin, although as little as 75 mg./100 ml. or as much as 200 to 300 mg./100 ml. may be required. The tolerance is directly dependent upon the ingestion of salt in the diet, 10 to 15 Gm. chloride being necessary for elimination of each gram of bromide ingested. A simple test for the presence of bromide is to add 1 Gm. of animal charcoal to 20 to 25 ml. urine and filter for a few minutes. To 5 ml. of the filtrate, add 1 ml. trichloracetic acid and 1 ml. 0.5% gold chloride. Brown color indicates the presence of bromides.

Prognosis. Good. In any patient with elevated blood bromide it is wise to withhold the final diagnosis of other psychosis until the blood bromide has returned to normal. Excretion is much slower than uptake. Mental symptoms may persist after the removal of bromide from the blood by as much as 2 weeks or more. With good chloride intake bromide level may fall 50% in 7 days. Excretion is principally via kidneys.

In general, the higher the blood bromide, the more intense are the symptoms. A routine blood bromide test can be of as great diagnostic value as a routine serological examination in patients admitted to a psychiatric service.

Treatment. Force fluids.

Give oral NH_3Cl, enteric-coated, up to 8 Gm. per day (in divided doses); 1000 to 2000 ml. physiological saline solution, I.V.

Sedate with chloral hydrate or paraldehyde if necessary. Chlorpromazine, 50 mg. I.M. q. 4 h., may be used cautiously.

SUGGESTED READINGS

Cornbleet, T.: Bromide intoxication treated with ammonium chloride, J.A.M.A. **146:**1116, 1951.

Hodges, H. H., and Gilmour, M. T.: The continuing hazard of bromide intoxication, Am. J. Med. **10:**459, 1951.

Levin, M.: Toxic psychoses. In Arieti, S., editor: American handbook of psychiatry, New York, 1959, Basic Books, Inc., Publishers, vol. 2.

Perkins, H. A.: Bromide intoxication. Analysis of cases from a general hospital, Arch. Intern. Med. (Chicago) **85:**783, 1950.

Sayed, A. J.: Mania and bromism: a case report and a look to the future, Am. J. Psychiatry **133:**338, 1976.

CARBON MONOXIDE INTOXICATION. Carbon monoxide combines with hemoglobin to form carboxyhemoglobin, which does not absorb oxygen; in carbon monoxide intoxication, the brain does not receive enough oxygen. Exhaust fumes, gas leaks, or suicide attempts account for most of the cases. Two-thirds of the patients pass from coma into delirium. One-third have a clear interval of a week and then develop apathy, confusion, and impairment of memory with confabulation. Chronic exposure to small amounts may lead to headache, emotional instability, depression, anxiety, vertigo, abdominal disturbances, and neuromuscular pains.

SUGGESTED READINGS

Garland, H., and Pearce, J.: Neurologic complications of carbon monoxide poisoning, Quart. J. Med. **36**:444, 1967.

Gilbert, G. J., and Glaser, G. H.: Neurologic manifestations of chronic carbon monoxide poisoning, N. Engl. J. Med. **261**:1217, 1959.

Ginsburg, R., and Romano, J.: Carbon monoxide encephalopathy: need for appropriate treatment, Am. J. Psychiatry **133**:317, 1959.

LEAD POISONING. Adults who inhale lead from paint spray, burning of lead batteries, or industrial use in enameling or glass manufacture develop acute delirium with confusion, insomnia, tremors, fear, persecutory delusions, visual halluncinations, and convulsions. Chronic exposure may lead to apathy, depression, memory loss with confabulation, weakness, dizziness, constipation, and vomiting. Black lines on the gums may be present.

SUGGESTED READINGS

Cheatham, J. S., and Chabot, E. F., Jr.: The clinical diagnosis and treatment of lead encephalopathy, South. Med. J. **61**:529, 1969.

Cummings, J. N.: Heavy metals and the brain, Springfield, Ill., 1959, Charles C. Thomas, Publisher.

Jenkins, C. D., and Mellings, R. B.: Lead poisoning in children, Arch. Neurol. Psychiatry **77**:70, 1957.

Karpinski, F. E., Rieders, F., and Gersh, L. S.: Calcium disodium versenate in the therapy of lead encephalopathy, J. Pediat. **42**:687, 1953.

MANGANESE POISONING. About 20% of manganese workers develop mental symptoms including elation, restlessness, and uncontrollable laughing or crying. Extrapyramidal symptoms, gait and speech disturbances, tremor of tongue, and muscular weakness occur.

MERCURY POISONING. Chronic mercury poisoning from inhalation of mercury occurs in certain trades (felt hat making, extraction of gold from silver amalgams, and painting ship hulls with antifouling plastic paint). Workers may become irritable with bursts of rage, and feel discouraged and afraid. Apathy, drowsiness, or loss of memory may occur. Methyl mercury from poisoned fish may lead to serious brain damage.

BARBITURATE INTOXICATION. In recent years the barbiturate compounds have been favorite chemical agents for suicide. *Acute barbiturate intoxication* occurs in 1 out of every 1,900 patients admitted to a general hospital and requires careful attention to medical as well as psychiatric factors, as death occurs in 7% to 15% of such cases.

Examination. The patient is brought to the emergency room in a coma with respiratory depression, followed by shock, a state clinically indistinguishable from uremia or opium poisoning. Hypothermia develops unless secondary pneumonitis has produced a rise in temperature. All neurological signs are sluggish, including pupillary reaction. Cyanosis and airway obstruction often supervene, followed by death from central respiratory inhibition.

Diagnosis. Diagnosis is usually made on the basis of history of ingestion of barbiturates plus finding barbiturates by chemical analysis of the urine. This method is preferable to testing the blood or stomach contents.

Treatment. If patient is seen within the first hour, remove any drug from the stomach by aspiration. Do not use emetics. Blood pressure, pulse, and respiration must be closely watched and frequently recorded. Suction apparatus and oxygen resuscitator should be at the bedside when symptoms indicate their usefulness. Good nursing care is essential with the emphasis on the prevention of complications. The patient should be kept warm, position frequently changed, and prophylactic antibiotics administered.

For stimulation of depressed respiratory center, use amphetamines; Benzedrine given intravenously at the rate of 1 mg./min. seems to be the drug of choice. Maintain an open airway and give oxygen as necessary to support respiratory exchange. Tracheotomy set should be quickly available. Maintain adequate cardiovascular circulation. Hypotension may be relieved by subcutaneous Neo-Synephrine, 1 to 5 mg., given when blood pressure falls below 90 mm. Hg systolic or 50 diastolic. Recent experience from Denmark seems to indicate that the treatment of choice relies upon maintenance of a stable cardiovascular state by the use of oxygen, blood, or plasma expanders and by forced diuresis in seriously ill patients. Osmotic diuretics (urea, mannitol) may be used intravenously. Hemodialysis may be accomplished by means of the artificial kidney or by the simpler procedure of intermittent peritoneal lavage with the addition of albumin to the peritoneal fluid to expedite the removal of barbiturate bound to the plasma protein.

SUGGESTED READINGS

Clemmeson, C., and Nilsson, E.: Therapeutic trends in the treatment of barbiturate poisoning, Clin. Pharmacol. Ther. **2:**220, 1961.

Cohn, R.: Barbiturate intoxication, a clinical EEG study, Ann. Intern. Med. **32:**1049, 1950.

Fraser, H. F., Wikler, A., Essig, C. F., and Isbell, H.: Degree of physical dependence induced by secobarbital or pentobarbital, J.A.M.A. **166:**126, 1958.

Fraser, H. F., and others: Chronic barbiturate intoxication, Arch. Intern. Med. (Chicago) **94:**34, 1954.

Matthew, H.: Acute barbiturate poisoning, Amsterdam, 1971, Excerpta Medica Foundation.

CORTISONE AND ACTH. A variety of mental symptoms may develop during the use of corticosteroids, such as depression, hypomania, depersonalization, hallucinations, delusions, and mutism.

IPRONIAZID. While treating patients for tuberculosis, mental symptoms may develop, including restlessness, disorientation, and auditory and visual hallucinations. There may be muscular twitching, troublesome urination, constipation, and convulsions.

SUGGESTED READING

Pleasure, H.: Psychiatric and neurologic side effects of isoniazid and iproniazid, Arch. Neurol. Psychiatry **72:**313, 1954.

OTHER. Delirium can also be produced by belladonna, chloral hydrate, paraldehyde, organic phosphorus insecticides, anticholinergic neuroleptics, and various plants.

SUGGESTED READING

Jacobziner, H.: Attempted suicide in adolescents by poisoning, Am. J. Psychother. **19:**247, 1965.

Childbirth

Psychosis with childbirth is classed among the psychoses associated with other physical conditions such as those of endocrine, toxic, infectious, or metabolic origin. However, pregnancy brings not only the internal stress of dramatic physiological changes but also the external stresses of new social responsibilities and emotional readjustments within the family. It is a natural breaking point for women with vulnerabilities of personality and is the situation in which up to 8% of psychoses in women occur. This category includes schizophrenic, manic-depressive, and toxic reactions which descriptively and from a therapeutic and prognostic point of view do not differ greatly from these disorders occurring in other life situations.

CLINICAL TYPES. Distribution is approximately as follows: schizophrenic (30% of cases), schizoaffective (20% to 25%), manic state (20%), depressive state (15%), and toxic psychoses (10%).

ANAMNESIS. The *chief complaint* is usually the observation by others that the patient has undergone a change in behavior 1 to 6 weeks following delivery, although in about one fifth of the cases the onset is before parturition. *History* reveals the onset of irritability, crying spells, insomnia, somatic complaints, and seclusiveness beginning in the first trimester. Except in toxic psychoses, no correlation exists with prolonged labor, toxemia of pregnancy, anemia, infection, or anesthetic complications, but in a sizeable percentage the child is basically unwanted or even illegitimate. Most studies do not indicate any correlation with the sex of the infant. Repeated pregnancies not uncommonly bring a repetition of symptoms. *Past* history may reveal a young woman who is not emotionally free from her mother, who was emotionally upset at the menarche, and who is sexually frigid with her husband. *Family* history reveals 14% with psychoses among parents or siblings.

Overall *behavior* does not differ from that in classic schizophrenic, manic, depressive, or toxic disorders except in content of thought. Fears of one's own and the baby's death, delusions of the baby's being deformed, dead, or not yet born—or even a complete denial of pregnancy and marriage—are not unusual. *Physical* examination frequently reveals signs of dehydration and malnutrition. As shown on *laboratory* tests, anemia, hypoproteinemia, and elevated nonprotein nitrogen may occur.

TREATMENT. Symptoms of mild or moderate emotional disturbance early in pregnancy should be treated immediately with psychotherapy as a preventive measure. Psychotic symptoms are treated with all the techniques of modern psychiatry, including phenothiazines, when the clinical picture includes agitation or schizophrenic symptomatology. Both during and after psychosis, psychotherapy is essential. It is a good rule to avoid leaving the mother alone with the new baby if the patient is delusional, as infanticide is not rare. Frequently social service work is of value at the time the patient leaves the hospital, in making plans for the new infant, or in case work with the family. Some authorities have recommended sterilization as a preventive measure after a careful evaluation of personality assets to determine the likelihood'of repeated psychosis with further pregnancies.

SUGGESTED READINGS

Brew, M. F., and Seidenberg, R.: Psychotic reactions associated with pregnancy and childbirth, J. Nerv. Ment. Dis. **111**:408, 1950.

Ekblad, M.: Induced abortion on psychiatric grounds; a follow-up study of 479 women, Acta Psychiat. Neurol. Scand. **99** (suppl.):1, 1955.

Gordon, J. E., Ingals, T. H., and Thomas, C. L.: Preventive medicine and epidemiology; psychosis after childbirth: ecological aspects of a single impact stress, Am. J. Med. Sci. **238**:363, 1959.

Hamilton, J. A.: Postpartum psychiatric problems, St. Louis, 1962, The C. V. Mosby Co.

Kendall, R. E., Wainright, S., Hailey, A., and Shannon, B.: The influence of childbirth on psychiatric morbidity, Psychol. Med. **6**:297, 1976.

Markham, S. A.: A comparative evaluation of psychotic and non-psychotic reactions to childbirth, Am. J. Orthopsychiatry **31**:565, 1961.

Melges, F. T.: Postpartum psychiatric syndromes, Psychosom. Med. **30**:95, Feb., 1968.

Rosenwald, G. C., and Stonehill, M. W.: Early and late post-partum illnesses, Psychosom. Med. **34**:129, 1972.

Thornton, W. E.: Folate deficiency in puerperal psychosis, Am. J. Obstet. Gynec. **129**:222, 1977.

Treadway, C. R., Kane, F. J., Jr., Jarrahi-Zadeh, A., and Lipton, M. A.: A psychoendocrine study of pregnancy and puerperium, Am. J. Psychiatry **125**:1380, 1969.

Wainright, W.: Fatherhood as a precipitant of mental illness, Am. J. Psychiatry **123**:40, 1966.

NONPSYCHOTIC ORGANIC BRAIN SYNDROMES
The epilepsies

These *seizure* disorders are important to the neuropsychiatrist not only because they are common afflictions (0.5% of the population) but also because they present a wide variety of deviations from normal behavior whose pathophysiology aids our understanding of the functioning of the central nervous system. The term "convulsive disorders" (introduced to avoid the odious label of "epilepsy") is misleading, because many seizures occur without motor (convulsive) manifestations. In the older terminology "grand mal" referred to seizures in which a major convulsion occurred, and the term "petit mal" was reserved for all lesser seizures. Observation of the seizure states by means of the electroencephalograph has disclosed that abnormal electrical disturbances of the brain (paroxysmal cerebral dysrhythmias) occur during all types of seizures and often in the resting record between seizures. The spread of such brain disturbance to the motor cortex can produce motor symptoms and generalized convulsions. Sensory, visceral, and other varieties of submaximal seizures occur when the brain disturbance remains focal in other then motor areas of the brain.

It is clinically useful to regard the seizure as a symptom, thus directing one's attention both to the possible etiological mechanisms and to the part of the brain involved. Thus seizures limited to one side of the body or, for example, characterized only by motor symptoms of one limb give definite evidence of focal brain involvement. The cause of a seizure, however, can be injury, neoplasm, infection, or other agent which so alters the cells as to induce a focus of abnormal electrophysiological discharge. The spread of such an electrical seizure to, or its origin in, diencephalic centers seems responsible for obliteration of conscious awareness. Seizure discharges which originate from the temporal lobes can produce a variety of behavior changes, often difficult to distinguish from symptoms occurring in some of the major psychotic reactions.

Studies made from electrodes inserted into brain tissue, at various depths below the cortex, have produced evidence that paroxysmal electrical storms can occur in the brain without being evident from conventional scalp or even from cortical recording electrodes. Reports have appeared relating such deep focal disturbance to the occurrence of hallucinations. *Psychic phenomena* in the form of lapses of consciousness are common to almost all seizures. Strange variations lasting a few seconds, minutes, or hours, such as dream states, a feeling of having experienced it all before (déjà vu), confusion, fugues, ecstasies, etc., are not uncommon. With focal, temporal lobe seizures the aura of the attack may consist of an illusion or hallucination which is related to the life experience of a patient (a remembered scene or dream experience), thus reaffirming that the acquired neuronal patterns of the temporal lobe have to do with the engrams of memories, thoughts, and feelings.

Postictal clouded states. After a seizure the patient may be confused and resistant, motor behavior returns but conscious control of it lags behind, and—if he is restrained—the patient may fight and injure those around him. With return of consciousness this behavior comes to an end.

Seizures in hysteria. Seizures may occur in hysterical patients without the usual widespread abnormal discharge in the EEG. The attacks usually begin in the presence of other persons and in a situation of emotional significance. The patient sinks to the ground without injury or tongue biting. Urinary incontinence is rare. The pupils usually react to light, consciousness is not entirely lost, and the patient responds to sensory stimulation. The duration of the attack may be prolonged, and its overall character is bizarre. One must not overlook the fact that the hysterics are not immune to epilepsy and that both types of attack can occur in the same individual.

Personality and intellectual changes with convulsive disorders. Although repeated severe seizures may be associated with mental changes, this is by no means always the case. Of the 90% of epileptics who are outside institutions, the majority show no gross evidence of peculiar personality or unusual behavior. Of clinic and private patients only about 1 in 10 shows recognizable intellectual deterioration.

Where mental symptoms do exist, common brain pathology may produce both the seizure and the mental defect. Abnormalities of thinking may be the result of drug treatment, as may personality alterations, particularly discouragement and loss of initiative.

ETIOLOGY. The immediate cause of the clinical seizure is the underlying cerebral dysrhythmia. Precipitating causes include trauma, brain tumors, infections (encephalitis, abscess, meningitis), toxins, anoxia, and metabolic diseases.

The role of heredity, though often overemphasized, is an important factor. Ten percent of epileptics have a family history positive for seizure disorder. In the case of children with febrile convulsions the family history is double this figure. The terms "idiopathic" and "cryptogenic" epilepsy refer to seizures of unknown cause and often to an inherited cerebral dysrhythmia.

TYPES. The most commonly seen seizures may be classified as (1) infantile spasms, (2) febrile convulsions, (3) petit mal, (4) petit mal variant, (5) grand mal, (6) focal motor and Jacksonian seizures, (7) myoclonic seizures, (8) focal sensory seizures, (9) thalamic and hypothalamic seizures, and (10) psychomotor seizures.

Infantile spasms. These are frequent, brief, jerking or quivering spells seen during the first year of life and lasting up to the fourth year. There may be eye rolling and an upward flinging of the arms. The accompanying brain wave disturbance of almost continuous high-voltage slow waves and spikes with shifting multiple foci has been termed hypsarrhythmia. The condition is seen in boys more frequently than in girls. Eleven percent die before the third year, and 87% of those who live are feebleminded. The usually ascribed causes are encephalitis, anoxia, and birth trauma.

Febrile convulsions. These are convulsions occurring during fevers associated with a variety of illnesses. This term is reserved for those cases in which repeated episodes occur. Seen in the third to tenth year, the condition carries a relatively good prognosis. The interseizure EEG is usually normal.

Petit mal. These seizures typically are brief (up to 15 seconds) lapses of consciousness, accompanied by rhythmic blinking of the eyes, nodding of the head, jerking of the arms, sudden loss of posture, or staring. Such attacks are accompanied by the classic 3/sec. spike and wave pattern in the EEG. Attacks occur frequently, from 5 or 6 to over 100 per day (pyknolepsy). Appearing before puberty, they tend to decrease and disappear with increasing age and rarely are carried into adult life. In those cases in which grand mal convulsions also occur or where the EEG shows a strong grand mal (spike) component the prognosis is more guarded, as the latter type of seizure may persist into adult life. Hereditary factors are the same as for other types of seizure. Encephalitis is believed to be a common cause.

Petit mal variant. This diagnosis is made from an EEG pattern in which the spike and wave complex is atypical and occurs at a frequency other than 3/sec. There occur tonic or tonic-clonic convulsions, brief attacks of impaired consciousness, or sudden losses of posture. It differs from petit mal by an earlier age of onset and is frequently associated with evidence of organic brain damage and the occurrence of intellectual impairment.

Grand mal. This term is applied to the generalized convulsive seizure. In usual sequence, with or without some premonition or transient sensory experience (aura), the patient loses consciousness, muscles become rigid (tonic), respiration is suspended, and he falls. Jerking (clonic) movements then occur, respiration returns, and consciousness is gradually recovered. Loss of sphincter control and minor injury such as tongue biting are common. During the seizure the EEG shows high-voltage spiking activity that is often indistinguishable from the electrical component of the muscle discharge; later the record becomes almost flat. Voltage returns with slow activity which increases in frequency as consciousness is gained. The interseizure records may show spiking activity, but more usually show high-voltage slow waves, often occurring paroxysmally. Forty percent of persons with grand mal seizures have relatively normal EEG tracings during the interseizure period. The etiology of this condition is varied and such seizures occur following trauma, oxygen lack, vascular disease, encephalitis, toxins, neoplasms, or metabolic disease, or they result from an inherited cerebral dysrhythmia.

Focal motor and Jacksonian seizures. These are sometimes called partial seizures and may occur with involvement of one extremity with or without loss of consciousness. A convulsion beginning locally and spreading on one side of the body is termed "Jacksonian." From such focal beginnings a spread to the opposite side of the body may occur, with production of a generalized seizure. The EEG may show localized spike discharges. Surgical intervention with removal of a focal lesion or focus of abnormally discharging brain tissue should be considered in these patients.

Myoclonic seizures. Sudden single jerking of the head, limbs, or trunk may occur, associated with multiple high-voltage spikes in the EEG, with or without mixed slow waves. Consciousness is not noticeably impaired. This phenomenon is commonly associated with major seizures (64%). Symptoms are aften accentuated upon awakening or on going to sleep.

Focal sensory seizures. These seizures may occur either as aurae (premonitory symptoms of a generalized seizure) or as an independent attack. Visual, auditory, or olfactory seizures may occur with focal involvement of the corresponding cortical area.

Thalamic and hypothalamic seizures. Paroxysmal brain disorder in these regions should be considered with the occurrence of attacks of vertigo, dizziness, cardiac palpitation, pain, or paresthesia, associated with loss of consciousness or convulsive phenomena. Sweating, vomiting, respiratory distress, and urge to micturate, as well as attacks of uncontrollable rage, have been described. Positive spike patterns of 14/sec. and 6/sec. may occur in the EEG associated with this clinical picture. These electroencephalographic patterns are seen most often in adolescents, are accentuated in light stages of sleep, and often have a temporal or occipital focalization. In patients with these symptoms, the paroxysmal nature of the complaint may be overlooked and the case be misdiagnosed as one of neurosis, gastric migraine, neurotic headache, behavior disorder, and the like. Trauma and encephalitis are among the commonest etiological factors.

Psychomotor seizures. The term "psychomotor" (psychic or epileptic equivalent) has been used to describe attacks of epilepsy in which the subject becomes confused but does not, as a rule, completely lose consciousness. There may be accompanying emotional displays of rage or fear and such behavior as negativism, staring, groping, chewing, swallowing, smacking of the lips, laughing, crying, rubbing, plucking, undressing, showing confusion in speech, or exhibiting other complex behavior for which the patient is later amnesic.

Neurophysiologically this type of epilepsy has been linked to the limbic system. The EEG may disclose a temporal spike focus which is sometimes seen only during the sleeping record. If the abnormal discharge remains localized in the anterior part of the temporal lobe, no clinical symptoms occur. When, however, it spreads, high-voltage 6/sec. and flat-topped 4/sec. waves are seen in distant cortical areas and the typical clinical manifestations occur.

This type of epilepsy occurs most commonly in adults but is found, rarely, in young children. It is often seen in combination with other types of convulsive disorder. It has been estimated that approximately half of the patients with anterior temporal foci have more or less continuous psychiatric symptoms, either as personality disorder or as psychosis. The etiology of the irritated temporal lobe focus may be traumatic, with birth trauma a common offender. Other types of focal lesions are less commonly found. Surgical intervention in selected cases may be of value.

DIAGNOSIS. The EEG is a definite aid to diagnosis in about 50% of cases. In an additional group, recording during sleep may elicit focal patterns, particularly anterior temporal spikes and 14/sec. and 6/sec. positive spiking. The precipitation of spike and wave activity, with or without a seizure, and less commonly the elicitation of other diagnostic patterns or convulsive phenomena by strong hyperventilation can be of distinct diagnostic aid. Other activation procedures (Metrazol, photo-Metrazol, and photic stimulation) are of questionable diagnostic significance. A search for the cause in every case of seizure should include complete neurological examination, x-ray films of the skull, spinal fluid examination, and—where indicated—arteriography and/or pneumoencephalography.

TREATMENT. In general it can be stated that no two cases of seizure disorder are alike; therefore, treatment must be individualized. Total management requires cooperation on the part of the patient and family, patience on the part of the doctor, and a mulifaceted treatment approach.

Anticonvulsant therapy. Drugs commonly used to control seizures are listed in Table 4. The safest drug with fewest side effects should be tried first and the dose rapidly increased to tolerance. If one is ineffective, another drug should be substituted; if partially effective, a second drug added and likewise systematically evaluated. Complete seizure control may require continued high dosage. Only when seizures are controlled is it wise to reduce the dosage of those drugs with annoying side effects.

Tranquilizers may be helpful to reduce hypermobility and agitation, especially in children and in patients with psychomotor seizures. In combination with anticonvulsants, tranquilizers may add to the somnifacient effects of phenobarbital, Mesantoin, Tridione, etc., such that dosages of the latter may be reduced. Be-

Table 4. Anticonvulsant drugs*

Seizure pattern	Drug	How supplied	Gm./day maximum Child	Gm./day maximum Adult	Dosage limited by‡	Idiosyncrasy§
Generalized convulsive, focal Jacksonian, or autonomic	Phenobarbital	Tab. 15, 30, and 100 mg. Elix. 15 mg/tsp.	0.1 Gm.	0.3 Gm.	—	Irritability
	Mebaral	Tab. 30, 100, and 200 mg.	0.2 Gm.	0.5 Gm.	—	Irritability
	Bromides	Tab. and sol.		3.0 Gm.	—	Bromide intoxication Nausea, giddiness
	Mysoline	Tab. 250 mg.	0.1 Gm.	2.0 Gm.	Unsteadiness	
	Mesantoin†	Tab. 100 mg.	0.1 Gm.	0.8 Gm.	Unsteadiness	Bone marrow depression, lymphadenopathy
	Dilantin	Cap. 30 mg., 100 mg. Enteric-coated 0.1 Gm. Cap. Loz. 50 mg.	0.1 Gm.	0.6 Gm.	Vomiting, unsteadiness	Gum swelling, hirsutism
	Valium	Tab. 2, 5, 10 mg. Sol. 5 mg./ml.	0.8 mg/kg	.040 Gm.	Respiratory depression	Paradoxical excitement
	Clonopin	Tab. 0.5, 1, 2, mg.	.03 mg/kg	.020 Gm.	Respiratory depression	CNS effects leukopenia, thrombocytopenia
Psychomotor attacks	Peganone	Susp. 100 mg./tsp. Tab. 250 mg., 500 mg.	1.0 Gm.	4.0 Gm.		

	Preparation	Initial dose	Maximum dose	Side effects	Toxic effects
Phenurone†	Tab. 500 mg.	1.0 Gm.	4.0 Gm.	Anorexia, insomnia	Hepatitis, psychosis
Tegretol	Tab. 200 mg.	200 mg.	1.2 Gm.	Side effects common	CNS, CV, Dermatologic, Hematopoietic
Celontin	Cap. 300 mg.	0.3 Gm.	2.5 Gm.	Headache, anorexia	
Milontin	Cap. 500 mg. Susp. 300 mg./tsp.	1.0 Gm.	3.0 Gm.		
Tridione†	Cap. 300 mg. Dulcet 150 mg. Sol. 150 mg./tsp.	0.9 Gm.	3.0 Gm.	Hiccups	Photophobia, bone marrow depression
Paradione†	Cap. 150 mg., 300 mg. Sol. 300 mg./ml.	0.9 Gm.	3.0 Gm.	Hiccups	Photophobia, bone marrow depression
Diamox	Tab. 250 mg.	0.2 Gm.	1.0 Gm.	Anorexia, thirst	Psychiatric symptoms, bone marrow depression
Zarontin	Cap. 250 mg.	0.5 Gm.	1.5 Gm.	Nausea	
Depakene	Cap. 250 mg.	30 mg./kg.			

Petit mal triad (absence, akinesia, myoclonus)

*Modified from table used by the Seizure Unit of the Children's Medical Center, Boston, Mass.

Mebaral (mephobarbital), Mysoline (primidone), Mesantoin (methylphenylethylhydantoin), Dilantin (dephenylhydantoin), Valium (diazepam), Clonopin (clonazepam), Peganone (ethytoin), Phenurone (phenacemide), Celontin (methsuximide), Tegretol (carbamazepine), Milontin (methylphenylsuccimide), Tridione (trimethyloxazolidinedione), Diamox (acetazolamide), Zarontin (ethosuximide), Depakene (valproic acid).

Dosages: Usually 25% to 50% of the maximum is prescribed initially and is given in two to three doses every day with meals. At 2- to 4-week intervals the dosage is increased by small steps as needed and tolerated until either seizures are eliminated or toxic symptoms appear.

Continued on p. 138.

ware of the occasional convulsant properties of some tranquilizers.

Antibiotics. Antibiotics should be given a trial in all cases with a history or question of encephalitis, and especially in those cases with a progressive worsening or multiple EEG foci. A course of 4 or 5 weeks of Achromycin, Terramycin, or Chloromycetin may be tried.

Surgical treatment. Surgical treatment consists of removal of epileptogenic focus localized by EEG.

Psychotherapy. Decisions regarding the type of psychotherapy used should be governed entirely by the needs of the patient. A type of supportive therapy is probably given by every doctor who treats epileptics and recognizes their need to accept the illness and to adjust to chronic medication and the limitation of certain activities. The adjustment to life in which the possibility of a convulsion is always potentially present may lead to a neurotic, chronic invalidism more restrictive than epilepsy. Some attempt should be made to discuss the emotional relationship of the patient to the physician and to encourage emotional expression as well as reeducation in life goals and patterns. Group therapy for epileptics has been found to be worthwhile and with the participation of relatives and employers can help in a reorientation of the attitudes of all concerned.

Footnote continued from p. 137.

Combinations: When drugs used singly fail to control seizures, combinations may succeed; e.g., Dilantin 3 parts, phenobarbital 1 part, or Dilantin 1 part, Tridione 3 parts. Amphetamines may be added as needed to combat mild sedation. Some believe that amphetamine has a beneficial effect on petit mal seizures. Occasionally Dilantin will aggravate petit mal seizures and Tridione or Atabrine, convulsive seizures. To simplify evaluation of therapy, *only one drug should be changed during a 2-week period.* Librium (chlordiazepoxide) and Valium (diazepam) have some anticonvulsant properties and are useful when given in combination with other anticonvulsants. They are preferred over phenothiazines, which lower convulsive threshold.

Essential observations:

†*Monthly* WBC count and differential smear are obligatory because of possible bone marrow depression.

‡Sedation or grogginess is usually the factor which limits dosage in all except Dilantin.

§Rash. All drugs have produced rash in sensitive patients, usually after 8 to 12 treatment days.

Complications: Bone marrow depression, erythematous rash, liver toxicity, or *psychosis* requires immediate withdrawal of the offending drug, and a maximal dose of phenobarbital is given daily for 2 weeks to prevent precipitation of status epilepticus.

The condition of *status epilepticus,* which occurs in about 8% of epileptics, requires vigilant nursing care, intravenous glucose and saline, and catheterization as necessary. Diphenylhydantoin (Dilantin sodium, Steri-Vial or ampule) is useful. Inject intravenously at a rate not to exceed 50 mg./min. Most episodes are controlled by 250 mg. This dose may be repeated or 250 mg. given intramuscularly at 4- to 6-hour intervals for 2 to 3 days. Continue orally when patient is conscious. Paraldehyde, 5 ml. (mixed with 10 ml. of vegetable oil), per 15 pounds of body weight, can be given by rectum. Barbiturates which may be used are sodium Amytal, 0.5 Gm. I.V., or Luminal sodium, 0.3 Gm. I.V. *Repeat only with great caution, as oversedation can be more dangerous than status.* Alternatively, magnesium sulfate, 10 ml. of 25% solution I.V., or Avertin with amylene hydrate in an anesthetic dose per rectum, 60 to 80 mg./kg. of body weight, may be given.

SUGGESTED READINGS

Barker, W., and Barker, S.: Experimental production of human convulsive brain potentials by stress-induced effects upon neural integrative function: dynamics of the convulsive reaction to stress, Proc. Assoc. Res. Nerve. Ment. Dis. **29:**92, 1950.

Cobb, S.: Borderlands of psychiatry, Cambridge, Mass., 1943, Harvard University Press.

Falconer, M. A.: Serafitinides, A., and Corsellis, J. A. N.: Etiology and pathogenesis of temporal lobe epilepsy, Arch. Neurol. (Chicago) **10:**233, 1964.

Flor-Henry, P.: Schizophrenic-like reactions and affective psychoses associated with temporal lobe epilepsy etiological factors, Am. J. Psychiatry **126:**400, 1969.

Gastaut, H., Jasper, H., Bancaud, J., and Waltregny, A.: The physiopathogenesis of the epilepsies, Springfield, Ill., 1969, Charles C Thomas, Publisher.

Gibbs, F. A., and Gibbs, E. L.: Borderlands of epilepsy, J. Neuropsychiatry **4:**287, 1963.

Lennox, W. G., and Lennox, M. A.: Epilepsy and related disorders, Boston, 1960, Little, Brown & Co. vols. 1 and 2.

Penfield, W., and Jasper, H.: Epilepsy and the functional anatomy of the human brain, Boston, 1954, Little, Brown & Co.

Rodin, E. A.: Psychomotor epilepsy and aggressive behavior, Arch. Gen. Psychiatry **28:**210, 1973.

Sherwin, I.: Temporal lobe epilepsy: neurological and behavioral aspects, Ann. Rev. Med. **27**:37, 1976.

Slater, E., Beard, A. W., and Glithor E.: The schizophrenia-like psychoses of epilepsy, Br. J. Psychiatry **109**:95, 1963.

Stevens, J. R.: Psychiatric implications of psychomotor epilepsy, Arch. Gen. Psychiatry **14**:461, 1966.

13

Psychoses not attributed to known physical condition

AFFECTIVE DISORDER

This chapter will follow the new APA Standard Nomenclature (DSM III), which divides affective disorders into three major categories—*episodic, chronic,* and *atypical.* However, it should be emphasized that the categorization of this group of illnesses is not yet definitive. Depression as an isolated mood symptom is universal and becomes a sign of illness only by degree. Thus in terms of severity of illness one can think of a continuum running from the normal griefs of bereavement to serious chronic anhedonic states unrelenting over many months or years. So, too, in terms of causative events, depressions may be thought of as *reactive* in terms of known precipitating social stress such as the loss of some valued person or thing. When such a precipitating event is absent or undetected, the term "endogenous" is frequently used, particularly for those forms of serious or "psychotic" nature based upon the theory that this type of depression results from constitutional factors or has an hereditary basis and includes such symptoms as guilt, psychomotor retardation, melancholia, feelings of hopelessness, nihilism, suicidal behavior, and sleep, appetite, and sexual disturbances.

On the basis of clinical and genetic data (Winokur, Perris, Angst, and others), these disorders have now been dichotomized into *bipolar* (manic-depressive) and *unipolar* (depressive) illnesses. Bipolar patients must have experienced an episode of mania, while in the unipolar group only depressions need have occurred. Over half of the patients with bipolar disorders become ill prior to 30 years of age; unipolar onsets reach their peak a decade later. Patients with bipolar disturbances have more episodes than those with the unipolar type.

Current biochemical work on brain amines correlated with patient response to different types of chemotherapeutic agents has suggested that in the near future it may be possible to categorize affective disorders on the basis of the type of underlying biochemical disturbance predominantly in the neurotransmittor system. Such a classification will enable a better selection of treatments matched to the specific biochemical cell disturbance.

While the term "affective disorder" implies a basic mood disturbance, changes in energy and activity level of the individual are of at least equal importance. The two do not necessarily vary in the same direction, as seen by such long-used terms as "agitated depression," "stuporous depression," and "rut depression." Occurring as it often does at the time of climacteric, in males as well as females, the term "involutional melancholia" has long been used to designate a typical affective disturbance occurring at a time when the body is undergoing physiological and psychological stresses. Similarly, depressions may occur with pregnancy and childbirth (postpartum depression) and during the stress periods of adolescence or old age. When accompanying paranoid symptoms occur at the time of menopause the terms "involutional paraphrenia" and "paranoid involutional psychosis" have been used. The role of endocrine changes as reflected in the alterations seen with life periods of major stress is reflected, too, in the hormonal variance of the menstrual cycle and with other circadian rhythms, the roles of which have not been as yet clearly elucidated.

In the DSM III classification the term "episodic affective disorder" is used to mean a period of illness clearly distinguished from previous functioning in which there is a mood disturbance, either depression or elation, which colors the whole psychic life. The term "chronic affective disorder" indicates a long-standing illness (at least 2 years). The term "atypical affective disorder" is reserved for cases which do not fulfill the criteria for episodic or chronic affective disorder or adjustment disorder—that is, such cases with an episode of illness with many features of a manic syndrome but without a persistent elevated expansive or irritable mood; or a depressive illness with symptoms of excessive somnolence, overeating, and absence of endogenous features; or a disorder that fulfills the criteria for chronic depressive disorder but with intermittent periods of normal mood lasting longer than 2 months at a time.

TYPES OF AFFECTIVE DISORDER
Episodic affective disorder
Manic episode

These are distinct periods in a person's life when the predominant mood is elevated, expansive, or irritable. Associated symptoms include: hyperactivity, pressure of speech, flight of ideas, inflated self-esteem, decreased need for sleep, distractibility, and, with seeming lack of good judgment, the excessive involvement in activity with high potential for legal, sexual, social, or economic embarrassment. The elevated mood is often described as euphoric and has an infectious quality. Expansiveness may appear as an unceasing and unselective enthusiasm, which may be replaced by irritability in some, especially when thwarted. Typically there is increased sociability, often with blatant sexuality, telephoning friends at all hours, buying sprees, reckless driving, etc. Often there is a bizarre flamboyant character to the activities, including colorful dress, excessive make-up, and giving away goods, money, and advice to perfect strangers. Manic speech is typically loud, rapid, and full of jokes, puns, and rhyming; it may become dramatic, with singing or with angry tirades if the predominant mood is irritable. These patients are easily distracted by passing stimuli, the examiner's dress, etc. When extreme the speech and thinking may be incoherent. Grandiose delusions may involve a special relationship to God or some well-known figure from the political or entertainment world. Absurd claims may be made and advice given on matters about which the individual has no special knowledge. The patient has great energy to carry out the above, often awakening in the early morning after only 2 or 3 hours of sleep or even going for days without sleep. The mood may, on occasion, shift rapidly; or depressive features (tearfulness, etc.) may appear intermixed with the mania. Hallucinations and delusions with religious and sexual content are common.

Depressive episode

The essential feature is a depressive mood or a pervasive loss of interest or pleasure. Accompanying symptoms include sleep disturbance (especially early-morning awakening), anorexia, weight change (usually loss), psychomotor retardation or agitation, cognitive disturbance, decreased energy level, feelings of worthlessness or guilt, and thoughts of death or suicide.

The mood may be described as sad, hopeless, discouraged ("down in the dumps"), or a painful inability to experience pleasure. There is a withdrawal from friends and family, and avocations as a source of pleasure are neglected. With severe agitation the patient may pace, wring hands, rub hair, or talk loudly or incessantly. With psychomotor retardation body movements may be slowed, and speech may be decreased or even absent. Cognitive disturbances may include inability to concentrate, indecisiveness, and slowed thinking. Decrease in energy level is experienced as fatigue. The sense of worthlessness may vary from mild inadequacy to inability to perform even the smallest task. Guilt may be expressed in terms of sinfulness or responsibility for some tragic event. Thoughts of suicide and death may be pervasive and lead to tragic consequences. Symptoms are often worse on awakening, with some slight improvement as the day progresses. Associated features may include tearfulness, anxiety, fearfulness, phobias, panic attacks, hypochondriacal delusions of cancer or other illness, or nihilistic beliefs of personal or world destruction. Hallucinations may occur but are transient and rare.

AGE-SPECIFIC FEATURES. Although manic and bipolar disorders typically begin prior to age 30, major depressive disorders may begin at any age. In childhood separation anxiety may lead to clinging, school refusal, and/or fears of self or parent's death. In boys especially adolescent depression may manifest itself in grouchiness, aggression, restlessness, uncooperativeness, withdrawal from social activities, desire to leave home, and other acting out. In elderly adults associated features such as apathy, memory loss, and mild disorientation have led to use of the term "pseudo-dementia."

COURSE. Manic episodes typically begin suddenly with a rapid escalation of symptoms over a few days; they last from a few days to months, are briefer, and have a more abrupt termination than depressive episodes. Most of these patients will eventually have depressive episodes and hence be reclassified as having bipolar affective disorder.

Depressive episodes have a more variable onset, rarely sudden, after some severe psychosocial stress, but more often developing over days or weeks. Predominant symptoms are generalized anxiety, phobias, panic attacks, or some of the physiological changes typical of the depressed state such as anorexia, sleeplessness, etc. Some 50% of individuals will have a recurrence of depression. Individuals with recurrent major depressive disorder are at greater risk of developing bipolar affective disorder than those having only a single episode of depression.

In bipolar affective disorder the initial episode is usually manic. Episodes are usually shorter and often one episode follows another with but brief intervening normal periods. At times there is a continuing alternation (cycling) without intervening periods of normalcy.

COMPLICATIONS. In approximately 20% of cases there is a chronic course with frequently recurring episodes and some residual impairment. With severe manic episodes impairment of social and occupational functioning may be so extreme that the individual requires protection from the consequences of his poor judgment and hyperactivity. With lesser degrees of illness the episode may be termed "hypomanic." In severe depressive episodes the individual may be unable to properly feed or clothe himself or maintain minimal personal hygiene. Common complications of manic episodes are substance abuse and the legal, financial, and social consequences of actions resulting from impaired judgment. The most serious complication of depression is suicide, the risk increasing with age.

INCIDENCE. Approximately 18% to 23% of females and 8% to 11% of males will have a depressive episode. Severity is such as to require hospitalization in 6% and 3%, respectively. Bipolar disorder is equally predominant in men and women. Episodes of manic disorder are less common than are episodes of depression. Episodic affective disorder, especially the bipolar type, is more common among family members than in the general population. Certain evdence suggests that bipolar illness is an inherited X-linked disorder.

DIFFERENTIAL DIAGNOSIS. *Manic episodes* must be distinguished from organic affective syndromes caused by substance abuse (amphetamines, steroids, etc.), multiple sclerosis, and other organic illnesses. Schizophrenics who are irritable and angry with paranoid or disorganized thinking may appear as manics. In schizoaffective psychosis there may, in addition, occur delusions of being controlled by some external forces and having one's thoughts taken away.

Depressive episodes may occur from the use of such substances as reserpine, benzodiazepines, and various antihypertensive substances or from the action of a virus (influenza), chemical, or food substance (cerebral allergy) upon the CNS. Senile, presenile, or multi-infarct dementia may show the mild disorientation, apathy, memory loss, and difficulty in concentration seen also with the "pseudo-dementia" of some depressions in the elderly. In the latter, however, these symptoms may promptly disappear with adequate antidepressant treatments which should in all such cases be seriously considered. Patients with schizophrenia may also have significant depressive symptoms preceding, following, or superimposed upon a schizophrenic episode. Patients with catatonic schizophrenia may appear suddenly withdrawn and depressed, thus resembling severe cases of retarded depression. The presence of a severe psychotic thinking disorder such as of being controlled by external sources would suggest the diagnosis of schizoaffective psychosis. It must be remembered that many chronic psychiatric and neurological disorders are accompanied by depression that can at times be severe. Mild depression is ubiquitous, a too common experience in the general population. Uncomplicated bereavement is transient and not considered a mental disorder even if associated with a full depressive syndrome.

Chronic affective disorder

This term is used for chronic conditions of at least 2 years duration; these are considered as nonpsychotic disturbances. *Chronic hypomanic disorder* involves elated, expansive, or irritable moods that are relatively persistent or intermittent and in which there are no normal periods of 2 months' or more duration. These persons are characterized by a change in behavior in which at least three of the following characteristics different from their usual premorbid self are present: (1) decreased need for sleep, (2) more energy, (3) inflated self-esteem, (4) increased productivity, (5) sharpened and unusually creative thinking, (6) extreme gregariousness, (7) hyper-sexuality, (8) restlessness, (9) increased talkativeness, (10) overly optimistic or exaggerating potential achievements, (11) inappropriate laughing, joking, or punning, and (12) excessive involvement in pleasurable activity without recognizing the high potential for painful consequences (e.g., buying sprees, foolish business investments, reckless driving, etc.).

In *chronic depressive disorder* the symptoms are less severe than in a depressive episode but may involve a continuing loss of interest or pleasure in almost all usual activities, together with a mood depression characterized by feeling constantly sad, blue, low, or down in the dumps, with no normal period lasting 2 months or more. Clear-cut changes from previous behavior should be present in at least three of the following categories: (1) insomnia or hypersomnia, (2) feelings of fatigue with low energy level, (3) feelings of inadequacy, (4) decreased productivity, (5) decreased ability to concentrate or think clearly, (6) social withdrawal, (7) loss of interest or enjoyment in sex, (8) guilt and brooding over past activities, (9) less involvement in pleasurable activity, (10) feelings of being slowed down, (11) less talkative than usual, (12) pessimism about the future, and (13) episodes of tearfulness and suicidal thoughts.

In *chronic cyclothymic disorder* there may be a mixture of symptoms of chronic hypomanic disorder and chronic depression, or the two may alternate with several months of normal behavior in between. In these disturbances there is never any evidence of delusions, hallucinations, incoherence, or loosening of associations (derailment).

Atypical affective disorder

The term "atypical affective disorder" is used for individuals with some manic, hypomanic, or depressive symptoms, yet of an insufficient amount to meet the criteria for either episodic or chronic disorder; examples may include persons with some factors of manic illness without a persistent elevated, expansive, or irritable mood, or persons with mild depression interspersed by normal periods of longer than 2 months or with recurrent short-lived depressive episodes following stress reactions, personal rejections, etc.

STUDY OF PATIENTS WITH AFFECTIVE DISORDER
Anamnesis

At the onset of manic episodes early rising, impatience with delay, good humor, and press of social and business duties characterize the hypomanic as a "live wire." As the manic tendency progresses, his family may notice his tendency to monopolize the conversation, increasing irritability, and intolerance of restraint. Poor judgment coupled with plans and schemes and increased sexual drive may lead to excesses that bring the family to seek a physician's aid.

In an episode of depression, insomnia and early awakening, failure to eat, and weight loss may precede the onset of extended mood disturbance, with self-accusation, slow thinking motor retardation, melancholia, feelings of guilt, self-accusation, and inability to accept responsibility and perform daily tasks. Libido is lost; there are suicidal ruminations and body- and self-preoccupation.

Of great importance is the recognition of cases of mild affective disorder in which symptoms of headache, blurry vision, dyspnea, palpitation, anorexia, weight loss, nausea, abdominal pain, weakness, and/or other generalized symptoms may bring the patient to his family physician. In such cases the history is not psychologically spectacular and the symptoms may remit without the true nature of the illness being recognized. Since such cases are commonly seen in the medical clinic and general hospital and are labeled as neurotic, the physician must be constantly alert for the minimal signs that clearly delineate the illness as an attack of affective disturbance. Such symptoms include insomnia, difficulty in concentration, obsessions and phobias (including the fear of insanity), suicidal ideas, and psychomotor retardation.

Family history is important, for it has long been accepted that heredity plays a role in this illness, particularly in those patients with bipolar disorder. Available figures indicate an occurrence in the general population of 0.4% (1 in 250 persons) with about 25% occurrence in parents and full siblings of the patient. According to one authority, if one parent is afflicted, the illness occurs in 25% of the children, whereas with both parents manic-depressive two-thirds of the children have definite manic-depressive illness and one-third show mild affective psychopathy. Kallmann's studies of monozygotic twins revealed a 95% co-twin involvement.

There is some acceptance that the illness occurs with greater frequency in those of pyknic build. It occurs about twice as frequently in women. The illness is said to occur more commonly in Irish and Jewish persons and those of higher socioeconomic strata. The disease is seen at ages from 15 to over 70 years but with a peak onset between 35 and 39. Attacks may occur coincidentally with the frequent disturbances of mood seen at puberty, pregnancy, menstruation, and menopause.

The family history may be of suicide rather than of manic or depressive attacks. The premorbid personality may be given to mood swings but otherwise seemingly well adjusted.

Examination

The essential feature of a *manic episode* is a distinct period when the predominant mood is elevated, expansive, or irritable. Other symptoms may include hyperactivity, excessive involvement in activities without recognizing the high potential for painful consequences, pressure of speech, flight of ideas, inflated self-esteem, decreased need for sleep, and distractibility. Rhyming, punning, and clang associations are seen. Bizarre dress, shameless hypersexuality, hallucinations, grandiose delusions, pressure of activity, and even delirium may occur. Physically the patient may appear exhausted. There may be fever and mild bodily injuries. Psychological examination in the early stages shows increased M and C on the Rorschach with lowered form-level and increased original productions.

The patient with *depression* shows cardinal symptoms of difficulty in thinking, psychomotor retardation, and emotional depression. These patients move slowly, and speak slowly, and in a low tone. They prefer to answer in monosyllables. Consciousness is not clouded and they are well oriented. They may describe their mood as sad, hopeless, discouraged, or down in the dumps. At times the mood disturbance is expressed as not caring any more, with an inability to experience pleasure. Typically there is withdrawal from friends and family with neglect of avocations that formerly gave pleasure. Early morning awakening is the most characteristic sleep disturbance, although initial insomnia, fitful sleep, or hypersomnia also occur. Anorexia may be accompanied by weight loss, which can be severe. Less commonly there is increased appetite with weight gain. Psychomotor agitation may take the form of pacing, hand-wringing, inability to sit still, pulling or rubbing of hair, skin, clothing, or other objects, outbursts of complaining or shouting, or talking incessantly. Psychomotor retardation may take the form of slowed speech, increased pauses before answering, low or monotonous speech, slowed body movements, or, when severe, a markedly decreased amount of speech or even muteness. One often sees a depressed countenance with downcast eyes and weeping.

Cognitive disturbance may manifest itself as inability to concentrate, indecisiveness, or slowed thinking. The decrease in energy level is experienced as sustained tiredness or fatigue even in the absence of any physical exertion. The sense of worthlessness varies from mild feelings of inadequacy to completely unrealistic negative evaluations of one's worth. The smallest task may seem difficult or impossible.

Self-accusation, hypochondriacal and nihilistic delusions, and hallucinations may occur, being more marked in cases of longer duration. Depressives accept the delusion as rightful punishment for their sins, whereas the paranoid resents his persecutors. The condition can progress to stupor. Constipation and danger of impaction and urinary retention can occur, and circulation may be poor. There is a decline in both potency and libido. Menstrual disorders are common. On the Rorschach psychological examination responses are few, reaction time is prolonged, and high F+% is seen, with Dd emphasis and low M and C. Test behavior is characterized by impoverishment of thought and action, with painful uncertainty, rejection, pedantic self-correction, self-deprecation, and qualification of responses. One fears suicide when the Rorschach protocol shows superior intelligence, color shock, deep conflict, and signs of depression. Macabre content on card IV may also be significant.

Research

Biochemical aspects of the affective disorders have received increasing attention and are contributing to our understanding of these illnesses. Early observations that monoamine oxidase (MAO) inhibitors reversed the depression caused by reserpine led to the hypothesis that depression was due to a depletion of brain serotonin or norepinephrine. As lithium, a good anti-manic agent, decreased such amines it seemed to follow that an excess of amines could produce manic symptoms. However, lithium has also been shown to be effective in treating some types of depression. There are also other exceptions; to date no simple theory explains the mechanism of these disorders.

Research today centers on studies of the amine-monoamine neurotransmittors, membrane electrolyte dysfunction, and neuroendocrine dysfunction—these are all interrelated. Key substances at the neural synapse are norepinephrine, serotonin, and dopamine. These amines are widely distributed in the brain and seem to serve some adaptive or regulatory function for, although small in number, the neurons in which these amines are specifically active synapse widely throughout the brain. Effective agents for the treatment of affective disorders include the tricyclics, which block the reuptake of neurotransmittors at the neural synapse; MAO inhibitors, which inhibit the depletion of neurotransmittors by catecholamine transferase enzyme; amphetamines, which enhance the release of amines into the synapse; and lithium, which, in addition to its effect on membrane electrolytes, may increase intraneuronal inactivation of norepinephrine and thus decrease the norepinephrine available to adrenergic receptors. Unfortunately much of the work to date has been done acutely and on animals, while the affective disorders are chronic illnesses occurring in humans. Thus there remains the question of applicability of animal observations to human illness. Recent work involving the measurement of MHPG has suggested that endocrine evaluations may eventually prove predictive of bipolar manic-depressive syndromes as yet clinically undetected.

TREATMENT OF PATIENTS WITH AFFECTIVE DISORDER

Depending upon the severity of the illness and the stage of recovery, electroshock (ECT), drug therapy, and psychotherapy will all be found useful.

Electroshock

Previous to the advent of effective antidepressant medication, ECT was the treatment of choice. Eight to twelve convulsive treatments given at the rate of three per week are usually sufficient for depression. One or two treatments per day are given as necessary to control manic excitement. Although there is little evidence to support claims of brain damage with ECT, public pressures have in some locations resulted in a restriction of this modality, which is now often applied only when the patient has failed to respond to a trial with antidepressant medication. Because ECT is thought to improve the movement of drug across the blood/brain barrier, some physicians initiate chemotherapy after four or five ECT treatments. Because of slower therapeutic response with drug treatment, ECT is the treatment of choice with suicidal depression or seriously disturbed manic patients. Transient memory loss does occur.

Drug therapy

The treatment of depression is usually begun with tricyclic medication. There is some evidence that retarded types of depression respond best to drugs affecting predominantly norepinephrine uptake; hence imipramine or its metabolite, desipramine, is commonly used. Treatment is usually started with 25 mg. t.i.d. and increased to 300 mg., often given as a single bedtime dose in order to minimize side effects of drowsiness. As persons metabolize the tricyclics differently, suggested doses are only a rule of thumb. Adequate dose level on an individual basis will be better controlled when serum tricyclic levels become generally available. The drug should be increased rapidly until anticholinergic side effects, dry mouth, constipation, urinary retention, and increased somnolence become limiting factors to which the patient may ultimately develop some tolerance. With agitated depressions the beginning drug of choice is amytriptyline or its metabolite nortriptyline, both of which have a maximum serotonin effect. A similar dosage schedule to that of imipramine is followed. Here, however, the increase in dosage must be at a slower pace as there appears to be a therapeutic window below and above which the drugs are less effective. Doxepin is a useful drug of this class with a more sedative action, which can be therapeutically useful. Onset of improvement with the tricyclics averages about 2 weeks, except in the case of protriptyline, when improvement is often seen within 1 week.

The trial with any tricyclic drug should not be considered a failure until after a full 6 weeks of treatment at maximal total dose. Often the family will notice an improvement in the patient's behavior such as more activity, socialization, etc., before the patient will himself talk of subjective improvement in mood. If there is no good response to the initial trial with either of these two major classes of tricylic drugs, one should shift to the other for a similar period and dose schedule as there is some evidence that depressions may be either of the predominantly norepinephrine or predominantly serotonin-deficient variety. Should there be a failure of therapeutic response with both types of tricyclics, then the monamine oxidase inhibitors such as tranylcypromine (Parnate), isocarboxazide (Marplan), nialamide (Niamid), and phenelzine (Nardil) should be tried. A slow build-up in dosage with later decrease to maintenance dose, morning administration to avoid problems of insomnia, and the necessity for dietary restriction are considerations with this medication. Although formerly thought to be contraindicated, there are now reports of particularly resistant depressions that have responded to a combination of tricyclics and MAO inhibitors.

Stimulants such as methylphenadate, 5 to 10 mg., or amphetamines, 5 to 10 mg., as single morning doses may be useful but these drugs cannot be substituted for specific antidepressant medications. Thyroid function tests should be run routinely and particularly in female patients a small dose (25 μg) of cytomel daily may permit an improved response to tricyclic medication. In selecting the proper antidepressant medication it is helpful to know if the patient or a relative has had a favorable or unfavorable response to that same drug. In clinically apparent episodic depressions a family history of manic attacks may suggest the possible use of lithium as a treatment or prophylactic agent for recurrent depressions. In patients with atypical depression, those with marked neurotic, anxiety, obsessive compulsive, or many somatic complaints. MAO inhibitors may be the drug of first choice. In depressed patients with delusions, amytriptylike is reportedly more effective than imipramine. The duration of treatment should be 9 to 12 months after a favorable response has been achieved and only then should the dose be slowly withdrawn. In some patients with recurrent depressions these medicines are given prophylactically for an indefinite period of time.

In *manic* states the phenothiazines may be initially useful. Large doses may be necessary. Such drugs can produce depressive symptoms and must be used with care in agitated depression. Large doses of phenothiazines may be successfully combined with ECT in the initial management of hyperactive manic patients. Lithium, however, is the treatment of choice and should be immediately started in all manic patients. The suggested dose range is 300 mg.-tablets given three times daily with larger doses up to 1.5 grams or more required initially but carefully monitored with blood levels to a suggested dose range of 0.75 to 1.5 mEg/L. Even after discharge from the hospital on maintenance lithium prophylactic therapy, the patient's blood levels must be carefully monitored to avoid toxic reactions, which can be fatal. Shifts in body sodium such as occur with extremes of temperature and changes in diet may affect the lithium level. Long-term adverse effects of lithium on thyroid and kidney functioning as well as effects on the fetus during pregnancy must be carefully considered.

During a manic episode nursing care should include spoon-feeding or tube-feeding if necessary. A high-calorie diet with vitamins, combined with measures to prevent constipation and urinary retention, are particularly necessary in depressed patients. Occupational therapy and ward management can be used to calm manic patients and to urge depressive ones to activity but with consideration of their diurnal mood rhythm (i.e., slowed in morning and more spontaneous in afternoon and evening). In excited manic patients one must guard against sudden exhaustive death. This develops with fall in blood pressure, rapid pulse, weight loss, profuse perspiration, and hyperthermia.

Psychotherapy

Establishment of psychotherapy is extremely difficult in severe cases; even in milder cases experienced therapists usually have achieved disappointing results. In this and other recurrent psychotic disorders, however, it is to be emphasized that the rapid symptomatic relief afforded by the physical therapies is only a part of the treatment plan, which should work toward an improved psychological condition. Such psychotherapeutic efforts may begin during abatement of the illness cycle and with the patient safely guarded in a watchful therapeutic institutional milieu. The value of such psychotherapy is as a prophylactic strengthening of defenses against future emotional stresses. Recent studies have indicated that psychotherapy in these patients can bring about significant improvements in self-image and interpersonal relationships but not in the physiological mood and energy level symptoms typical of these illnesses. Likewise, psychopharmacology can dramatically affect the latter while having no impact upon improving self-image or interpersonal relationships. Thus in the proper management of these patients pharmacotherapy and psychotherapy both can play important roles.

SUGGESTED READINGS

Akiskal, H. S., and others: Cyclothymic disorder: validating criteria for inclusion in the bipolar affective group, Am. J. Psychiatry **134:**1227, 1977.

Davis, J. M.: Overview: maintenance therapy in psychiatry: II. Affective disorders, Am. J. Psychiatry **133:**1, 1976.

Dunner, D. L., Fleiss, J. L., and Fieve, R. R.: The course of development of mania in patients with recurrent depression, Am. J. Psychiatry **133:**905, 1976.

Johnson, G. F. S., and Leeman, M. M.: Analysis of familial factors in bipolar affective illness, Arch. Gen. Psychiatry **34:**1074, 1977.

Kraepelin, E.: Manic depressive insanity and paranoia, (Barclay, E., translator), Edinburgh, 1921, E. & S. Livingstone, Ltd.

Lund, R.: Personality factors and desynchronization of circadian rhythms, Psychosom. Med. **36:**224, 1974.

Mendels, J.: Lithium in the treatment of depression, Am. J. Psychiatry **133:**373, 1976.

Mendelo, J., Stern, S., and Frazer, A.: Biochemistry of depression, Dis. Nerv. Syst. **37:**5, 1976.

Morrison, J. R.: Bipolar affective disorder and alcoholism, Am. J. Psychiatry **131**(10):1130, 1974.

Munoz, R. A.: Treatment of tricyclic intoxication, Am. J. Psychiatry **133:**1085, 1976.

Perris, C.: A study of bipolar (manic-depressive) and unipolar recurrent depressive psychoses, Acta Psychiat. Scand. (Suppl.) **194:**1, 1966.

Raskin, A., and Crook, T. H.: Antidepressants in black and white inpatients, Arch. Gen. Psychiatry **32:**643, 1975.

Rosser, R.: Thyrotoxicosis and lithium, Br. J. Psychiatry **128:**61, 1976.

Shaw, D. M.: The practical management of affective disorders, Br. J. Psychiatry **130:**432, 1977.

Weissman, M. M., and Klerman, G. I.: Sex differences and the epidemiology of depression, Arch. Gen. Psychiatry **34:**98, 1977.

Wheatley, D.: Potentiation of amitriptyline by thyroid hormone, Arch. Gen. Psychiatry **26:**229, 1972.

Winokur, G., Clayton, P., and Reich, T.: Manic-depressive illness, St. Louis, 1969, The C. V. Mosby Co.

Wood, D., and others: Primary and secondary affective disorder. I. Past social history and current episodes in 92 depressed inpatients, Compr. Psychiatry **18:**201, 1977.

SCHIZOPHRENIC DISORDER

In 1849, Conolly in England recognized that some young persons developed a melancholia without grief and become apathetic. In 1860, Morel in Belgium described a brilliant 14-year-old boy who fell into melancholia, threatened to kill his father, and deteriorated into a state of inactivity. He first used the term "dementia précoce" (dementia praecox). He saw the condition as a hereditary type of mental deficiency with arrest of mental development in youth. In 1871, Hecker in German described "hebephrenia" as a progressive disease of puberty and adolescence. In 1874, Kahlbaum in Germany described "catatonia" as "tension insanity" with the patient sitting mute, motionless, immovable, and in severe cases with cerea flexibilitas. In 1896, Kraepelin in Germany differentiated between manic-depressive psychosis and dementia praecox (schizophrenia). He noted onset early in life with chronic course and combined "hebephrenia," "catatonia," and certain paranoid psychoses into a single classification. Dementia means deteriorating course and praecox means literally "parboiled," or premature. In 1906, Meyer in the United States said dementia praecox was not a disease but a faulty adaptation with accumulation of faulty habits ending in deterioration. In 1911, Eugen Bleuler in Switzerland published "Dementia Praecox or the Group of Schizophrenias." The fundamental symptoms include disturbances in associations (loosening, blocking), affect (disharmony between ideas and affect), ambivalence, and autism; the accessory symptoms include hallucinations, delusions, and bizarre behavior. Often the intensity of the accessory symptoms overshadowed the primary or fundamental symptoms. In examining a patient, it was important not to overlook the fundamental symptoms and miss the diagnosis, since the accessory symptoms were often intense and dramatic, they obscured the essential symptoms. Bleuler described fundamental (primary and pathognomonic) symptoms and accessory (seen in other diseases) symptoms.

That same year, 1911, Freud published his analysis of the famous "Schreber case," based on the "Memoirs of a Neurotic," published by Daniel Paul Schreber in 1903. Freud's publication was entitled "Notes upon an Autobiographical Account of a Case of Paranoia (Dementia Paranoides)." He gave a psychoanalytic view of paranoid delusions. However, Freud always felt the psychosis had an organic basis.

Schizophrenia constitutes the largest group of severe behavior disorders in our culture. One person in 100 will be hospitalized for schizophrenia, and, due to an increase in marriage and reproduction among schizophrenics, this number is increasing. Usually experiencing the onset of personality disorganization in adolescence or in early adult life, the schizophrenic patient has a lifelong struggle to gain internal security and to maintain relationships with other persons. Although often unrecognized, severe emotional problems, including a tendency to react to stress by withdrawal into a world of fantasy, arise early in life and often are associated with a failure to establish security with parental figures.

Although seen throughout the world and among persons of all cultures, schizophrenia occurs most frequently in individuals from lower socioeconomic groups. As demonstrated by Faris and Dunham, it occurs in areas of high mobility and social disorganization. Although occurring in persons of all ages, it is seen primarily in persons between 20 and 40 years of age, with a peak in the 25- to 34-year-old group.

The etiology of schizophrenic conditions is today unknown. Many theories abound, including genetic, biochemical, psychological, and social formulations.

Major genetic evidence has come from twin studies of Kallman and others which show identical twins both affected in 60% to 85% of instances, whereas with fraternal twins, both are affected in only 14% of cases, or about the same as sibling expectancy. In the general population, the incidence approaches 1%. Currently, geneticists propose "a specific inherited disease due to a single mutant inherited gene, either recessive, dominant, or intermediate." *Incomplete penetrance* and *constitutional resistance* are mentioned.

Some propose that the genetic factor is manifested through an "inborn error of metabolism," and Heath and co-workers speak of "taraxein" as a substance which ". ... impairs enzymatic activity in a pathway related to the metabolism of amines." Injected into the body, it produces abnormal electrical potentials from the limbic area or other brain areas.

Osmond and others predicted an abnormal pathway of epinephrine metabolism, with the production of psychotomimetic substances, adrenochrome, and adrenolutin. Another unproven report related schizophrenia to serum copper in the form of the metalloprotein ceruloplasmin, a test for which was developed by Akerfeldt. Wooley and Gaddum proposed, and later abandoned, a theory of central serotonin deficiency in schizophrenia.

A number of workers have demonstrated the adverse effects of schizophrenic serum and urine upon rope climbing and other task-learning and retention abilities of rats, upon web spinning of spiders, and upon behavior of tropical fish, tadpole larvae, and cells in tissue culture. Considerable work has been done in an attempt to identify such substances in blood and other body fluids (Heath, Gottleib, Martin, Bercel). An odorous substance has been found in the sweat of schizophrenic patients by Kathleen Smith, while Kety and others, working on an intoxication theory, have studied possible disturbances in transmethylation as related to exacerbation of schizophrenic symptoms.

Psychodynamic formulations since Freud's suggestion of a narcissistic psychosis have focused on ego disturbance, on an inability to achieve self vs. object differentiation, and on the disruptive effect on ego development resulting from unusual sensitivity to sensory input. Mednick and Schulsinger have studied children with schizophrenic mothers and have suggested that, in addition to heredity, factors that are predisposing to a "high risk for schizophrenia" include a history of severe paranatal distress and a poorly controlled hyperresponsive autonomic nervous system. A further hypothesis is that the latter comes about from damage to the hippocampus from anoxia at birth. Shakow pointed out perceptual problems with the inability to long maintain a major set. Mahler demonstrated in children a "symbiotic schizophrenic-like psychosis" in which the child was unable to differentiate from the mother, while others speak of the schizophrenogenic mother as a rejecting or an overprotecting person or as one unable to understand her child. Social psychiatrists impugn the total family as manifesting disturbed communication and interaction, marital schism, and placing the child in the double bind so that he or she "can't win."

To date the search for biochemical concomitants of behavior in schizophrenia has failed to demonstrate a constitutional, endocrine, or metabolic defect. At present interest centers on the "dopamine hypothesis," which suggests that schizophrenic symptoms result from overactivity of dopamine (a neurotransmitter, a biogenic amine of the catecholamine type) at the synapse in the brain. Such overactivity could explain stereotyped behavior, paranoid delusions, and auditory hallucinations but not anhedonia, withdrawal, flatness of affect, and autism. It has been postulated that the latter group of symptoms could result from a lessened activity of norepinephrine at the synapse. An imbalance of the two mechanisms could explain combinations of the two sets of symptoms. Interference with an enzyme at the synapse (dopamine-hydroxylase, which converts dopamine to norepinephrine) is being investigated.

Lacking today is a single coherent, well-formulated, and testable hypothesis; it continues to be widely accepted that schizophrenic conditions result from some genotypically determined traits that are either suppressed or elicited by other genotypic or environmental factors to produce the symptoms of schizophrenia.

The term "schizophrenia" is commonly used therefore to include a group of psychoses with a course which is at times chronic and marked by intermittent attacks and which can stop or retrogress at any stage but does not permit full *restitutio ad integram.*

The "disease" or syndrome is characterized by a specific type of alteration of thinking, feeling, and relation to the external world. The term "splitting of psychic functions" includes the lack of integration of different strivings and complexes. Rather, one set of complexes or ideas dominates the personality for a time, while other groups of ideas or drives are split off and seem partly or completely impotent. Often ideas are only partly worked out, fragments of ideas are connected in an illogical way to constitute a new idea, and concepts lose their completeness. The process of association often works with mere fragments of ideas and concepts. This results in associations which appear incoherent, bizarre, and utterly unpredictable. Often thinking stops in the middle of a thought (blocking), at least as far as it is a conscious process. Instead of a continuing thought, new ideas crop out which neither the patient nor the observer can bring into connection with the previous stream of thought (so-called tangential thinking). Genuine interference with perception, concentration, or memory is not demonstrable, although these functions suffer qualitative distortions. In the most severe cases emotional and affective expression seems to be completely lacking; in other cases the feelings expressed are inappropriate or of less than ordinary intensity (flattening). Ambivalence of emotion with the simultaneous occurrence of good and evil thoughts is common.

In addition to the above *primary features,* many accessory or *secondary symptoms* are present: hallucinations, delusions, confusion, stupor, manic or melancholic fluctuations, and catatonic symptoms. It is to be remembered that in schizophrenic patients outside hospitals these secondary symptoms are less apparent and may be absent altogether.

Psychoanalytic theory considers the logic of schizophrenic associations to be closely related to the associative patterns in dreams, fantasies, and the imaginative productions of young children. This type of thinking, which is believed to be present at the preverbal stage of personality development before the child has socialized concepts of interpreting the world, has been called *primary process thinking.* In it, important wishes, self-attitudes, and communication of even very mundane needs may be in highly symbolic form; this form tends to be consistent for each individual, so that intuitive, observant hospital personnel may gradually learn that a certain bizarre gesture or word actually is a distorted but specific request.

The question is not one of defining and delimiting different entities but of grouping symptoms. Type classification is not static, for a case which begins as hebephrenic may be classified as paranoid several years later.

Types of schizophrenic disorder
Schizophrenia–simple type

In simple schizophrenia the accessory symptoms are absent. The patients simply become affectively and intellectually weaker; will power and the capacity for work and caring for themselves diminish. They appear stupid and finally show the picture of severe dementia. The condition progresses slowly over the years and may never be seen as a medical problem. Eventual adjustment is more commonly that of a vagabond, transient laborer, or alcoholic than of a hospital inmate.

Schizophrenia–hebephrenic type

The term "hebephrenic" is used to designate those acute psychoses with subsequent deterioration and without catatonic or paranoid characteristics. Onset is usually between ages 12 and 25 years. The picture is sometimes characterized by pronounced feelings of mental and physical incapacity, various pathological sensations, and areas of hypochondriacal concern which gradually induce the patients to renounce all activities. There may be sexual preoccupation, emotional dulling, and clowning or grotesque silliness; there is concern with abstruse philosophical problems but without formation of clear-cut delusional symptoms.

Schizophrenia—catatonic type

Catatonic schizophrenia is distinguished by symptoms of stupor, mutism, negativism, impulsivity, and peculiar motility. In hyperkinetic phases (catatonic type, excited) patients are given to random impulsive activity, cursing, self-disregard, sleeplessness, and much repetitious overactivity. In akinetic phases (catatonic type, withdrawn) they may manifest cerea flexibilitas, failure to swallow, and command automaticity. Onset is usually acute and may alternate between mania and melancholia. There is marked improvement in over half of the cases followed eventually by new thrusts, with more deterioration each time.

Schizophrenia—paranoid type

In the beginning, patients state that things seem different. They do not feel as they used to; they become suspicious and overuse projection to the point that completely indifferent events are referred to themselves; they believe there is a conspiracy against them; voices talk about them and finally to them. This may lead to violent action, as in turning upon or fleeing from supposed tormentors. As the disorder tends toward chronicity patients may experience diminishing affective disturbances, ideas of omnipotence, and delusions of grandeur.

Acute schizophrenic episode

The term "acute schizophrenic episode" is used for patients who show an acute onset of schizophrenic symptoms, often associated with confusion, perplexity, ideas of reference, emotional turmoil, dreamlike dissociation, and excitement, depression, or fear. These attacks frequently subside in a few weeks. Usually such remissions are followed by recurrences, or the illness may take on the characteristics of catatonic, hebephrenic, or paranoid schizophrenia, and then the diagnosis should be accordingly changed.

Meduna and McCulloch delimited from the group of acute schizophrenics those patients who showed confusion and disorientation, raised body temperature, and a pseudodiabetic glucose tolerance curve. The prognosis of this condition (labeled oneirophrenia) is good, but the finding of a defect in sugar metabolism has not been replicated by some workers. Mayer-Gross described an oneiroid dreamlike state of clouded consciousness occurring in acute schizophrenic breakdown.

Previously these conditions were included under the term "acute undifferentiated schizophrenia."

Schizophrenia—latent type

The latent category is used for those patients who have clear symptoms of schizophrenia but no history of a previous psychotic schizophrenic episode. Terms sometimes used for this group of patients include "prepsychotic," "pseudopsychopathic," or "borderline" schizophrenia.

Schizophrenia—residual type

The residual category is for patients who show signs of schizophrenia but who, following a psychotic episode, are no longer psychotic.

Schizoaffective type

The schizoaffective category is intended for those cases showing significant admixtures of schizophrenic and affective reactions. The mental content may be predominantly schizophrenic, with pronounced elation (schizoaffective, excited) or depression (schizoaffective, depressed). Patients may show predominantly affective changes with schizophrenic-like thinking or bizarre behavior. The prepsychotic personality may be at variance with expectations based on the presenting psychotic symptomatology. On prolonged observation, such patients usually prove to be basically schizophrenic in nature.

Schizophrenia—childhood type

The diagnosis of schizophrenia in children is being made with increasing frequency. The prognosis of this condition diagnosed before puberty is poor. This illness presents as atypical and withdrawn behavior (autistic child), alteration of motor behavior, failure to develop identification separate from the mother (symbiotic psychosis of Mahler), and as general unevenness, gross immaturity, and inadequacy in development. Communication is poor. There is difficulty in establishing good relationship with persons around them, and behavior is often repetitive and stereotyped. This may result in a picture of general mental retardation.

Schizophrenia—chronic undifferentiated type

The term "chronic undifferentiated" has been used to describe the disorder in patients who show mixed schizophrenic symptoms and definite schizophrenic thought, affect, and behavior but who cannot be clearly classified under one of the other types of schizophrenia.

Schizophrenia—other types

It is not unusual in a disease group as complex as schizophrenia that a variety of terms have been used as various workers emphasize different aspects of the multiple symptom pattern. Thus the term "periodic relapsing schizophrenia," has been applied to a group of cases originally studied by Gjessing. These patients are subject to exacerbations of the disease, occurring at more or less regular intervals and accompanied by alterations in nitrogen balance. Some of these cases have been reported to respond to treatment with thyroxin.

Another term widely used is "pseudoneurotic schizophrenia." This concept was introduced by Hoch and Polatin to identify a large group of patients who frequently are misidentified as psychoneurotic but who in reality show the autistic and dereistic approach to life that is characteristic of schizophrenia. A diffuse withdrawal from life and an ambivalence are seen. These patients have an all-pervading anxiety, with many hysterical and bodily or vegetative symptoms. Phobias are often present. The patient may have psychotic episodes, between which the personality is well integrated; in such intervals diagnosis is difficult. The Rorschach test is reported to be of help in pointing out the thinking disorder in these cases. A sodium amytal interview may release unexpected psychotic material.

EXAMINATION. There appears *behaviorally* to be a defect in the patient's awareness of social or interpersonal realities. It is helpful to think of the symptom picture as composed of (1) fundamental and (2) accessory symptoms.

1. Fundamentally, the disease process shows a defect in *associative* function: Associations lose their continuity; two ideas are combined into one (condensation); there are clang associations, blocking, dearth of ideas, and pressure of thoughts; paralogical thinking occurs in which ideas are linked by mere grammatical form, similarity, habit, etc., rather than by logical ordering. There is stereotypy, a clinging to one idea, senseless naming or touching of all visible objects, and echolalia (repeating over and over what someone else has said). In the realm of *affectivity* there may be marked emotional indifference, even to a complete imperviousness to pain and discomfort in severe cases; in milder cases there is seeming oversensitivity of emotion but a lack of depth. Affective expression may be inconsistent with thought or action or may alter rapidly because of haphazard accidental associations. Emotional deterioration is apparent rather than real, as after decades of emotional indifference affect can be produced in all its original vividness, even to long-past events. *Ambivalence* is commonly seen, often as the simultaneous appearance of thought and counterthought. The simple functions of sensation, perception, memory, orientation, consciousness, and motility are intact. Apparent alteration of these functions is based upon negativism, indifference, reluctance to think, or randomness of responses. Activity and behavior are marked by lack of interest, initiative, and definite goals and by inadequate adaptation to the environment. Stereotypy is characteristic and unpleasant stubbornness frequent. There is a limitation of contacts with the outside world, often with an apparently complete absorption with autistic fantasy. Despite the latter, outside events may register in memory with remarkable clarity, and patients may later answer questions which they did not seem to comprehend when asked.

2. It is the accessory symptoms that usually lead to social difficulties and give the disease its external stamp. *Hallucinations* are most frequently auditory and of a persecutory nature. Hallucinations of body sensations, taste, and smell are common

but tactile and visual uncommon. *Delusions* are usually persecutory, but commonly seen too are those of grandeur, of inferiority,
or of being loved or defiled or diseased. These are rarely well systematized. Mutually contradictory beliefs can be held and, although the self remains alien to the delusion, they are impervious
to logic. *Memory disturbances* may include amnesias, hyperes-
thesia, and déjà vu type phenomena. The patient may act as two
persons, either simultaneously or alternately, or may incorporate
all or part of the behavior of some other person. *Speech* and *writing* show abnormalities such as blocking, poverty of ideas, incoherence, clouding, delusional content, and emotional anomalies. Mutism may last for decades. Speech may show affected mannerisms. There may be verbigeration, distortions, similar to
dreams, with fusion of ideas (condensation), substitutions, distortions, accidental associations, and word salad. Writing shows
bizarre changing of margins, random repetition of words, letters,
and sentences, queer designs, shapes and curliques. The so-called
catatonic symptoms of behavior can occur in any type of schizophrenia and consist of catalepsy (rigidity and waxy flexibility of
psychic quality); stupor (intense inhibition, blocking, lack of interest, loss into own autisms); hyperkinesis; stereotypies of speech,
movement, expression, an even of hallucinations (all of which
tend to become abbreviated with time); mannerisms (stilted,
pompous, mocking, etc.); negativism (which may be passive,
active, or a denial of own inner striving and functions); and
echopraxia and command automatism (in which patient feels his
thoughts, actions, etc., are being forced by someone else).

The findings of the *physical* examination are nonspecific, but it
is not uncommon that schizophrenics have an asthenic habitus,
with pale blotchy skin, and poor oily complexion. They are un-
kempt and frequently underweight but may show either anorexia
or bulimia. There is not infrequently autonomic instability shown
by cardiovascular variations and hyper- or hypoactivity of sweat
glands. Impotence and menstrual irregularities are common.
There are poor motor coordination, awkward gait, laughing and
crying spells, and fits of rigidity. *Laboratory* evidence of mild
thyroid, adrenal, or liver dysfunction is variable. *Psychological*
tests, when confirmed clinically, are of great assistance. Disturbances in abstract thinking with a tendency to overgeneralization
may be noted on intelligence tests. Projective tests may speed

thorough clinical understanding by uncovering bizarre or contaminated (e.g., "moss growing on a dog") associations, delusions, fears, motivations, and ways of handling sexual or aggressive feelings toward specific individuals in the patient's life. Psychological testing may clearly bring out the highly symbolic nature of the patient's mental productions. Psychological testing may also uncover the failure to distinguish between what is self and not self (loss of ego boundaries).

PROGNOSIS. Langfeld has proposed that there are two types of schizophrenia: *process schizophrenia,* in which the illness progresses inevitably toward a final state of deterioration, and *reactive schizophrenia,* with onset in temporal relationship to a traumatic event in persons with better premorbid adjustment and with more favorable outcome of the illness. In patients ill less than 1 year, most clinicians believe that a history of an acute onset, the presence of catatonic symptoms, or the presence of much affective disturbance augurs a good deal of hope for the future. On the other hand, a sickness beginning at a young age and progressing slowly without much overt anxiety bodes ill for the future. The following data are illustrative.

	Remissions
Hospitalized less than 3 months, first illness	75%
Hospitalized less than 1 year, first illness	50%
Hospitalized 1 to 2 years	10%
Hospitalized over 2 years	1% to 2%

TREATMENT. As the etiology of schizophrenia is not known, so the treatment must remain empirical. Experience has demonstrated, however, that many patients will improve with a combined approach utilizing organic, psychological, and environmental treatments tailored carefully to the individual needs of each patient. No truly satisfactory remedy exists to repair the devastating personality damage encountered in many of these individuals. With the exception of those hospitalized schizophrenics who make a rapid improvement with nursing care, pharmacological treatment, electroshock, or insulin and those ambulatory schizophrenics who happily discover a properly supportive environment, these patients require long supportive care. Great skill is often needed to establish and maintain the close doctor-patient relationship necessary for successful management of these patients.

Many a psychiatrist becomes discouraged, however, by the slow progress, deep hostility, and strong self-punishing tendencies seen in schizophrenics. There is impressive evidence that highly structured psychotherapy is of very little use with schizophrenic patients. At times when the schizophrenic is freely communicative, the psychotherapist must beware lest fascination with deciphering the intricate and emotionally rich implications of his patient's words distract attention from the often more important interpersonal feelings being masked by the delusions.

In evaluating disturbed psychiatric patients, too much weight must not be placed upon any single symptom. Thorough anamnestic study of the case with attention to special personality assets as well as liabilities will lead to a more successful therapeutic plan than will rules of thumb.

General agreement exists in regard to the importance of therapy as a "growing up" experience during which the patient gains a firmer grasp of the real nature of human relationships, gives up his severe distortions of the world about him, and achieves a more honest appreciation of his own latent capacities. Throughout months of therapy, frightening sexual or aggressive fantasies may form the main content of interviews. Opinions vary as to the proper technique for dealing with this material. Followers of Rosen advocate active participation in the patient's delusional system, forming an immediate intimacy with the patient and using schizophrenic symbolic language in disagreeing, questioning, or interpreting. Fromm-Reichmann advocated a more conservative, patient approach, in which the therapist attempts to understand the changing meaning and goals of the patient's pathological behavior as the latter tests whether the therapist will abandon him, show disrespect, or confirm his fears in other ways. Interpretation with schizophrenics focuses heavily upon the genetics of symptomatic behavior rather than its meaning. Unlike neurotics, these patients tend not to repress the meaning of their symptoms. Still another approach is to view the patient's distorted behaviors and fantasies as products of the disease, to be forgotten as soon as possible. In this role the therapist, while empathizing with and accepting the patient's bizarre feelings, takes a very down-to-earth attitude about them and continually encourages the patient in a supportive manner to begin to deal more directly with the world around him.

An aspect of therapy which many a time determines success or failure is the way the patient's environment is handled. Where indicated, the physician should not fail to help friends, relatives, or employers to react with understanding to the patient's behavior; more often than not, thorough treatment will involve at some time social case work with an important member of the schizophrenic's own family.

Aid should be provided toward an increasingly healthy schedule of living. In keeping with the patient's capacities, some type of supervised activity and socialization program should be instituted. Occupational therapy and group therapy aimed at actively working through the behavior aberrations at the moment they occur are valuable.

The phenothiazine tranquilizers and other ataractics have produced as marked a change in the management of schizophrenic patients as did ECT with psychotic depression. Although these drugs seem to have some antipsychotic action, they act as nonsedative tranquilizers. With relief from agitation and anxiety, the disturbing secondary symptoms of the illness become less prominent and patients are able to better adapt their behavior to the demands of the environment. In some reported cases the quieting effect has permitted the patient to live a sheltered life in the community despite the continued presence of delusions and hallucinations. In other cases as the patient becomes less agitated, delusions and hallucinations seem to diminish in importance and ultimately disappear. Due to the fluctuant nature of the illness control studies of drug therapy are difficult, but they are at this point a necessity if a rational approach to chemotherapy is to develop. Certainly today every schizophrenic patient should be given an adequate trial on pharmacological treatment. For example, chlorpromazine may be given in doses of 600 to 2000 mg. daily, later tapered off to 600 to 800 mg., and continued for several months or years, as need be. Other phrenotropic drugs are used in similar fashion. (See tables, pp. 326 to 334.)

Although there is considerable talk about target symptoms and the therapeutic merits of one phenothiazine over another, there is little to guide one in selecting from among the various phenothiazines for the specific symptom picture of any given patient. Usually the drug preference is the physician's, and a change is made only if untoward complications arise. The usual error is failure to give a sufficiently large dose for a sufficient length of time. Another common mistake is to add a similar drug to one inadequately administered, and another to that, etc. ("polypharmacy").

During periods when the disorder is aggravated, somatic therapies are often of value. Electroconvulsive therapy (up to 20 to 25 treatments) has been used. Regressive shock treatments (1 to 3 convulsions daily until the desired state of regression is achieved), electronarcosis, and insulin coma therapy (40 to 100 comas) have been used in the past but are seldom used today.

Electroconvulsive therapy has the greatest hope of success in recent illnesses which display depressive or catatonic symptoms. Lobotomy is occasionally tried in patients incapacitated over 2 years who have failed to respond to other techniques. Such surgery, however, has for the most part fallen out of favor and, in any case, should not be used in the absence of facilities for thorough rehabilitation.

SUGGESTED READINGS

Arieti, S.: Interpretation of schizophrenia, New York, 1975, Basic Books, Inc.

Bolles, M., and Goldstein, K.: A study of the impairment of "abstract behavior" in schizophrenic patients, Psychiatr. Q. 12:42, 1938.

Burt, D. R., Creese, I., and Snyder, S. H.: Antischizophrenic drugs: chronic treatment elevates dopamine receptor binding in brain, Science 196:326, 1977.

Davis, J. M.: Overview: Maintenance therapy in psychiatry: I. Schizophrenia, Am. J. Psychiatry 132:1237, 1975.

Fowler, R. C., Tsuang, M. T., and Cadoret, R. J.: Parental psychiatric illness associated with schizophrenia in the siblings of schizophrenics, Compr. Psychiatry 18:271, 1977.

Goldberg, S. C., Schooler, N. R., Hogarty, G. E., and Roper, M.: Prediction of relapse in schizophrenic outpatients treated by drug and sociotherapy, Arch. Gen. Psychiatry 34:171, 1977.

Goldstein, G.: Cognitive and perceptual differences between schizophrenics and organics, Schizophrenia Bull. 4:160, 1978.

Gottesman, I. I., and Shields, J.: A critical review of recent adoption, twin, and family studies of schizophrenia: behavioral genetics perspectives, Schizophrenia Bull. 2:360, 1976.

Hamilton, M., editor: Fish's schizophrenia, ed. 2, Bristol, 1976, John Wright and Sons, Ltd.

Helm, D.: Psychodynamic and behavior modification approaches to the treatment of infantile autism: empirical similarities, J. Autism Child Schizo. 6:27, 1976.

Hoch, P. H., and Polatin, P.: Pseudoneurotic forms of schizophrenia, Psychiatr. Q. 23:248, 1949.

Keith, S. J., and others: Special report: schizophrenia 1976, Schizophrenia Bull. 2:510, 1976.

Kety, S. S., and others: Studies based on a total sample of adopted individuals and their relatives: why they were necessary, what they demonstrated and failed to demonstrate, Schizophrenia Bull. 2:413, 1976.

Koehler, K., Guth, W., and Grimm, G.: First-rank symptoms of schizophrenia in Schneider-oriented German centers, Arch. Gen. Psychiatry 34:810, 1977.

Kornetsky, C.: Hyporesponsivity of chronic schizophrenic patients to dextroamphetamine, Arch. Gen. Psychiatry 33:1425, 1976.

Levenson, A. J., and others: Speed and rate of remission in acute schizophrenia: a comparison of intramuscularly administered fluphenazine HCl with thiothixene and haloperidol, Current Psychotherapeutic Research 20:695, 1976.

Murphy, D. L., Donnelly, C. H., Miller, L., and Wyatt, R. J.: Platelet monoamine oxidase in chronic schizophrenia: some enzyme characteristics relevant to reduced activity, Arch. Gen. Psychiatry 33:1377, 1976.

Polonowitz, A., and James, N. M.: Fluphenazine decanoate maintenance in schizophrenia: a retrospective study, New Zealand Medical Journal 83:316, 1976.

Reich, W.: The schizophrenia spectrum: a genetic concept, J. Nerv. Ment. Dis. 162(1):3, 1976.

Sartorius, N., Jablensky, A:, and Shapiro, R.: Two-year follow-up of the patients included in the WHO international pilot study of schizophrenia, Psychol. Med. 7:529, 1977.

Schulsinger, H.: A ten-year follow-up of children of schizophrenic mothers; clinical assessment, Acta Psychiat. Scand. 53:371, 1976.

Strauss, J. S., and Gift, T. E.: Choosing an approach for diagnosing schizophrenia, Arch. Gen. Psychiatry 34:1248, 1977.

Tsuang, M. T., Dempsey, M., and Rauscher, F.: A study of "atypical schizophrenia," Arch. Gen. Psychiatry 33:1157, 1976.

Welner, A., and others: The group of schizoaffective and related psychoses: a follow-up study, Compr. Psychiatry 18:413, 1977.

Wender, P. H., and others: Schizophrenics' adopting parents, Arch. Gen. Psychiatry 34:777, 1977.

Wyatt, R. J.: Biochemistry and schizophrenia. IV. The neuroleptics. Their mechanism of action: a review of the biochemical literature, Psychopharmacol. Bull. **12**:5, 1976.

PARANOID STATES

The paranoid conditions are disorders of thinking characterized by suspiciousness, blaming others (projection), and paralogical reasoning to the point of delusion formation. Such thinking is seen at times in many persons (paranoid personalities) and may occur as a prominent symptom in all of the major psychoses and occasionally in the psychoneuroses and character disorders. When paranoid symptoms occur in the course of some other psychosis (senile psychosis, paranoid type; schizophrenia, paranoid type; alcoholic psychosis, paranoid type; etc.) the symptoms of the accompanying psychosis blend with the paranoid features. In the schizophrenic and organic types of paranoid conditions derogatory hallucinations may be an outstanding feature. To designate those paranoid schizophrenics who fail to show diffuse personality dilapidation, the term "paraphrenia" was used by Kraepelin.

Paranoia. True paranoia (monomania or litigious paranoia) designates only those rare cases in which highly systematized delusions of insidious onset exist along with the preservation of other personality functions. The intricate and elaborate paranoid system of these patients often develops insidiously, proceeding at first logically from the misinterpretation of an actual event. Individual patients may exhibit both persecutory and grandiose traits and often believe themselves to be endowed with superior abilities. In spite of the chronic course, the condition does not seem to interfere with the rest of the patient's thinking.

Involutional paranoid state. This term is used to designate delusion formation having its onset in the involutional period. The characteristic thought disorders of schizophrenia are lacking although depressive content may indicate that it is in reality only a paranoid variety of the involutional psychosis.

Other paranoid states. Characterized by paranoid delusions, these may occur lacking the logical nature of systematization seen in paranoia and yet not manifesting the bizarre fragmentation and deterioration of the schizophrenic reactions. Such states are likely to be of relatively short duration although they may become persistent and chronic.

ETIOLOGY. The etiology of the paranoid reactions is not known, although constitutional factors have been believed to be important. In Freudian theory, developed from the famous Schreber case, paranoid reactions have been considered to be defenses against unconscious homosexuality. Recent studies have not supported this point of view. Freud has hypothesized a mechanism in which "I love him" is denied by "No, I hate him" and the projective accompaniment "He hates me." More recently others have conjectured that paranoid symptoms may be a defense against the wish to kill, the wish to receive passively oral or anal pleasures, the fear of being damaged, or a variety of other such unconscious attitudes.

These syndromes occur more frequently in males than females, having an onset usually during or after the third decade of life. They make up no more than 10% of mental hospital admissions.

PROGNOSIS. In early cases prognosis is guarded; in longstanding cases it is poor.

TREATMENT. These patients in general are resistant to psychotherapy although in mild cases remissions may apparently follow an explanatory supportive type of psychotherapy by a physician who can engage the patient's trust. Hospitalization is necessary for those who become intensely litigious, assaultive, or homicidal. Treatment with tranquilizers may be of use in relieving anxiety, agitation, drive to assaultiveness, and diminuation in paranoid ideation.

SUGGESTED READINGS

Arthur, A. Z.: Theories and explanations of delusions: a review, Am. J. Psychiatry **121**:105, 1964.

Freedman, N., Cutler, R., Engelhardt, D. M., and Margolis, R.: On the modification of paranoid symptomatology, J. Nerv. Ment. Dis. **144**:29, 1967.

Freud, S.: Psychoanalytic notes upon an autobiographical account of a case of paranoia. In Collected papers, London, 1950, Hogarth Press, Ltd., vol. 3.

Kitay, P. M.: Symposium on reinterpretations of the Schreber case: for its theory of paranoia, Int. J. Psychoanal. **44**:191, 1963.

Klaf, F. S.: Female homosexuality and paranoid schizophrenia, Arch. Gen. Psychiatry **4**:84, 1961.

Leonhard, K.: Prognosis of paranoid states in relation to the clinical features, Acta Psychiat. Scand. **51:**134, 1975.

Retterstol, N.: Paranoid and paranoiac psychoses, Springfield, Ill., 1966, Charles C Thomas, Publisher.

Revitch, E.: The problem of conjugal paranoia, Dis. Nerv. Syst. **15:**271, 1954.

Rosen, H., and Kiene, H.: Paranoia and paranoiac reaction type, Dis. Nerv. Syst. **11:**330, 1946.

Rosen, H., and Kiene, H.: Early reversible paranoic reaction, J. Nerv. Ment. Dis. **109:**291, 1949.

Tanna, V. L.: Paranoid states: a selected review, Compr. Psychiatry **15:**453, 1974.

14

Neuroses

DEFINITION. Psychoneuroses are personality disturbances which show neither gross disturbances of reality testing nor severely antisocial behavior and which seem determined mostly by environmental factors. These factors may be separated for convenience into two categories: those environmental influences acting on the infant or child, which produce a defect in personality development, and those influences immediately preceding an exacerbation of psychoneurotic symptoms, i.e., the precipitating stress.

With onset often in early adult life, these conditions tend to be chronic, the patient usually from very early life presenting evidence of periodic or constant maladjustment of varying degree. Symptoms are at their peak in the period of active reproductive activity and social responsibility. Men and women are affected about equally, although, for specific psychoneurotic syndromes, sex differences exist. Disturbances related to interpersonal conflict or sexual functioning are common. Many of the symptoms seen in this group are expressed through the autonomic nervous system. The degree to which symptoms interfere with activities varies. Some patients retreat into complete invalidism; others lead an outwardly healthy existence, successfully concealing their illness from acquaintances. Although most never require hospitalization, at times a stay within the hospital may be advisable to alleviate severe tensional crises.

Although Sigmund Freud, father of dynamic psychiatry, postulated constitutional and biological factors underlying neurotic illness, the nature and importance of such organic neurotic predisposition have only recently been investigated. It is now known from both animal and human studies that genetic and fetal conditions can influence later tension level, irritability, and other behaviors, such as degree of persistence in overcoming obstacles, related to adaptation. For the present, therapy of these conditions is based almost entirely upon attempts to modify neurotic behavior patterns through psychotherapy founded upon theoretical notions of the importance of previous life experience and current social stress as the etiological determinants. These postulations concern the psychiatrist with modifying learned patterns of feelings, attitudes, defenses against anxiety, and modes of problem solving which developed during infancy and childhood and which appear inappropriately as neurotic or immature adjustments to the demands of adult life.

CLASSIFICATION. There is considerable variance in the classification systems used to describe psychoneurotic disorders, although a dozen or more separate categories have found some acceptance. Anxiety neurosis, hysteria, obsessive-compulsive neurosis, and neurotic depression seem to be the most universally accepted forms in practice; even these may at times have sufficient symptoms in common to warrant a more general term. Formerly the label *mixed psychoneurosis* was utilized, qualified by additional terms such as "with hysterical features," "with obsessive features," or "with depression and anxiety," etc. Somewhat more recently the A.P.A. used the concept of neurotic reactions to life stress and specified a classification based upon (1) anxiety reaction, (2) phobic reaction, (3) dissociative reaction and conversion reaction, (4) obsessive-compulsive reaction, and (5) depressive reaction. Currently the A.P.A. nomenclature has reverted to the classical notion of neurosis, specifying eight major types with two subtypes within hysterical neurosis.

The defense mechanisms serve as a basis for symptom formation. For, although anxiety may be dispelled in this manner, the mechanism of defense itself now forms a means by which the conflict is expressed and neurotic symptoms develop.

The subject of neurosis is usually discussed within the framework of psychoanalytic theory. In this view, *anxiety reaction* (in Freud's original thinking "anxiety hysteria") is the simplest kind of psychoneurosis, in which uncomfortable inner tension appears in the presence of certain objects, places, persons, or animals. It is seen in childhood as the first neurotic reaction that children experience. It has been postulated that unclear or partial memories of events which arouse intense emotion but are not understood, as, for example, the sexual act between the parents (the primal scene), observation that girls lack a penis (the castration fears), etc., form permanent unconscious fixations which lie at the basis of these displacements.

The concept of "actual neurosis," now very rarely used, refers to Freud's early oversimplified notion—later discarded—that some cases of anxiety reaction are caused by lack of sexual gratification or other meaningful emotional outlets.

Conversion hysteria is felt to have its origin in the childhood Oedipal conflict (child's love fixated on one parent, with jealousy toward parent of opposite sex). It differs from anxiety hysteria in that the anxiety is "converted" into a dysfunction that symbolically represents the conflicts; for example, a paralyzed limb may act as a defense against feared or secretly desired hostile aggressive action. Hysterics may also experience episodes of *dissociation,* in which confusion, amnesia, or multiple personality serves to defend against awareness of the anxiety-laden conflicts.

Closely related to hysteria is the *phobic neurosis,* in which the anxiety, instead of being converted into a physical symptom, is experienced as fear but as fear removed (displaced) in space and time and related to apparently innocuous objects or places. Although similar to anxiety hysterics, phobic patients are distinguished by their prominent use of avoidance (avoidance of the feared objects or places) as a way of escaping the experience of anxiety.

Obsessive-compulsive neuroses arise as an outcome of fixation in the anal stage of development. The anal character traits of orderliness, frugality, and obstinacy are clearly seen.

In patients with psychoneurotic *depression,* deeply helpless and dependent feelings are common, although hysterical or obsessive-compulsive dynamisms—or both—may be observed also. The diagnosis is based primarily upon the prominence of depressive symptoms.

SUGGESTED READINGS

Denker, P. G.: Results of treatment of psychoneuroses by the general practitioner. A follow-up study of 500 patients, Arch. Neurol. Psychiatry 57:504, 1947, including the discussion.

English, O., and Pearson, G.: Emotional problems of living, ed. 3, New York, 1963, W. W. Norton & Co., Inc.

Eysenck, H. J., editor: Behavior therapy and the neuroses, New York, 1960, Pergamon Press, Inc.

Fenichel, O.: The psychoanalytic theory of neurosis, New York, 1945, W. W. Norton & Co., Inc.

Freud, S.: The basic writings of Sigmund Freud (translated by A. A. Brill), New York, 1938, Modern Library, Inc., p. 1001.

Freud, S.: Collected papers, London, 1924-1952, Hogarth Press, Ltd., vols. 1 to 5.

Hilgard, J. R., and Newman, M. F.: Anniversaries in mental illness, Psychiatry **22:**113, 1959.

Ross, T. A.: The common neuroses, Baltimore, 1937, The Williams & Wilkins Co.

Ulett, P. C., and Gildea, E. F.: Survey of surgical procedures in psychoneurotic women, J.A.M.A. **143:**960, 1950.

Anxiety neurosis

Symptoms of anxiety occur when the subject is faced with real or symbolic danger. This apprehension is expressed through widespread autonomic discharge. Although it occurs from time to time in all human beings, a diffuse free-floating anxiety or readiness for anxiety may in some patients lead to the syndrome of continuous tension or recurrent exacerbations. This is usually seen in young adults and is known as anxiety neurosis. Beginning with Beard's description of nervous exhaustion in 1869, over the years various terms have been applied to the symptom complex: "neurocirculatory asthenia," "hyperventilation syndrome," "effort syndrome," "vasomotor neurosis," and "anxiety tension state."

It is usual to discover that these patients early learned to fear intense affects of anger, hate, love, or erotic attraction. In the course of daily living when these feelings would tend to be aroused the substitutes of intense confusion and a sense of loss of self-control, as well as autonomic discharge phenomena, were utilized.

ANAMNESIS. The patient comes to the doctor with the *chief complaint* being spells of dyspnea, palpitation, irritability, dizziness, insomnia, faintness, weakness, chest pain, trembling, headache, or "attacks." *Past history* reveals that first symptoms usually appear in the second decade of life and may be of dramatic onset associated with stress situations, muscular exertion, pregnancy, or military service. Often beginning with a choking sensation, these attacks precede fears of fainting, dying, or "losing the mind." Crowded busses, movies, or public gatherings are often the setting for the attacks. Increasing irritability and intolerance for noises and for children and spouse may precipitate the need for hospitalization. *Family history* may reveal a high incidence of this disorder in the immediate family. It is important to differentiate anxiety neurosis from acute reactions to intense life stress in otherwise well-adapted persons as well as from schizoid or borderline schizophrenic patients. In the former condition, an acute onset close in time to severe trauma (death of a loved one, wartime fear, exposure to tornado or other sudden unanticipated natural disaster) in a previously adequate personality is characteristic. An anxious schizoid personality, on the other hand, may require careful study over an extended period to distinguish it from anxiety neurosis.

EXAMINATION. The patient, *behaviorally,* is fidgety and apprehensive and often mildly depressed. His conversation is filled with worries and concerns over heart, lungs, inability to concentrate, and other symptoms. *Physically,* slight inconstant tachycardia, tachypnea, flushed face and neck, moist cool palms, tremor of fingers, and brisk tendon reflexes are seen. *Laboratory* examination shows that basal metabolic rate is normal or raised due to motor restlessness; sighing respirations may be visualized on a breathing tracing.

PROGNOSIS. In only a small percentage does the neurosis interfere with general life pursuits. The illness may be of brief duration or proceed for many years with exacerbations or remissions.

TREATMENT. Complete medical work-up to reassure the patient and physician at the beginning of the treatment.

Explain the nature of the disease and symptoms to the patient.

Encourage the patient to return to a regular balance of work and play.

Provide psychotherapy with the working through of anxiety-provoking conflicts in the context of present meaningful relationships.

Make judicious use of sedatives and such psychopharmacological agents as meprobamate (Miltown, Equanil), chlordiazepoxide (Librium), diazepam (Valium), and others.

SUGGESTED READINGS

DiMascio, A., and Barrett, J.: Comparative effects of oxazepam in "high" and "low" anxious student volunteers, Psychosomatics **6:**298, 1965.

Freud, S.: The problem of anxiety, Albany, N.Y., 1936, The Psychoanalytic Quarterly Press, and New York 1936, W. W. Norton & Co., Inc.

Gellhorn, E.: The neurophysiological basis of anxiety. A hypothesis, Perspect. Biol. Med. **8:**488, 1965.

Hoch, P., and Zubin, J.: Anxiety, New York, 1950, Gruen & Stratton, Inc.

Lehmann, H. E., and Ban, T. A.: Pharmacotherapy of tension and anxiety, Springfield, Ill., 1970, Charles C Thomas, Publisher.

Leighton, D., and others: The character of danger, New York, 1963, Basic Books, Inc., Publishers.

Levitt, E., Persky, H., and Brady, J.: Hypnotic induction of anxiety, Springfield, Ill., 1964, Charles C Thomas, Publisher.

Masserman, J. H.: Anxiety: protean source of communication. In Masserman, J. H., editor: Science and psychoanalysis, New York, 1965, Grune & Stratton, Inc., vol. 8.

Meares, A.: The management of the anxious patient, Philadelphia, 1963, W. B. Saunders Co.

Uhlenhuth, E. H., Covi, L., and Lipman, R. S.: Indications for minor tranquilizers in anxious outpatients. In Black, P., editor: Drugs and the brain, Baltimore, 1969, The Johns Hopkins Press.

Wheeler, E. O., White, P. D., Reed, E. W., and Cohen, M. E.: Neurocirculatory asthenia (anxiety neurosis, effort syndrome, neurasthenia): a twenty-year follow-up study of 173 patients, J.A.M.A. **142:**878, 1950.

Wittenborn, J. R.: The clinical psychopharmacology of anxiety, Springfield, Ill., 1969, Charles C Thomas, Publisher.

Hysterical neurosis

Hysteria (Briquet's syndrome) is the name applied to a disease or personality disorder characterized by an involuntary psychogenic loss or disorder of function. Symptoms characteristically begin and end suddenly in emotionally charged situations and are symbolic of the underlying conflicts. Often they can be modified by suggestion alone. It apparently occurs more frequently in women and the symptoms are limited typically to impairment of motor or sensory functions (blindness, paresthesia, paralysis, etc.) but may also include pyschological dysfunction (dissociation) and autonomic disturbance. The term "hysterical" is not uncommonly applied to describe the occurrence of isolated conversion symptoms appearing either alone or in company with other types of psychiatric disorder.

TYPES. The major types of hysterical neurosis include *psychogenic amnesia, psychogenic fugue, multiple personality,* and *depersonalization disorder.* In the conversion type special senses or voluntary nervous system are affected, causing such symptoms as blindness, deafness, anosmia, anesthesias, paresthesias, paralyses, ataxias, akinesias, and dyskinesias. The patient often shows an inappropriate lack of concern about these symptoms which may actually provide secondary gains by winning him sympathy or relieving him of unpleasant responsibilities. This type of hysterical neurosis must be distinguished from psychophysiological disorders, which are mediated by the autonomic nervous system, from malingering, which is done consciously, and from neurological lesions, which cause anatomically circumscribed symptoms. In the other major type of hysterical neurosis, the dissociative type, the alterations may occur in the patient's state of consciousness or in his identity, with production of such symptoms as amnesia, somnambulism, fugue, and multiple personality.

Hysterical disorders in which elements of injury and compensation seem to play a role in producing and maintaining the symptoms have been termed "compensation neurosis" by some authors. In these patients the symptoms seem to be maintained or exaggerated by the fact that the social environment rewards the symptoms; they are often found in Veterans Hospitals and among Workmen's Compensation cases.

ANAMNESIS. Despite the fact that the *complaints* elicited by a careful history are extremely numerous, paradoxically the patient may come to the clinic only under the pressure of relatives and frequently shows a strange indifference ("la belle indifférence") to usually dramatic handicaps. The *history* is one of recurrent accidents, illnesses, operations, sexual and menstrual difficulties, as well as gross interpersonal abnormalities. A majority suffer from frigidity, dyspareunia, and difficulties during pregnancy. A previously conditioned sensitivity to illness often leads to prolonged convalescence and tendency to invalidism. Unlike obsessional patients, hysterics tend to be unaware of the ideas underlying their feelings and actions. Symptoms usually have onset in early adolescence or soon after marriage although history of sexual misunderstanding and conflict arising before the age of 7 years may be eventually elicited during psychotherapy.

The overt interpersonal difficulties and sexual symptoms of the hysteric stem from defensive manipulation of others, which is experienced as safer (more under control by the patient) than free expression of feelings directly. Underlying these difficulties, it is usual to discover a type of basic distrust of friendship, love relations, or comfortable intimacy with another. This deep distrust of closeness, while somewhat similar to that observed in the borderline or schizophrenic patient, is accompanied by less disorganization of the personality.

EXAMINATION. In *behavioral* terms in the doctor's interview these patients (usually young girls) tend to dress in a naively seductive fashion; in conversation they seem to escape the experience of anxiety by avoidance mechanisms such as amnesia and dissociation of ideas. In these patients the mood, popularly known as "hysterical," is characterized by lability and poor emotional control. In addition to conversion symptoms, there may occur anxiety attacks, periods of indifference, or depressive episodes accompanied by suicidal gestures. Hysterical attacks may vary from episodic histrionic loss of emotional control to motor seizures which are differentiated from epilepsy only with difficulty. In *physical* examination certain diagnostic tricks may be found useful in distinguishing conversion symptoms. In hysterical blindness visual fields remain the same when tested at varying distances from the eye and the patient does not collide with the furniture. Anesthetic areas are frequently of stocking and glove type, not coinciding with sensory nerve distribution. Paralyses may be shown to alter in degree when the patient's attention is directed elsewhere. The Rorschach *psychological* test may show overemphasis on color responses, with "blood" seen in card II, and the content shows excessive preoccupation with the body.

PROGNOSIS. Prognosis for the relief of presenting complaints through dramatic suggestion or patient psychotherapy is good; psychotherapeutic efforts at modifying the hysterical character are believed well worthwhile by most psychotherapists but long-term follow-up studies are few and difficult to carry out in a valid manner.

TREATMENT. Medical concern directed toward the symptoms tend to fix them more firmly and impede therapy.

Therefore, repeated examination of the affected part and hospitalization are to be avoided.

Removal of presenting symptoms in the emergency room can sometimes be effected by such means as suggestion and persuasion, hypnotism, and intravenous sodium Amytal (particularly good for amnesia).

Psychotherapy must overcome resistances through the development of a positive relationship. Analysis of blocks to affectional feelings and broad reeducation of interpersonal attitudes are of value. In the psychoanalytic approach, material stemming from unresolved Oedipal and oral feelings is found to be genetically important and appears prominently in the transference. Basic distrust of self and others and deep inadequacy feelings tend to underlie severe hysteria.

SUGGESTED READINGS

Abse, D. W.: Hysteria and related mental disorders: an orientation to psychological medicine, Bristol, 1966, John Wright & Sons, Ltd.

Aring, C. D.: Observations on multiple sclerosis and conversion hysteria, Brain 88:663, 1965.

Breuer, J., and Freud, S.: Studies in hysteria, New York, 1936, Nervous & Mental Diseases Publishing Co.

Deckert, G. H., and West, L. J.: Hypnosis and experimental psychopathology, Am. J. Clin. Hypn. 5:256, 1963.

Easser, B. R., and Lesser, S. R.: Hysterical personality: a re-evaluation, Psychoanal. Q. 24:390, 1965.

Farber, L.: Will and willfulness in hysteria. In the ways of the will, New York, 1968, Basic Books, Inc., Publishers.

Guze, S. B., and Perley, M. J.: Observations on natural history of hysteria, Am. J. Psychiatry 119:960, 1963.

Halleck, S. L.: Hysterical personality traits, Arch. Gen. Psychiatry 16:750, 1967.

Janet, P.: The major symptoms of hysteria, ed. 2, New York, 1920, The Macmillan Co.

Lehmann, L. S.: Depersonalization, Am. J. Psychiatry 131:1221, 1974.

Lesser, R. P., and Fahn, S.: Dystonia: a disorder often misdiagnosed as a conversion reaction, Am. J. Psychiatry 135:349, 1978.

Lindemann, E.: Hysteria as a problem in a general hospital, Medical Clinics of North America, Philadelphia, 1938, W. B. Saunders Co.

Ludwig, A. M., Brandsma, J. M., Wilbur, C. B., Bendfeldt, F., and Jameson, D. H.: The objective study of a multiple personality, Arch. Gen. Psychiatry 26:298, 1972.

McGill, V. J., and Welch, L.: Hysteria as a conditioning process, Am. J. Psychother. **1:**253, 1947.

Rabkin, R.: Conversion hysteria as social maladaptation, Psychiatry **27:**349, 1964.

Slater, E.: The thirty-fifth Maudsley lecture: "Hysteria 311, J. Ment. Sci. **107:**359, 1961.

Vieth, I.: Hysteria, the history of a disease, Chicago, 1965, University of Chicago Press.

Woerner, P. I., and Guze, S.: Family and marital study of hysteria, B. J. Psychiatry **114:**161, 1968.

Phobic neurosis

Phobic neurosis (anxiety hysteria) is a concept initiated by Freud to refer to cases where the anxiety is connected with a particular object or situation which symbolically represents the neurotic conflict. Neurotic reactions in children are frequently of this kind and involve the appearance of anxiety attacks associated with phobic objects, castration fears, and other symbols of danger. The phobic syndrome was classified by Janet with obsessive-compulsive neurosis under the term "psychasthenia."

Phobias occur in many psychoneuroses but only in a very small percentage of cases predominate the symptom picture. In these patients anxiety appears when the patient finds himself in places which tend to threaten the sense of self-control. The patient thus must avoid such distressing situations, and his life becomes increasingly sequestered. Types of phobias encountered include acrophobia (high places), agoraphobia (open places), algophobia (pain), astraphobia (thunder and lightning), claustrophobia (closed places), coprophobia (excreta), hematophobia (blood), hydrophobia (water), lalophobia (speaking), mysophobia (dirt), necrophobia (dead bodies), nyctophobia (darkness), pathophobia (disease), peccatiphobia (sinning), phonophobia (speaking aloud), photophobia (strong light), sitophobia (eating), taphephobia (being buried alive), thanatophobia (death), toxiphobia (being poisoned), xenophobia (strangers), zoophobia (animals).

TREATMENT. Although traditional psychotherapeutic techniques are often used, more recently there appears greater promise of favorable outcome with the technique of reciprocal inhibition. Presumably the successful outcome of short-term psychotherapy depends upon whether the phobic neurosis is mild and of recent origin in a personality with many areas of competence. In patients with chronic, multiple progressively worsening phobias, the symptoms often represent an attempt to reduce intense disorganizing inner conflict by participating in few life situations. Removing through reeducation and conditioning this simple defensive life strategy may bring a measure of relief while other serious conflicts are being resolved. Forced exposure to the feared object or situation, such as in flooding, has met some success.

SUGGESTED READINGS

Arieti, S. A.: A re-examination of the phobic symptom and of symbolism in psychopathology, Am. J. Psychiatry **118:**106, 1961.

Buglass, D., and others: A study of agorophobic housewives, Psychol. Med. **7:**73, 1977.

Freud, S.: Analysis of a phobia in a five-year-old boy. In Collected papers, London, 1950, Hogarth Press, Ltd., vol. 3.

Gelder, M. G., and Marks, I. M.: Desensitization and phobias: a crossover study, B. J. Psychiatry **114:**323, 1968.

Kazdin, A. E., and Wilcoxon, L. A.: Systematic desentization and nonspecific treatment effects: a methodological evaluation, Psychol. Bull. **83:**729, 1976.

Rachman, S.: Phobias: their nature and control, Springfield, Ill., 1968, Charles C Thomas, Publisher.

Terhune, W.: The phobic syndrome, Arch. Neurol. Psychiatry **62:**162, 1949.

Wolpe, J.: The experimental foundations of some new psychotherapeutic methods. In Abracha, C. H., editor: Experimental foundations of clinical psychology, New York, 1962, Basic Books, Inc., Publishers, p. 554.

Wolpe J.: Psychotherapy by reciprocal inhibition, Stanford, Calif., 1958, Stanford University Press.

Zitrin, C. M. Klein, D. F., and Woerner, M. G.: Behavior therapy supportive psychotherapy, imipramine, and phobias, Arch. Gen. Psychiatry **35:**307, 1978.

Obsessive-compulsive neurosis

Obsessive or anancastic thoughts are those which perseverate and cannot be put out of consciousness. When translated into action they are known as compulsions. These symptoms may occur in the course of psychotic illness but alone may be the most noticeable symptom of an incapacitating neurosis.

ANAMNESIS. Indecisiveness may prevent an early visit to the physician by a patient who as his *chief complaint* constantly ruminates about avoiding dirt or germs, has recurring sexual thoughts, and spends his time in such elaborate rituals as hand washing, object touching, and prolonged dressing. *Past history* is that of a rigid, orderly person, perhaps of superior intellectual capacity. Maternal overconcern about bowel training, table manners, and cleanliness is felt to be a conditioning factor. Traits such as penuriousness and stubbornness are believed to develop in the anal sadistic (retentive) phase of childhood as a defense against open or implied parental threats. When present in mild degree, conscientiousness and adherence to strict ethical codes may be valuable character traits of these individuals. This form of neurosis usually appears in adolescence and advances during adult life, but obsessional rituals may occasionally be seen as early as 2 years of age in children of disturbed families.

EXAMINATION. The individual, *behaviorally,* is clean, neat, and overly polite and speaks in a guarded way about his symptoms rather than his personal feelings. Often indecisive, these patients show a striving for perfection and superiority with symptoms expressive of guilt. Anxiety and depression may be present in various degrees, particularly if rituals are prevented. Unjustified fear of their own dangerous impulses may be admitted. The compulsive rituals have been said to represent a caricature of masturbation which expresses a variety of psychological urges. In contrast to the visual daydreams of the hysteric, the fantasies of the compulsion neurotic tend to be verbalized and bring back the archaic attitudes that accompanied the first use of words. The compulsion neurotic, being afraid of his emotions, is afraid of things that arouse emotions. His defenses are intellectual and verbal. *Psychological* tests reveal paucity of imaginative productions, great attention to detail and a tendency toward a stereotyped, overcontrolled approach to the solution of tasks. These patients may conventionalize responses excessively and deny disturbing feelings aroused by the test.

TREATMENT. Problems in therapy arise from the patient's overintellectualizations and inability to experience feelings and to free-associate. Countertransference problems may result from the patient's inability to accept formulations other than his own and from the ambivalence and stubbornness of this character type. Some therapists advise gradual prohibition of compulsions as a means of producing anxiety, which in turn leads to new behavior. In mild cases psychotherapy may be of value, and techniques of reciprocal inhibition should be considered. Long-term psychotherapy may be recommended if feasible for the patient. In chronic severe cases, lobotomy has been used combined with an active postoperative rehabilitation program. Insulin and electroshock therapy are not indicated.

SUGGESTED READINGS

Dowson, J. H.: The phenomenology of severe obsessive-compulsive neurosis, B. J. Psychiatry **131**:75, 1977.

Goodwin, D. W., Guze, S. B., and Robins, E.: Follow-up studies in obsessional neuroses, Arch. Gen. Psychiatry **20**:182, 1969.

Ingram, I. M.: The obsessional personality and obsessional illness, Am. J. Psychiatry **117**:1016, 1961.

Ingram, I. M.: Obsessional illness in mental hospital patients, J. Ment. Sci. **107**:382, 1961.

Pollitt, J. D.: Natural history studies in mental illness: a discussion based on a pilot study of obsessional state, J. Ment. Sci. **106**:93, 1960.

Wolpe, J.: Pychotherapy by reciprocal inhibition, Stanford, Calif., 1958, Stanford University Press.

Depressive neurosis

Depression as a symptom is seen in varying degree in nearly all psychoneurotics, but in some it is the predominant symptom. With complaints including insomnia, anorexia, decreased sexual drive, weight loss, constipation, fatigue, and menstrual disturbances, the entity somewhat resembles manic-depressive psychosis but differs from it in the depth of guilt and depression, degree of retardation, and in the absence of delusions or hallucinations. It is important to keep in mind that suicide can occur.

As in all psychoneuroses, psychotherapy is the usual mode of treatment. Electroshock, however, may be used to dispel the depression, but, in the usual case, it does not affect the other psychoneurotic symptoms favorably, and anxiety may even be increased. Antidepressant drugs are often of benefit and both the iminodibenzyl derivatives and the monoamine oxidase inhibitors have been advocated.

The terms "neurotic depression," "neurotic depressive reaction," and "mixed psychoneurosis with depression" have been used to describe the above condition. The term "reactive depression" is often used synonymously with these. Actually "reactive depression" is a purely descriptive term, implying that the symptoms of depression, whether in a neurosis or psychosis, have arisen in response to a known environmental problem (loss of loved ones, financial difficulty, marital discord, etc.). The use of this term usually implies an illness of short duration that is amenable to psychotherapy. The term does not accurately define a distinct disease entity, for in modern dynamic psychiatry every depression is reactive in the sense that it is a reactivation of infantile mood disturbances, in response to current life stresses which symbolically resemble earlier traumatic relationships. Actually one can think in terms of a continuum from a minor to a grossly traumatic precipitating factor—from one detectable only after careful analysis of mental content to a precipitating factor evident to all. The former is classed as endogenous depression, the latter exogenous or reactive. It is apparent that the better prognosis of the latter (i.e., reactive depression) should but emphasize the fact that the personality that succumbs with depression only to a maximum trauma must be better adjusted than one developing symptoms to a minimal or hidden stress.

SUGGESTED READINGS

Ayd, F. J.: Recognizing the depressed patient, New York, 1961, Grune & Stratton, Inc.

Clayton, P., Desmarais, L., and Winokur, G.: A study of normal bereavement, Am. J. Psychiatry **125**:168, 1968.

Derogatis, L. R., Klerman, G. L., and Lipman, R. S.: Anxiety states and depressive neurosis, J. Nerv. Ment. Dis. **155**:392, 1972.

Devaul, R. H., and Zisook, S.: Unresolved grief: clinical considerations, Postgrad. Med. **59**:267, 1976.

Greenblatt, M.: The grieving spouse, Am. J. Psychiatry **135**:43, 1978.

Kubler-Ross, E.: On death and dying, New York, 1969, The Macmillan Co.

Lindemann, E.: Symptomatology and management of acute grief, Am. J. Psychiatry **101**:141, 1944.

Mendels, J.: Depression: the distinction between syndrome and symptom, B. J. Psychiatry **114**:1549, 1968.

Parkes, C. M., and Brown, R. J.: Health after bereavement: controlled study of young Boston widows and widowers, Psychol. Med. **34**:449, 1972.

Prusoff, B., and Klerman, G. I.: Differentiating depressed from anxious neurotic outpatients, Arch. Gen. Psychiatry **30**:302, 1974.

Ward, A. W. H.: Mortality of bereavement, Br. Med. J. **1**:700, 1976.

Neurasthenic neurosis

The term *neurasthenia* (neurasthenic neurosis) predates psychoanalytic theory and refers to a severe chronic anxiety neurosis, often accompanied by obsessive or depressive features, which seem fixed and less labile or responsive to changes in life situation than is true of most anxiety neurosis. Fatigue is a prominent symptom, accompanied by an inability to participate in active work and social relationships.

Depersonalization neurosis

When inner conflicts are not being adequately defended against by neurotic mechanisms, a patient may begin to exhibit anxiety and markedly disruptive changes in personality. One such symptom, which in many cases never leads to any more severe symptoms, is depersonalization.

Depersonalization neurosis is a term for individuals who experience parts of their bodies as not belonging or as suddenly expanding greatly or changing in size or shape. Face, hands, head, or genitals are commonly selected, and the experience is usually transient and uncanny and may be identifiably in response to a meaningful event or encounter. This condition illustrates the fact that, as any neurosis increases in severity, experiences and symptoms resembling psychotic behavior may be reported. Nevertheless, it is not usual for neuroses to transmute into true psychoses. Rather the borderline or schizoid neurotic tends to be more difficult to treat than other psychoneurotic patients. Although such symptoms may occur either alone or as part of some other primary mental disorder, such as an acute situational reaction, brief experiences of depersonalization are not necessarily a symptom of illness.

Hypochondriacal neurosis

The term *hypochondriacal neurosis* refers to individuals chronically and obsessively preoccupied with fancied bodily sensations and dysfunctions. Depending upon the particular case, elements of hysterical neurosis, obsessive-compulsive neurosis, depressive neurosis, or even psychosis may be identified. In addition to these standard diagnostic categories, several others may be mentioned because of their past common usage.

The term *traumatic neurosis* refers to those cases in which symptoms emerge immediately following a violently disturbing life experience. Fenichel states that probably many individuals classified under this heading are really psychoneurotics in whom the neurotic predisposition was unrecognized and the trauma actually only a contributory cause.

15

Personality disorders and certain other nonpsychotic mental disorders

PERSONALITY DISORDERS

Every person exhibits certain habitual attitudes and reaction patterns in human relationships which have existed since early years and may be designated as his character structure. When these ways of behaving become inappropriately exaggerated, the individual may be said to suffer a character disorder. In most cases these patterns of behavior cause the individual little or no anxiety or sense of distress. These disorders are manifested by lifelong patterns of action or behavior rather than by mental or emotional symptoms.

Attempts at classifying these disorders have resulted in no acceptable scheme. Yet the outworn, all-inclusive, wastebasket category *psychopath* is no longer considered useful, since it referred to *all* deviate behavior patterns not frankly psychotic or psychoneurotic. Persons with character disorders tend to create in a sterotyped fashion particular interpersonal conflicts which arise from the individual's own style of of thinking, valuing, and feeling about specific life situations. An adequate scheme for categorizing character disorders will have to consider systematically multivariate verbal, motor, and physiological pathways for emotional release and also diverse but highly influential structural aspects of situations and relationships. Former attempts at classification have included such types as the following: excitable, explosive, irritable, quarrelsome, anxious, depressive, phlegmatic, artistic, egocentric, schizoid, hysterical, impulsive, litigious, etc.—terms which may describe the behavior of any of us at some time or other. Perhaps in the broadest sense we all have personality disturbances, in that we overwork some defense or reactive mechanism. The transient and not the prolonged and incapacitating nature of these idiosyncracies, however, spells the difference between a normal person and one showing a character disorder.

Formerly in the American Psychiatric Association terminology, the term "personality trait disturbance" was used to describe individuals unable to maintain their emotional equilibrium and independence under minor or major stress, because of disturbances in emotional development. The term "personality pattern disturbance" was applied to persons who function in a disturbed fashion rigidly in all situations and in whom the core personality type could rarely be altered by any kind of therapy. A variety of terms has been used to describe personality disorder. Some of the more common are described in the following paragraphs.

Paranoid personality. Individuals of this type show a propensity for projection mechanisms expressed by suspiciousness, envy, irritability, extreme jealousy, and stubbornness. Reality-testing, however, is not grossly impaired, and stable, well-formulated delusions are absent.

Cyclothymic personality (atypical affective disorder). These persons are characterized by outgoing adjustment to life situations, with apparent warmth and friendliness and ready enthusiasm for competition. They are frequently alternating between moods of elation and sadness without obvious relation to external events or with a grossly exaggerated intensity of emotion.

Schizoid personality (schizotypal, latent, borderline). Showing avoidance of close interpersonal relationships and lack of aggressiveness, with inability to express hostility and with autistic thinking, these cold, aloof, fearful individuals exhibit emotional detachment and avoidance of competition with consequent solution of problems in daydreaming. They are described in childhood as quiet, shy, obedient, sensitive, and retiring and at adolescence receive the appellation of introvert.

Explosive personality (epileptoid personality disturbance).

These persons have periodic outbursts of rage with verbal and/or physical aggressiveness. They differ from normals in the unexpectedness and intensity of such behavior and their inability for control. At times they may be regretful and repentant. Such persons are excitable and overresponsive to environmental pressures. If the patient is amnesic for the outburst, a diagnosis of hysteria or convulsive disorder should be considered.

Obsessive-compulsive personality (anancastic personality). Characterized by chronic excessive or obsessive concern with adherence to standards of rationalism, conscience, or conformity, these individuals are rigid, overconscientious, and have an inordinate capacity for work. There is a reduced capacity for relaxation and for experiencing emotions. The self is experienced as being monitored and directed rigidly by a set of inner directives or moral principles.

Hysterical personality (histrionic personality disorder). These persons demonstrate excitability and emotional instability. They tend to overreact and to dramatize. Their behavior is attention getting and seductive. Immature, self-centered, and often vain, such persons may appear entertaining but are willfully manipulative and dependent on others.

Asthenic personality. These persons are of low energy level and show an incapacity for enjoyment. They are easily fatigued, lack enthusiasm, and are oversensitive to physical and emotional stress.

Antisocial personality. (sociopathic personality disturbance). The group with this problem includes those individuals with chronic or lifelong disturbance who are ill primarily in forms of behavior conflict with the customs, rules, and laws of society. The failure to conform to the rules of prevailing cultural milieu may often be symptomatic of other severe personality disorder, neurosis, psychosis, organic brain injury, or other disease, and so the likelihood of such conditions should also be considered. One subgroup of such disorders has been referred to in psychoanalytic parlance as *impulse neurosis.*

The inability of these patients to deny themselves wished-for pleasures or to inhibit aggressive impulses has been understood as a means of avoiding severe depression or anxiety. The inability of many of these patients to form an adult sexual relationship has led to studies relating symptoms to primitive sexual expression.

Such formulations have been developed for kleptomania (compulsion to steal), gambling (sexual excitement with compulsion to gamble), and pyromania (compulsion to set fires, often with masturbation).

Under this category fall persons who are chronically in trouble with society. They seem to suffer a defect in concept of time relating to self, with no concern for either past or future; hence, they show concern only with the present and have been called hedonistic. They have no concern for the consequences of their actions and profit neither from experience nor from punishment, maintaining no real loyalties to any person, group, or code. They are often chronic liars, show marked emotional immaturity with poor judgment, and lack any sense of responsibility. Their manner is frequently disarming, they have the ability to ingratiate themselves with others, and they may appear likeable although superficial. They often have an ability to rationalize their behavior so that it appears reasonable and justified. The group intended here includes individuals often referred to by such terms as "psychopath," "psychopathic personality," or "constitutional psychopathic inferior."

Some individuals manifest disregard for the usual social codes and come into conflict with them as a result of having all their lives lived in an abnormal environment. They may be capable of strong loyalties. These individuals typically do not show significant personality deviations other than those implied by adherence to the values or codes of their own predatory, criminal, or other social group.

Passive-aggressive personality. In this type the picture may be characterized predominantly by helplessness and indecisiveness (with a tendency to clinging, pouting, stubbornness, and passive obstructionism) or by oscillation from this to a persistent reaction to frustration with irritability, temper tantrums, and destructive behavior. These persons may be adept at covertly and "innocently" fomenting crises between others.

Inadequate personality. This type is one in which the individuals show inadequate response to intellectual, emotional, social, and physical demands. Grossly they are neither physically nor mentally deficient on examination but show lack of adaptability, ineptness, poor judgment, social incompatibility, and lack of stamina.

SUGGESTED READINGS

Aichorn, A.: Wayward youth, New York, 1955, Meridian Books, Inc.

Brody, F. B.: Borderline states, character disorders and psychotic manifestations—some conceptual formulations, Psychiatry **23**:75, 1960.

Cleckley, H.: The mask of sanity, ed. 5, St. Louis, 1976, The C. V. Mosby Co.

Craft, M., and others: 100 admissions to a psychopathic unit, J. Ment. Sci. **108**:564, 1962.

Gibbens, T. C. N., Pond, D. A., and Stafford-Clark, D. A.: A follow-up study of criminal psychopaths, J. Ment. Sci. **105**:108, 1959.

Gurr, T. R.: Why men rebel, Princeton, N. J., 1970, Princeton University Press.

Guze, S. B.: A study of recidivisim based upon a follow-up of 217 consecutive criminals, J. Nerv. Ment. Dis. **138**:575, 1964.

Jenkins, R. L.: The psychopathic or antisocial personality, J. Nerv. Ment. Dis. **131**:318, 1960.

O'Neal, P., Robins, L. N., King, L. J., and Schafer, J.: Parental deviance and the genesis of sociopathic personality, Am. J. Psychiatry **118**:1114, 1962.

Redl, F., and Wineman, D.: Children who hate, Glencoe, Ill., 1951, The Free Press.

Reich, W.: Character analysis, ed. 3, New York, 1949, Orgone Institute Press.

Rifkin, A., and others: Lithium in emotionally unstable character disorder, Arch. Gen. Psychiatry **27**:519, 1972.

Robins, L. N.: Deviant children grown up: a sociological and psychiatric study of sociopathic personality, Baltimore, 1966, The Williams & Wilkins Co.

Schneider, K.: Psychopathic personalities, Springfield, Ill., 1958, Charles C Thomas, Publisher.

Thompson, G. N.: Sociopathic personality, its neurophysiology and treatment. In Rinkel, M., editor: Biological treatment of mental illness, New York, 1966, L. C. Page & Co.

Tooth, G.: The aggressive psychopathic offender, Lancet **1**:42, 1969.

SEXUAL DEVIATIONS

Deviant sexual behavior may be a symptom of other fundamental psychiatric disorder, such as schizophrenia, psychoneurosis, or senile psychosis, or it may occur as a predominant behavior aberration of a disordered personality. The term "deviation" suggests behavior counter to custom or accepted cultural mores. In the light of studies by Kinsey and others, however, much that we have formerly termed aberrant is found to be rather common behavior. Therefore, we must evaluate symptoms of sexual deviation in the light of current and regional social approval as well as potential danger to society and the production of discomfort in the patient. Freud has defined *perversion* as a reaction to castration fear, with regression to infantile sexuality as the only possible sexual outlet.

What are and what are not considered perverse sexual acts depend greatly on time and society. For example, homosexuality, which for years was classified as deviant sexual behavior, has in recent years been more openly practiced and hence is by many considered acceptable social behavior. The same is true of fellatio and cunnilingus, which are today openly talked about and widely practiced despite the fact that in some parts of the country such acts are technically considered illegal. Types of sexual behavior that have traditionally considered deviant include: *homosexuality*, attraction for or sexual relations with persons of the same sex, which may be either passive or active in character; *fetishism*, in which some object substitutes for the genitals; and *transvestitism*, in which the subject wears clothes of persons of the opposite sex. In *exhibitionism* sexual pleasure is obtained by exposing one's genitals; *voyeurism* (scoptophilia) is a perversion in which the individual enjoys sexual excitement from watching naked men, naked women, and naked children, normal or perverse sexual acts, or excretory acts; sometimes the subject watches himself in a mirror during sexual intercourse. *Bestiality* (erotic zoophilia) involves use of an animal as a sex object. This may be partly determined by the environment and is common among persons brought up on farms. *Pedophilia* is an attraction to children as sex objects and *pederasty* refers to anal intercourse with small children. In the oral acts of *fellatio* and *cunnilingus* the mouth becomes a substitute for the genitals. *Sadism* (active algolagnia) is a perversion in which cruelty to others is substituted for the sex act or in which cruelty may accompany the sex act, as in *flagellation*, where satisfaction is achieved through whipping the partner; in *masochism* (passive algolagnia) the patient must experience pain himself in order to enjoy the sex act, or he seeks out suffering as a substitute for sexual enjoyment. Patients with *gerontophilia* need an elderly sexual partner, and this can be regarded as a displacement of incestuous wishes. *Necrophilia* is defined as sexual intercourse with the dead. Some authors have suggested that the choice of a chronically sick or crippled partner is really a modified form of necrophilia. *Transsexualism* is a type of abnormality in which patients believe that they have the mind of the opposite sex in the wrong body. Male patients, for example, claim they are changing their sex and are frightened of all male activity, including erections. *Masturbation* is one form of autoerotism; practically all men masturbate to some degree during adolescence, and although it creates no physical harm, it may produce much guilt and shame.

SUGGESTED READINGS

Baittle, B., and Kobrin, S.: On the relationship of a characterological type of delinquent to the milieu, Psychiatry **27**:6, 1964.

Baker, H. J., and Stoller, R. J.: Sexual psychopathology in the hypogonadal male, Arch. Gen. Psychiatry **18**:631, 1968.

Becker, H. S.: Outsiders: studies in the sociology of deviance, New York, 1964, The Free Press of Glencoe, Inc.

Becker, H. S., editor: The other side: perspectives on deviance, New York, 1964, The Free Press of Glencoe, Inc.

Belleau T., and Arsenian, J.: Homicide and hospitalization: a case report, Psychiatry **30**:73, 1967.

Bieber, I., and others: Homosexuality, a pyschoanalytic study, New York, 1962, Basic Books, Inc., Publishers.

Groth, A. N., Burgess, A. W., and Holmstrom, L. L.: Rape: power, anger, and sexuality, Am. J. Psychiatry **134**:1239, 1977.

Hendin, H.: Marijuana abuse among college students, J. Nerv. Ment. Dis. **156**:259, 1973.

Karpman, B.: The sexual offender and his offenses; etiology, pathology, psychodynamics and treatment, New York, 1954, Julian Press, Inc.

Kenyon, F. E.: Studies in female homosexuality, Br. J. Psychiatry **114**:1337, 1968.

Kinsey, A., Pomeroy, W., Martin, C., and Gebbard, P. H.: Sexual behavior in the human female, Philadelphia, 1953, W. B. Saunders Co.

Kinsey, A., Pomeroy, W., and Martin, C.: Sexual behavior in the human male, Philadelphia, 1948, W. B. Saunders Co.

Kramer, W., Meyer, L. C., and Carroll, N. E.: Victims of rape, Washington, D.C., 1977, DHEW Publication No. 017-024-00683-1.

Masters, W. H., and Johnson, B. E.: Human sexual response, Boston, 1966, Little, Brown & Co.

Masters, W. H., and Johnson, B. E.: Human sexual inadequacy, Boston, 1970, Little, Brown & Co.

Rosen, I., editor: The pathology and treatment of sexual deviation, London, 1964, Oxford University Press.

ALCOHOLISM

"Alcoholism" is the general term to designate the condition in which alcohol intake is great enough to damage physical health and personal or social functioning or when it has become a pre-requisite to normal functioning. The term "episodic excessive drinking" is used when alcoholism is present and the individual becomes intoxicated as frequently as four times a year. *Intoxication* is defined as a state in which the individual's coordination or speech is definitely impaired or his behavior is clearly altered. Persons who become intoxicated more than twelve times a year or are recognizably under the influence of alcohol more than once a week, even though not intoxicated, are classified under the term "habitual excessive drinking." The term "alcohol addiction" is used when there is direct or strong presumptive evidence that the patient is dependent upon alcohol. This may be demonstrated either by withdrawal symptoms or by an inability to go 1 day without drinking. When heavy drinking continues for 3 months or more, it is reasonable to presume addiction to alcohol.

Alcoholism affects 10 million individuals in the United States today and is a major social, economic, and medical problem in many countries throughout the globe. It is found as part of the symptom complex in character disorders or borderline psychotic individuals as well as in neurotic and other psychiatric disorders. The search for a common etiology has not been entirely rewarding. A marked sense of inferiority and helplessness with strong dependency needs may be combined with fantasies of self-importance and belief in a right to be taken care of. Alcohol can temporarily drown the frustration of inferiority feelings and the conflict of impossible ambitions.

The World Health Organization has defined alcoholism as a chronic behavioral disorder manifested by repeated drinking of alcoholic beverages in excess of the dietary and social uses of the community and to an extent that interferes with the drinker's health or his social or economic function. Dr. Ebbe Hoff states that in alcoholism there is: (1) loss of controlled alcohol intake—the victim finds himself drinking when he intends not to drink or drinking more than he has planned; (2) functional or structural damage—physiological, psychological, domestic, economic, or social; (3) use of alcohol as a kind of universal therapy—a psychopharmacological substance by which the problem drinker attempts to keep his life from disintegrating.

Despite common belief, alcoholism is not a skid row problem. More than 70% of alcoholics reside in respectable neighborhoods. The risk rate among drinkers in the United States is approximately 1 in 10. The estimated ratio of female to male alcoholics is 1 to 3. The life expectancy of an alcoholic is approximately 12 to 14 years less than average life expectancy. The estimated cost in the United States is 43 billion dollars annually. Alcoholism contributes heavily to suicide, crime, and to at least 50% of traffic accidents.

DIAGNOSIS. The warning signs of alcoholism include frequent drinking sprees, a steady increase in intake, solitary drinking, early morning drinking, Monday morning absenteeism, frequent disputes about drinking, and the occurrence of blackouts (a period of time in which, while remaining otherwise fully conscious, the person undergoes a loss of memory). An individual may probably be considered an alcoholic if he continues to drink despite the fact that his drinking causes physical illness, headache, gastric distress, or hangover and repeatedly causes trouble with spouse, employer, or police.

TREATMENT. The successful therapeutic approach is often a multifaceted one involving psychotherapeutic, social, and medical methods in both hospital and community settings. Countertransference problems in the psychotherapist are often major. The psychotherapist may be tricked or provoked by the patient into retaliatory or rejecting responses or may in a contagious fashion begin to feel as hopeless about the patient as the patient does about himself. These patients tend to be experts in self-destructive acting out as a defense against experiencing tension or disappointment. The conditioned reflex treatment of alcoholism (which develops an aversion to drink by negative conditioning) and/or disulfiram (Antabuse, 0.5 Gm. daily for 1 to 3 weeks, then maintenance on 0.25 to 0.5 Gm. daily) serves only to help the patient resist alcohol during ongoing psychotherapy. The goals of psychotherapy should be consistent with the resources of the patient and his environment and must be tailored to the needs of the individual. Denial is a major mental mechanism seen in most alcoholics and should be dealt with in therapy.

The A.A. (Alcoholics Anonymous) is reputed to be helpful to about 50% of its members. Its "12-step" program is built around principles of comradeship, self-help, and a Good Samaritan attitude toward other alcoholics. It combines the therapeutic principles of activity groups with a revival type of religious identification and a service club appeal. It helps to elevate the patient's self-esteem by making him useful to other alcoholics, as well as to strengthen his resistance to temptation by moral suasion and group pressure. It requires the selfadmission of the individual that he is powerless over alcohol and that his life has become unmanageable. Al-Anon and Ala-Teens are parallel organizations developed to help the spouse and children of alcoholics.

SUGGESTED READINGS

Alcoholics Anonymous: The story of how many thousands of men and women have recovered from alcoholism, New York, 1955, Works Library Publications.

Alcoholics Anonymous: Twelve steps and twelve traditions, New York, 1953, Alcoholics Anonymous Publishing Co.

A.M.A. Committee on Alcoholism and Addiction and Council on Mental Health: Dependence on barbiturates and other sedative drugs, J.A.M.A. **193:**673, 1965.

Catanzaro, R. J.: Alcoholism—the total treatment approach, Springfield, Ill., 1968, Charles C Thomas, Publisher.

Chafetz, M. E.: Liquor: the servant of man, Boston, 1965, Little, Brown & Co.

Chafetz, M. E., and Demone, H. W., Jr.: Alcoholism and society, New York, 1962, Oxford University Press, Inc.

Charuvatra, C. V., Panell, J., Hopper, M., Ehrmann, M., Blakis, M., and Ling, W.: The medical safety of the combined usage of disulfram and methadone, Arch. Gen. Psychiatry **33:**391, 1976.

Gordon, J. E.: The epidemiology of alcoholism. In Kruse, H. D., editor: Alcoholism as a medical problem, New York, 1956, Paul B. Hoeber, Inc.

Hart, W. T.: A comparison of promazine and paraldehyde in 175 cases of alcohol withdrawal, Am. J. Psychiatry **118:**323, 1961.

Himwich, H. E.: Alcohol and brain physiology and alcoholism, Springfield, Ill., 1956, Charles C Thomas, Publisher.

Jellinek, E. M.: The disease concept of alcoholism, New Haven, Conn., 1960, Hill House Press.

Kaim, S. C., Klett, C. J., and Rothfeld, B.: Treatment of the acute alcohol withdrawal state: a comparison of four drugs, Am. J. Psychiatry **125:**1640, 1969.

Kissin, B., Rosenblatt, S. M., and Machover, S.: Prognostic factors in alcoholism, Psychiat. Res. Rep. Amer. Psychiat. Assoc. **24**:22, March, 1968.

McCord, W., and McCord, J.: Origins of alcoholism, Palo Alto, Calif., 1960, Stanford University Press.

Pittman, D. J., and Gordon, C. W.: Revolving door: a study of the chronic police case inebriate, Yale University Center of Alcohol Studies, monograph no. 2, Glencoe, Ill., 1958, The Free Press.

Tamerin, J. S., and Mendelson, J. H.: Psychodynamics of chronic inebriation: observations of alcoholics during process of drinking in experimental group setting, Am. J. Psychiatry **125**:886, 1969.

Thomas, D. W., and Freedman, D. X.: Treatment of alcohol withdrawal syndrome: comparison of promazine and paraldehyde, J.A.M.A. **188**: 316, 1964.

Wilson, W. P., and Wolk, M.: The treatment of delirium tremens, N. Carolina Med. J. **26**:552, 1965.

DRUG DEPENDENCE

Drug abuse is the term generally employed to refer to the use, usually by self-administration, of any drug in a manner that deviates from approved medical and social patterns. The term *drug dependence* refers to a *physical* dependence on drugs other than alcohol, tobacco, and ordinary caffeine-containing beverages. Dependence on medically prescribed drugs is also excluded as long as the drug's use is indicated and the intake is proportionate to the medical need. *Habituation (psychic dependence)* refers to the situation in which a person desires and becomes accustomed to a drug but is not physically dependent upon it. *Tolerance* refers to that state in which the body's tissues become accustomed to the presence of the drug and fail to respond to concentrations ordinarily effective; thus increasingly large quantities are required to produce the desired effect. *Addiction* is a condition of physical dependence habituation, and tolerance.

The abuse of and addiction to different drugs varies from time to time and from country to country. At this time in the United States, it is estimated that perhaps 10 million individuals have used marijuana, although only one-tenth of this number are heavy users. There are an estimated 250,000 to 500,000 nonnarcotic drug abusers and perhaps 100,000 hard narcotics addicts. Although drug abuse occurs in all strata of society, it is most prevalent in the slum districts of large highly urbanized areas. Seventy percent of all narcotics addicts in the United States live in ten big cities.

The reason given for taking drugs by nearly half of the addicts is to obtain the desired euphoria, to feel "normal," and to overcome a state of depression. Other reasons cited are curiosity and the influence of friends or the environment. Narcotics addicts have a wide range of personality characteristics, with perhaps 10% having sociopathic personality disorders. The majority are described as emotionally unstable, immature, impulsive, unreliable, angry against society, and unable to establish long-range goals or meet the demands of the environment. Four out of five narcotics addicts are male, with Negroes and Caucasians being about equal in number. Eighty percent of narcotic drug users are between 20 and 40 years of age with an increasingly large number of teenagers involved with marihuana and hallucinogens. In the last few years deaths associated with drug addiction, most often from acute reaction or overdosage, have markedly increased.

The argot of the addict is colorful and includes such phrases as the following: *acid*, LSD; *bennies,* amphetamines; *blow a stick*, to smoke a marijuana cigarette; *cold turkey*, abrupt withdrawal from narcotics without medication; *fix*, an injection of narcotics; *goofballs*, barbiturates; *grass*, marijuana; *head (acid head, pothead)*, one high on LSD, marijuana, or hashish; *hooked*, to be dependent on drugs; *joypot*, the intermittent use of heroin by a nonaddict; *junkie*, a narcotics addict; *kick the habit*, to stop using the drugs; *mainline*, to take drugs intravenously; *nod*, to behave in a lethargic or somnolent manner, or, when under the influence of drugs; *O.D.*, overdose of drugs, often lethal; *pusher*, a seller of drugs; *score*, to obtain drugs; *skin pop*, to inject drugs under the skin; *stoned*, to be high on drugs; *trip*, a hallucinogenic experience; *turned on*, excitement or sensory experience after taking drugs; *weed*, marijuana.

OPIUM, OPIUM ALKALOIDS, OR THEIR DERIVATIVES. Addiction to opium is a chronic physiological intoxication in which the drug injection is maintained· by an individual suffering from personality disorder. The particular difficulties of an addict are determined not only by physiological and psychological factors but also by cultural attitudes toward the addict who, after his funds are gone, may be led to criminal means of obtaining the drug. Opiate addiction occurs most frequently in persons who are immature or self-centered, or in dependent persons who tend to have a psychoneurotic or psychopathic life pattern. In general, it

Table 5. Drug dependence

Class of drug	Psychic dependence	Physical dependence	Tolerance	Characteristics of intoxication	Characteristics of withdrawal
Cannabis sativa (marijuana, hashish)	Moderate to strong	No	Not demonstrated	Milder preparations induce drowsy, euphoric state with inappropriate laughter and disturbances in perception of space and time; stronger preparations (hashish) induce psychotic reaction with hallucinations; pupils normal, conjuntivae injected	No specific withdrawal symptoms
Psychostimulants (amphetamines)	Variable	Mild to absent	Slowly developed, not equal for all components of central nervous system	Agitation, tachycardia, paranoid thought disturbances with high doses; pupils dilated and sluggishly reactive with high doses; acute brain syndrome common; convulsive seizures may occur	Lethargy, somnolence, general malaise, psychic depression, often with suicidal tendency; acute brain syndrome may persist for weeks

Opiates (morphine, heroin, etc.)	Strong	Develops early	Yes	Pinpoint pupils; analgesia with or without depressed sensorium; patient may be alert and appear normal; respiratory depression with overdose	Dilated and reactive pupils, gastrointestinal disturbances, low back pain, rhinorrhea, lacrimation, gooseflesh
Hallucinogens (psychostimulants, psychomimetics; LSD, mescaline, morning glory seed, etc.)	Varies greatly, usually not intense	No	High degree, develops rapidly	Unpredictable psychic disturbance, extreme lability of affect, chaotic disruption of thought, danger of uncontrolled behavior, pupils dilated and reactive to light	No specific symptoms; effects may persist for indefinite period after discontinuation of drug
Barbiturates	Yes	Yes	Yes	Drowsiness, with nystagmus on lateral gaze; ataxia; slurred speech; respiratory depression with overdose; pupil size and reaction appear normal	General agitation, tremulousness, insomnia, gastrointestinal disturbances, blepharoclonus, hyperpyrexia, acute brain syndrome, convulsive seizures

Continued.

Table 5. Drug dependence—cont'd

Class of drug	Psychic dependence	Physical dependence	Tolerance	Characteristics of intoxication	Characteristics of withdrawal
Cocaine	Yes	No	Moderate	Apprehension, tremulousness, tachycardia, hyperventilation, mydriasis; large doses produce toxic psychosis with visual, auditory, and tactile (formication) hallucinations; paranoid delusions and resistant behavior may occur	Should be immediately withdrawn; depression and delusions may persist for weeks

should be looked upon as a symptom of these disorders; it is noteworthy that psychotics are rarely attracted to opiates.

Therapeutic introduction to opiate addiction in the United States occurs in less than 5% of cases; most begin opiates experimentally though association with addicts (although those who handle the drug—medics and nurses—may also be tempted). Regular administration of opiates produces tolerance, leading to steadily increasing dosage, with withdrawal symptoms if the drug is stopped. The drug is taken for its effect of "false euphoria" which includes a sexual-like pleasure experienced over the whole body, not accompanied by any diminution of intellectual functions or disturbance of behavior. Side effects of nausea, itching, miosis, anorexia, and constipation are borne willingly, and the addict's life becomes one of nonproductivity, socioeconomic and family problems, apathy, lowered sex drive, and frequently criminal activities to support a costly habit.

Examination. Because of legal restrictions, the problem of obtaining opiates is a difficult one for the addict, who may become adept at feigning acute medical conditions, such as coronary occlusion, kidney stone, or acute abdomen, to receive morphine. Because of this unreliability, close examination is important. Scars from unsterile hypo abscesses may have a black tinge from sterilization of the needle by matches. Objective signs of the *morphine abstinence syndrome* include yawning ("the yaps"), lacrimation, rhinorrhea, and perspiration; these appear in 10 to 15 hours, followed by gooseflesh, mydriasis, and tremors. In more severe cases there are insomnia, restlessness, hyperpnea, and a rise in systolic blood pressure followed by the appearance of vomiting, diarrhea, and weight loss (as much as 5 pounds per day).

Prognosis. With an adequate rehabilitation and follow-up program, about 20% of addicts remain abstinent; many others obtain a worthwhile remission lasting several years.

Treatment. The treatment of addiction to drugs is far from satisfactory. Traditional commitment of narcotics users to federal prison hospitals resulted in an increasingly high rate of relapse. In fact, a lasting cure was the rare exception with many addicts using such periods of hospitalization merely to reduce the cost of their habit by a decrease in the level of drug tolerance. More recently treatment of the drug abuser and addict in his home community has given greater promise of success. *Medical-psychiatric* hospital-based programs admit heroin and other addicts on a voluntary basis for detoxification, attention to medical problems, and psychiatric treatment. Other programs use group pressure, interpersonal confrontation, and a therapeutic community to help drug abusers change their behavior. *Addicts Anonymous* is a voluntary program modeled after Alcoholics Anonymous, providing group meetings and interpersonal support. *Periodic testing* with nalorphine (Nalline) injections, plus thin-layer chromatography and other methods of urine examination, may be used to test for evidence of readdiction. *Substitute programs* in which methadone (cyclazocine or dolophine-*dl*-4, 4-diphenylamino-3-heptanol) is substituted for heroin are now widely used but still on an experimental basis. In the methadone treatment programs, 1 mg. of methadone has an abstinence-suppressing potency of 3 to 4 mg. of morphine or 1 mg. of heroin. Ordinarily 10 to 20 mg. of methadone orally twice daily is sufficient. When the patient is psychologically ready for participation in the total rehabilitation program, methadone may be gradually withdrawn.

BARBITURATES. The conservative employment of barbiturates as a temporary relief from tensional symptoms is a blessing to many so afflicted, but persons suffering from insomnia, tension headaches, anxiety attacks, or other manifestations of anxiety may gradually become *physiologically dependent upon* these drugs. Since the introduction of the benzodiazepines barbiturates are less widely used. *Tolerance* to the barbiturates may develop, but it is less noticeable than with opiates.

Examination. Regular ingestion of large doses leads to *intoxication*, marked by signs of cortical and cerebral dysfunction, such as increased emotional lability, impairment of intellect, disorientation, dysarthria, ataxia, and nystagmus. Abrupt withdrawal of barbiturate or a marked reduction of dosage in a chronically intoxicated individual leads to an *abstinence syndrome.* More threatening to life than the opiate abstinence syndrome, this condition is characterized by weakness, tremors, feelings of intense panic, increase in pulse, respiration, temperature, and blood pressure accompanied by nausea, vomiting, and rapid weight loss. After about 30 hours grand mal convulsions may appear. This phase may be followed in 3 to 7 days by delirium similar to delirium tremens with agitation, confusion, and hallucinations. The total syndrome may last 2 to 3 weeks, and recovery can occur with no permanent changes.

Treatment. Gradual withdrawal of the addicting barbiturates is indicated, with the substitution of short-acting pentobarbital in place of the longer-acting barbiturate to which the patient has become addicted. Once the patient's tolerance level has been determined, the pentobarbital can be withdrawn at the rate of about 10% of total dosage per day.

Prescribe Dilantin, 0.1 Gm. t.i.d., for 2 weeks.

Provide vigilant therapeutic attention to nutrition, fluid balance and prevention of infection. After 2 to 4 weeks a well-rounded psychological, social, and occupational rehabilitation program is indicated and preferably is commenced within a closed ward where the patient's activities can be supervised.

OTHER HYPNOTICS, SEDATIVES, OR TRANQUILIZERS. Addiction to a variety of chemical agents comes about through a complex interaction of physiological, pharmacological, socioenvironmental, and personality factors. This dependence may be in the form of addiction (physiological and psychological dependence) or habit formation (mostly psychological dependence). Agents involved include meprobamate (Miltown and Equanil), chlordiazepoxide (Librium), paraldehyde, chloral hydrate, ethchlorvynol (Placidyl), glutethimide (Doriden), methyprylon (Noludar), methaqualone (Quaalude, Sopor), diazepam (Valium), or destropropoxyphene (Darvon).

COCAINE. This drug produces habituation. Continued stimulation leads not only to euphoric excitement and pleasant hallucinations but also to dangerous paranoid delusions, digestive disorders, emaciation, and even convulsions. Perforation of the nasal septum can occur from snuffing cocaine powder ("snow").

CANNABIS SATIVA (HASHISH, MARIJUANA). This drug is also known as pot, hemp, charge, gear, kef, Mary Jane, stuff, tea, weed, and grass. It is widely taken by teen-agers and others in search of an escape from reality. The World Health Organization—Expert Committee on Addiction-Producing Drugs has pointed out that physical dependence on this drug does not occur. Temporary psychoses have been reported. The major danger seems to be that the use of this drug frequently leads to use of other addicting and more dangerous agents.

OTHER PSYCHOSTIMULANTS. The excessive intake of amphetamines for their exhilarating effects has become a major problem. Such drugs may be inhaled or taken orally ("pep pills," "goofballs") or by injection ("mainlining").

HALLUCINOGENS. A variety of psychedelic drugs, including lysergic acid diethylamide (LSD), mescaline, stramonium, nutmeg, and banana peels, have been used to produce hallucinatory and psychotic-like states. Similar "jags," consisting of euphoria and excitement, have been produced by the sniffing of glue, gasoline vapors, lacquers, paint thinners, ether, catnip, and lighter fluid.

Treatment. The treatment of these conditions involves not only hospitalization with immediate removal of the offending agent but also a thorough exploration of the personality problems leading to the use of such agents, with therapy aimed at the underlying characterological and environmental problems.

SUGGESTED READINGS

Ackerly, W. C., and Gibson, G.: Lighter fluid "sniffing," Am. J. Psychiatry **120:**1056, 1964.

Cohen, S.: Amphetamine abuse, J.A.M.A. **231:**414, 1975.

Cohen, S., and Ditman, K. S.: Prolonged adverse reactions to lysergic acid diethylamide, Arch. Gen. Psychiatry **8:**475, 1963.

Cohen, S.: Suicide following morning-glory seed ingestion, Am. J. Psychiatry **120:**1025, 1964.

Cole, J. O., and Wittenborn, J. R.: Drug abuse: social and psychopharmacological aspects, Springfield, Ill., 1969, Charles C Thomas, Publisher.

Connell, P. H.: Amphetamine psychosis, London, 1958, Chapman & Hall, Ltd.

Essig, C. H.: Addiction to non-barbiturate sedative and tranquilizing drugs, Clin. Pharmacol. Ther. **5:**334, 1964.

Ewing, J. A., and Grant, W. J.: The bromide hazard, Southern Med. J. **58:**148, 1965.

Farnsworth, D. L.: Hallucinogenic agents, J.A.M.A. **185:**878, 1963.

Freedman, A. M.: Treatment of drug addiction in a community general hospital, Comp. Psychiatry **4:**199, 1963.

Hendin, H.: College students and LSD: who and why?, J. Nerv. Ment. Dis. **156:**249, 1973.

Isbell, H.: Addiction to barbiturates and the barbiturate abstinence syndrome, Ann. Intern. Med. **33:**108, 1950.

Jackson, B., and Reed, A.: Catnip and the alteration of consciousness, J.A.M.A. **207:**1349, 1969.

Jaffe, J. H., Zaks, M. S., and Washington, E. N.: Experience with the use of methadone in a multimodality program for the treatment of narcotics users, Int. J. Addict. **4:**481, 1969.

Massengale, O. N., and others: Physical and psychologic factors in glue sniffing, N. Engl. J. Med. **269:**130, 1963.

Maurer, D. W., and Vogel, V. H.: Narcotics and narcotic addiction, ed. 3, Springfield, Ill., 1967, Charles C Thomas, Publisher.

McGlothlin, W. H., and West, L. J.: The marihuana problem, an overview, Am. J. Psychiatry **125:**126, 1968.

Post, R. M.: Cocaine psychosis: a continuum model, Am. J. Psychiatry **132:**225, 1975.

Rockwell, D. A., and Ostwald, P.: Amphetamine use and abuse in psychiatric patients, Arch. Gen. Psychiatry **18:**612, 1968.

Schultes, R. E.: Hallucinogens of plant origin, Science **163:**245, 1969.

Thacore, V. R., and Shulda, S. R. P.: *Cannabis* psychosis and paranoid schizophrenia, Arch. Gen. Psychiatry **33:**383, 1976.

Stimmel, B., editor: Heroin dependence: medical, economic and social aspects, New York, 1975, Stratton Intercontinental Medical Book Corp.

Ungerleider, J. F., and others: "The bad trip"—the etiology of the adverse LSD reaction, Am. J. Psychiatry **124:**1483, 1968.

Wikler, A.: Opioid addiction. In Friedman, A., and Kaplan, H., editors: Comprehensive textbook of psychiatry, Baltimore, 1967, The Williams & Wilkins Co.

Wikler, A.: Diagnosis and treatment of drug dependence of the barbiturate type, Am. J. Psychiatry **125:**758, 1968.

16

Miscellaneous—psychiatric conditions not in standard nomenclature

Munchausen's syndrome (chronic factitious illness). This term is used for patients who consciously distort their medical history, produce misleading physical findings and laboratory results through self-inflicted lesions, and wander from one hospital and one city to another seeking medical care. Sometimes the motive is simply the desire for free board or haven from the police, some patients are drug addicts using the method to satisfy their craving, and in others psychological motives include a grudge against physicians or desire to be the center of attention.

Ganser's syndrome (prison psychosis). This rare illness, most frequently observed in prisoners, has been referred to as "hysterical pseudostupidity." Characteristically, these patients give utterly incorrect and often ridiculous replies to questions, although there is usually no doubt that they are alert and not confused in the usual sense; they behave, other than verbally, as persons oriented to their environment. It has been described as a dissociative state, intermediate between psychosis and psychoneurosis, and between malingering and disease. The patient usually recovers within a few days or weeks.

Gilles de la Tourette's disease (tic convulsif). Symptoms begin in childhood with an increasing display of motor tics, from spasmodic grimacing to violent movements of the body; pathognomonic is the compulsive coprolalia in which the patients are compelled to utter obscenities, accompanied by compulsive coughing, spitting, blowing, and barking sounds. Physical examinations, including neurological tests and EEG, are usually negative and strong elements of self-punishment may be present. Although previously reported to have a poor outcome, recent therapy with Haloperidol has given promising results.

Folie à deux (double insanity). This term, coined by Lasèque and Falret in 1873, refers to the transfer of delusions from one partner to another by association. When the active partner imposes his delusions on the passive one, the term "folie imposée" is used. When the passive partner resists the influence of suggestions but later develops a full-fledged psychosis, including delusions and hallucinations and perhaps eventually showing a psychotic picture totally different from that of the dominant partner, the term used is "folie communiquée. "Folie simultanée" develops when transmission and suggestibility are negligible and the delusions occur simultaneously. The terms "folie à trois," "folie à quatre," and "folie à cinq" have also been reported. Care should be taken in diagnosis to determine whether there is a genetic factor involved, for the term should be used only in cases where the partners are not consanguineous, there is no history of schizophrenia on either side, and there is a definite alleviation of symptoms in at least one partner in a longitudinal study.

Capgras syndrome. The Capgras syndrome is a rare condition characterized by the delusional conviction that certain persons in the environment are not their real selves but instead are doubles, impersonating and behaving like persons known to the patient.

Malingering. Simulation of disability or illness is sometimes used consciously with the motive of some secondary gain (e.g., by soldiers and prisoners). Some authors state that normal individuals do not malinger and that the condition is either a forerunner of some more serious mental illness or else a symptom of some disorder of personality. Differential diagnosis includes consideration of various neurotic conditions in which secondary gain is often a feature but on a level beyond the conscious control of the patient. Proof of malingering may require a bit of detective work.

· · ·

Culture-specific syndromes. Amok. In sudden unprovoked outbursts of rage occurring in natives of the Malay peninsula the afflicted person, usually armed with a knife, attacks, maims, or kills indiscriminately all who come within his path. Although originally considered a reaction due to frustration and humiliation, in recent reports this behavior has been associated with toxic conditions and delusional psychoses.

Koro. An acute anxiety attack among men of the Malay Archipelago and southern China, characterized by fear that the penis is shrinking and that it will disappear into the abdomen, resulting in death.

Latah. A disorder generally seen among Malaysians in which a sudden stimulus provokes an involuntary reaction in one of two forms: a startle reaction with unusual and inappropriate motor and verbal manifestations, such as coprolalia; or an echo reaction with the imitation of another's words (echolalia) or actions (echopraxia).

Piblokto. Attacks in Eskimo women with screaming, crying, running naked through the snow, sometimes with suicidal or homicidal components.

Susto. Panic reactions in Latin Americans, with fear of the evil eye, black magic, and possession by spirits.

Windigo (Wihtiko). A psychosis with agitated depression and a craving for human flesh because of possession by a cannabalistic monster (Windigo, Wihtiko), which is a supernatural being feared by primitive Indian tribes (Ojibwa, Chippewa, Cree).

SUGGESTED READINGS

Bankier, R. G.: Capgras syndrome: the illusion of doubles, Can. Psychiat. Assoc. J. **11**:10, 1966.

Bruun, R. D., and others: A follow-up of 78 patients with Gilles de la Tourette's syndrome, Am. J. Psychiatry **133**:944, 1976.

Bursten, B.: On Munchausen's syndrome, Arch. Gen. Psychiatry **18**:261, 1965.

Caine, E. D., Margolis, D. I., and Brown, G. L.: Gilles de la Tourette's syndrome, tardive dyskinesia, and psychosis in an adolescent, Am. J. Psychiatry **135**:241, 1978.

Challas, G., Chapel, J. L., and Jenkins, R. L.: Tourette's disease: control of symptoms and its clinical course, Int. J. Neuropsychiatry 3(Suppl. 1):95, 1967.

Christodoulou, R. N.: Syndrome of subjective doubles, Am. J. Psychiatry **135**:249, 1978.

Cramer, B., Gershberg, M. R., and Stern, M.: Munchausen syndrome; its relationship to malingering, hysteria, and the physician-patient relationship, Arch. Gen. Psychiatry **24:**573, 1971.

Davidson, G. M.: The syndrome of Capgras, Psychiatr. Q. **19:**513, 1945.

Dow, T. W., and Silver, D.: A drug-induced Koro syndrome, J. Florida Med. Assoc. **60:**32, 1973.

Enoch, M. D., Trethowan, W. H., and Barker, J. C.: Some uncommon psychiatric syndromes, Bristol, 1967, John Wright & Sons.

Goldfarb, A. I., and Weiner, M. B.: The Capgras syndrome as an adaptional maneuver in old age, Am. J. Psychiatry **134:**1434, 1977.

Goldin, S., and MacDonald, J. E.: The Ganser state, J. Ment. Sci. **101:**267, 1955.

Kamal, A.: Folie a cinq, Br. J. Psychiatry **111:**583, 1965.

Klempe, K.: False recognition on the pattern of the "Capgras syndrome" and related phenomena, Psychiat. Clin. **6:**17, 1973.

Kallman, F. J., and Mickey, J. S.: Genetic concepts and folie a deux: a re-examination of "induced insanity" in family units, J. Hered. **37:**298, 1946.

Lennox, W.: Amnesia, real or feigned, Am. J. Psychiatry **99:**732, 1943.

Lucas, A. R., and Rodin, E. A.: Electroencephalogram in Gilles de la Tourette's disease, Dis. Nerv. Syst. **43:**85, 1973.

Spiro, H. R.: Chronic factitious illness: Munchausen's Syndrome, Arch. Gen. Psychiatry **18:**569, 1968.

Stern, K., and MacNaughton, D.: Capgras syndrome: a peculiar illusionary phenomenon considered with special reference to the Rorshach findings, Psychiatr. Q. **19:**139, 1945.

Todd, J.: The syndrome of Capgras, Psychiatr. Q. **31:**250, 1957.

Tsoi, W. F.: The Ganser syndrome in Singapore: a report on ten cases, Br. J. Psychiatry **122:**604, 1973.

Whitlock, F. A.: The Ganser syndrome, Br. J. Psychiatry **113:**19, 1967.

Yap, P. M.: Mental disease peculiar to certain cultures, a survey of comparative psychiatry, J. Ment. Sci. **97:**313, 1951.

17

Psychophysiological disorders

Psychophysiological (psychosomatic) disorders include those in which psychological factors are of importance in the initiation, exacerbation, or perpetuation of the disorder. Actually the term encroaches upon every branch of medicine because it is now well recognized that psychosocial factors such as prevailing environmental stresses, family and job tension, habitual modes of coping, patient's interpretation of his symptoms, experiential factors, etc., are important in the development, modification, and chronicity of any organic illness. While dealing with such factors may not "cure" the disease, they are often of such importance that the wise physician will seriously consider them in developing the plan of treatment.

While the interaction of mind and body was known to Hippocrates, psychosomatic theories are still in a state of flux but with increasing elucidation from current research. Early research followed classic psychoanalytical lines and focused on Franz Alexander's "holy seven" (bronchial asthma, rheumatoid arthritis, ulcerative colitis, essential hypertension, neurodermatitis, thyrotoxicosis, and duodenal peptic ulcers), with the implication that one could differentiate between these specific diseases on the basis of specific psychological patterns associated with each item. Draper, Alvarez, and Dunbar also noted relationships among certain emotions, personality types, and certain diseases. Such early hypotheses have not, however, been well supported by research of the last two decades, which has indicated that, apart from the Type A behavior and the development of coronary heart disease, a wide range of personality types and conflicts can be seen in most "psychosomatic" illnesses. Mahl and Brady are identified with the "nonspecific" hypothesis, in which it is proposed that a multitude of stresses, rather than a specific psychological stress, is important in the genesis of psychosomatic illness and that heredity, constitution, and conditioning are crucial in determining which organ becomes the site of disease.

The latter concept is in keeping with the original hypothesis of Cannon, who thought that bodily changes were caused by stress and that involvement of the thalamus, autonomic nervous system, and adrenals prepared the animal for "fight or flight." Hans Selye further classified the body's organized reaction to stress, which he labeled "general adaptation system," built upon the pituitary adrenocortical axis with ACTH in the role of mediator.

Other workers (Malmo, Lacey) have postulated an individual response specificity hypothesis in which individuals are classed as "cardiac reactors," "gastric reactors," etc., invoking genetic, prior conditioning and exposure to illness and stress, operant conditioning, individual coping strategies, attitudes, and personality to explain enduring psychological and physiological response characteristics and individual susceptibility to disease.

Following Schilder, Bruch, Taylor, and others have suggested that a person's perception of his own body image may help predict the type of illness or symptom he will develop in response to stress. Holmes and Rahe suggested that the stress of adjusting to change is an important predisposing factor and predictor of illness. They have listed commonly experienced life changes in a scale (Table 6), measured in "life change units" (LCU). An accumulation of over 200 such LCU in a year has, in their research, been found to be associated with a high incidence of reported illness.

While clinicians have theorized from patient material, basic researchers have increasingly clarified the neurophysiological and endocrine links between the CNS and other bodily systems that explain the mechanism of psychophysiological disorders.

The neurobiological basis of bodily and emotional dysfunction has been described on the basis of a reciprocal balance (homeostasis) between ergotrophic and trophotropic systems with CNS, ANS, and neuro-endocrine components. A developing body of data seems to indicate that norepinephrine and dopamine are neurotransmitters for the ergotrophic system, with 5-hydroxytryp-

Table 6. Social readjustment rating scale*

Rank	Life event	Mean value
1	Death of spouse	100
2	Divorce	73
3	Marital separation	65
4	Jail term	63
5	Death of close family member	63
6	Personal injury or illness	53
7	Marriage	50
8	Fired at work	47
9	Marital reconciliation	45
10	Retirement	45
11	Change in health of family member	44
12	Pregnancy	40
13	Sex difficulties	39
14	Gain of new family member	39
15	Business readjustment	39
16	Change in financial state	38
17	Death of close friend	37
18	Change to different line of work	36
19	Change in number of arguments with spouse	35
20	Mortgage over $10,000	31
21	Foreclosure of mortgage or loan	30
22	Change in responsibilities at work	29

*From Holmes, T. H., and Rahe, R. H.: J. Psychosom. Res. **11:**216, 1967.

tamine and acetylcholine playing the role for the trophotropic system. The anatomical substrate for these reactions includes primarily the reticular formation, hypothalamus and limbic system.

Selye's work highlighted the importance of homeostatic endocrine mechanisms in our adaptation to the environment. Viewed phylogenetically, endocrine mechanisms would appear to be an evolutionary development from the simplest forms of chemical signaling of one cell to another that allowed the survival of primitive multicellular organisms prior to development of the nervous system.

Even the nervous system with cells specialized for rapid conduction depends upon such chemical transmitters at the synaptic junctions between cells. An understanding of psychophysiological disorders depends upon rapidly conducting systems for emotion-

Table 6. Social readjustment rating scale—cont'd

Rank	Life event	Mean value
23	Son or daughter leaving home	29
24	Trouble with in-laws	29
25	Outstanding personal achievement	28
26	Wife begin or stop work	26
27	Begin or end school	26
28	Change in living conditions	25
29	Revision of personal habits	24
30	Trouble with boss	23
31	Change in work hours or conditions	20
32	Change in residence	20
33	Change in schools	20
34	Change in recreation	19
35	Change in church activities	19
36	Change in social activities	18
37	Mortgage or loan less than $10,000	17
38	Change in sleeping habits	16
39	Change in number of family get-togethers	15
40	Change in eating habits	15
41	Vacation	13
42	Christmas	12
43	Minor violations of the law	11

ally engendered signals of thalamus and cortex, autonomic responses from hypothalamus and reticular areas, and the hormonal neuroendocrine mediating systems. Of importance to the latter is the recently clarified concept of releasing hormones—polypeptide messengers synthesized by the hypothalamic neurocirculatory cells and carried by the pituitary portal system to the anterior pituitary, which in turn releases various trophic hormones (growth, ACTH, LD, FSH, TSH). These act upon the endocrine glands, which in turn through hormonal release (cortisol, androgens, estrogens, thyroxin, epinephrine, norepinephrine, vasopressin, oxytocin, aldosterone) affect the target tissues.

Thus the response of the individual to stressful stimuli involves a complex physiological (neuroendocrine) mechanism of defense for adapting the individual to his environment. When this process malfunctions, overreacts, or otherwise escapes the control of normal homeostasis, disease occurs.

The picture is of course not quite so simply explained, because each subsystem has its own feedback or control mechanism. The hypothalamus thus senses the need for more or less releasing substance by the products of end organ activity releasing into the circulation that reaches the brain. In addition, an exciting new chapter is being written as these new peptide releasor substances have, in addition, a direct influence upon CNS metabolism.

Successful diagnosis and therapy of psychophysiological disorders demand cooperation among internist, surgeon, and psychiatrist; teamwork among nurses, social workers, occupational therapists, and physiotherapists is frequently important. Initial understanding of symptoms may be attained by a careful history which seeks temporal correlations between the appearance of symptoms and life crises, or symbols of such crises.

The physician does well to bear in mind that many patients have initial difficulty in comprehending that emotional and social forces do contribute to their illness—for this reason, thorough physical and laboratory work-up is best completed early; findings and their interpretation should be presented frankly; and adequate time should be spent with the patient to help him understand his illness sufficiently to cooperate in treatment. In the care of patients with psychosomatic illness the role of the psychiatrist is often adjunctive. The diagnosis is not "either-or"; but rather, psychological factors should have a demonstrated presence as well as those physical findings of the disturbed organ or body system.

When patients doubt the role of important causative factors, it is often helpful to gain intimate grasp of the patient's own private formulation to explain his sysmptoms. Then, as the patient begins to feel that the physician is really interested in *his* point of view, he will more freely divulge those hidden feelings and attitudes which provide valuable diagnostic and psychotherapeutic clues.

Reference to expressions of "organ language," long recognized in our daily speech through such terms as "pain in the neck," "he gripes me," "I can't stomach that," or "my heart was broken," may serve as an introduction to a discussion of psychophysiological mechanisms with the patient.

A flexible, supportive type of psychotherapy is useful in these disorders. The frequency, length, and number of interviews can be varied to suit the circumstances. When symptoms are severe, several brief interviews may be held in a single day. Under other conditions widely spread contacts held at the time of return visits for medical treatment may suffice. Interviews held in a private room, although desirable, may be replaced by bedside chats in the case of hospitalized ward patients.

In addition to psychotherapy, the management of the psychosomatic patient may also include the use of psychotropic medication and a variety of behavior—modifying and anxiety—lessening techniques. Medications specific for depression and anxiety may be very helpful, especially initially, but should be viewed as a crutch from which the patient is gradually weaned. A wide variety of relaxation techniques, autogenic training, meditation, hypnosis, biofeedback, and acupuncture has been used with varying success in managing the disturbances in these disorders.

SUGGESTED READINGS

Alexander, F.: Psychomatic medicine, New York, 1950, W. W. Norton Co., Inc.

Cannon, W. B.: Bodily changes in pain, hunger, fear and rage, ed. 2, New York, 1929, Appleton-Century-Crofts.

Dunbar, F.: Emotions and bodily changes, New York, 1954, Columbia University Press.

Gersten, J. C., and others: An evaluation of the etiologic role of stressful life-change events in psychological disorders, J. Health Soc. Behav. **18**:228, 1977.

Holmes, T. H. and Rahe, R. H.: The social readjustment rating scale, J. Psychosom. Res. **11**:212, 1967.

Kampmeier, R. H.: Diagnosis and treatment of physical diseases in the mentally ill, Ann. Intern. Med. **86**:637, 1977.

Lacey, J. I., and Lacey, B. C.: The law of initial value in the longitudinal study of autonomic constitution: reproducibility of autonomic responses and response patterns over a four-year interval, Ann. N.Y. Acad. Sci. **98**:1257, 1962.

Lipowski, Z. J. Psychosomatic medicine in the seventies: an overview, Am. J. Psychiatry **134**:233, 1977.

Lipowski, Z. J., Lipsitt, D. R., and Whybrow, P. C.: Psychosomatic medicine, current trends and clinical applications, New York, 1977, Oxford University Press.

Malmo, R. B.: Activation. In Bachrach, A. J., editor: Experimental foundations of clinical psychology, New York, 1962, Basic Books, Inc.

Rahe, H., McKean, J. D., Jr., and Arthur, R. J.: A longitudinal study of life changes and illness patterns, J. Psychosom. Res. **10**:355, 1967.

Selye, H.: Stress without distress, Philadelphia, 1974, Lippincott Press.

Wittkower, E. D., and Warnes, H.: Psychosomatic medicine: its clinical applications, New York, 1977, Harper & Row, Publishers.

Skin disorders

Embryologically the skin and central nervous system arise from ectoderm, and, like the nervous system, the skin serves as a means of communications between a person's inner and outer worlds (for example, blushing with shame or embarrassment and blanching with fear). Some authors have correlated urticaria with suppressed weeping, pruritus with inhibited or vicariously gratified sexual excitement, and neurodermatitis with obsessive-compulsive traits. There is, however, no general agreement that a specific personality profile or unconscious conflict can be identified with any skin disease; rather it appears that a variety of psychosocial stresses antedate the flareup of skin diseases. Hereditary factors, allergy conditioning endocrine imbalance, disturbance in autonomic regulation of skin physiology, and—at the cortical level—conversion mechanisms may all play a part in producing these disorders.

It is well to evaluate each new case with an unprejudiced, observant eye. In patients with *dermatitis factitia, pruritus, neurodermatitis,* and *trichotillomania* psychic factors predominate. For example, history of pleasure in physical exhibitionism has been reported in cases of neurodermatitis, and urticaria in inhibited sexual excitement or disturbed sexual functioning. In such conditions as *hyperhidrosis, urticaria, rosacea, psoriasis, herpes, warts, lichen planus,* and *alopecia* psychic factors may or may not be significant.

SUGGESTED READINGS

Ely, N. F., Veehey, J. W., and Holmes, T. H.: Experimental studies of skin inflammation, Psychosom. Med. **25**:264, 1963.

Goldberg, E. L., and Comstock, G. W.: Life events and subsequent illness, Am. J. Epidemiol. **104**:146, 1976.

Macalpine, I.: Pruritus ani, Psychosom. Med. **15**:499, 1953.

Muspah, H.: Itching and scratching; psychodynamics in dermatology, Basel, 1964, S. Karger.

Schoenberg, B., and Carr, A. C.: An investigation of criteria for brief psychotherapy of neurodermatitis, Psychosom. Med. **25**:253, 1963.

Taylor, B. W., Litin, E. M., and Litzow, T. J.: Psychiatric considerations in cosmetic surgery, Mayo Clin. Proc. **41**:608, 1966.

Wittkower, E. D., and Edgell, P. G.: Eczema: a psychosomatic study, Arch, Derm. Syph. **63**:207, 1951.

Musculoskeletal disorders

That anxiety and fear are often accompanied by increase in muscle tone is commonly recognized. Chronically increased muscle tone becomes especially important as an aggravating factor in various forms of arthritis, backache, tension headache, and any other condition in which muscle irritation or spasm may play a role.

Tension headache is usually described as a dull constant pain or "pressure feeling" beginning gradually and lasting from a few minutes to days, weeks, or even years. The headache may be occipital, frontal, or over the top of the head and it is often associated with noticeable muscular tension. This type of headache may be relieved by treating the underlying emotional disorder, although temporary relief usually is attained by combination doses of sedatives and mild analgesics.

Attempting to elucidate the common observation that exacerbations of *rheumatoid arthritis* follow emotional stress, a number of psychoanalytical studies have discovered a history of development as a child under excessively restricting parental attitudes. While immunological abnormalities apparently play a role in rheumatoid arthritis it should not be forgotten that stress acting through the hypothalamus can also affect immune mechanisms.

Back pain is a common psychophysiological affliction. Interscapular tension can produce upper back pain in anxious persons. Low back syndrome following trauma often persists in the absence of physical signs when factors of litigation or secondary gain are present.

Occupational cramp may occur in an obsessionally perfectionistic individual faced with conflicting and frustrating circumstances.

EMG, biofeedback, and Jacobsen's "progressive relaxation" routine may be helpful in these conditions. Temporary relief from muscle relaxants should be followed by physical therapy and muscle retraining. An important mode of discharging tension and relieving frustration is muscle activity (e.g., hard work, sports, gardening).

SUGGESTED READINGS

Brenner, C., Friedman, A. P., and Carter, S.: Psychologic factors in the etiology and treatment of chronic headache, Psychosom. Med. **11**:53, 1949.

Cleveland, S. E., and Fisher, S.: Behavior and unconscious fantasies of patients with rheumatoid arthritis, Psychosom. Med. **16**:327, 1954.

Gottschalk, L. A., Serota, H. M., and Shapiro, L. B.: Psychological conflict and neuromuscular tension; I, Preliminary report and method as applied to rheumatoid arthritis, Proc. Ass. Res. Nerv. Ment. Dis. **29**:735, 1950.

Holmes, T. H., and Wolff, H. G.: Life situations, emotions and backache, Psychosom. Med. **14**:18, 1952.

Moos, R. H.: Personality factors associated with rheumatoid arthritis: a review, J. Chronic Dis. **17**:41, 1964.

Scotch, N. A., and Gieger, H.: The epidemiology of rheumatoid arthritis: a review with special attention to social factors, J. Chronic Dis, **15**:1037, 1962.

Sternbach, R. A., Wolf, S. R., Murphy, R. W., and Akeson, W. H.: Aspects of chronic low back pain, Psychosomatics **14**:52, 1973.

Respiratory disorders

HYPERVENTILATION SYNDROME. Hyperventilation (panting) is a basic physiological accompaniment of excitement. Such forced respiration, even when unnoticed by the patient, can produce biochemical changes in the blood, resulting in reflex alterations of cerebral circulation; reduction of consciousness or syncope may follow. Clinically this phenomenon is used as a test to induce slowing and abnormal discharge in the EEG. Prolonged hyperventilation can result in shifts in CO_2 and $H+$ ion concentration, alkalosis, tingling and coldness of the extremities, tachycardia, palpitation, carpopedal spasm, and tetany.

Tense, anxious, or depressed patients may hyperventilate without realizing it when placed in difficult situations; frequently they report some or all of the signs noted above without mentioning overbreathing. Voluntary hyperventilation can be used to demonstrate to patients the origin of their symptoms.

BRONCHIAL ASTHMA. This is a lifelong, often life-threatening disorder, in which a chronic predisposition interacts with a variety of life circumstances to produce a variable and fluctuating pattern of illness. Although its cause is not clear there is often a genetic predisposition as well as immunological sensitization to specific antigens. Recent biological evidence suggests that there are mechanisms whereby emotional conflicts can influence the pulmonary processes involved in asthma. Psychological factors can influence pulmonary function in asthma either adversely or beneficially. As with most psychophysiological reactions, it is important to define the relationship of the psychic to the allergic, infectious, and endocrine factors specifically in each case.

VASOMOTOR RHINITIS (HAY FEVER). Since the nasal mucus membrane is continuous with that of the bronchi, significant functional changes can occur with any type of respiratory disorder. Altered morphology can occur during stressful interviews; like changes also can be produced by pollen in allergic individuals, and sufficient pollen can produce this reaction in any subject. Experiments have shown that during exposure to emotional conflict, relatively low concentrations of pollen for short periods of time can lead to rhinitis.

SUGGESTED READINGS

Doust, J. W. L., and Leigh, D.: Studies on the physiology of awareness. The interrelationships of emotions, life situations, and anoxemia in patients with bronchial asthma. Psychosom. Med. **15:**292, 1953.

Groen, J. J., and Pelser, H. E.: Experience with and results of group psychotherapy in patients with bronchial asthma, J. Psychosom. Res. **4:**191, 1960.

Guze, S. B., Gabbard, J., Roos, A., and Saslow, G.: Chronic psychogenic hyperventilation, Arch. Neurol. Psychiatry **67:**434, 1952.

Knapp, P. H., and Nemitz, I. S.: Personality variations in asthma, Psychosom. Med. **19:**443, 1957.

Knapp, P. H., Mathe, A. A., and Vachon, L.: Psychosomatic aspects of broncial asthma. In Weiss, E. B., and Segal, M. S., editors: Bronchial asthma, its nature and management, Boston, 1976, Little, Brown & Co.

Rubenstein, H. S.: Behaviour in a medical clinic of patients with well-controlled bronchial asthma, Lancet **I:**1011, 1976.

Schiavi, R. C., Stein, M., and Sethi, B. B.: Respiratory variables in response to a pain-fear stimulus and in experimental asthma, Psychosom. Med. **23:**485, 1961.

Cardiovascular disorders

VASOMOTOR INSTABILITY AND DISTURBANCES OF HEART ACTION. Cardiovascular changes accompany most emotional reactions as concomitants of the neuroendocrine response to stress. The quickening of the pulse in response to passion or to fear is a common observation. Existing cardiac arrhythmias such as occur in Wolf-Parkinson-White syndrome can be aggravated by stress. Many psychiatric disorders manifest one or more symptoms or cardiovascular instability (e.g., spontaneous vasodepressor syncope, paroxysmal auricular tachycardia). Although few psychological generalizations can be made about these ubiquitous symptoms, such individuals tend to give a history of childhood neurotic traits and as adults often experience severe anxiety attacks and nightmares. The patient's equating of cardiac sensations with danger of imminent death may lead to a vicious circle (anxiety–vasomotor disturbance–cardiac sensation–anxiety), which can threaten medical management of true heart lesions. The cardiovascular system may also be indirectly influenced by stress through changes in electrolytes, clotting mechanisms, and fat levels. Psychological stress is mediated through an imbalance between the sympathetic and parasympathetic tone of the heart and has been demonstrated to produce EKG changes, tachycardia, as well as increased levels of triglycerides, free fatty acids, and plasma noradrenalin.

ESSENTIAL HYPERTENSION. Essential hypertension is characterized by a sustained rise in systemic blood pressure above 140 mm. Hg systolic and 90 mm. Hg diastolic. It is the end result of a still incompletely defined group of physiological and psychological dysfunctions. Heredity predisposes to hypertension, but environmental, neurogenic, humoral, and vascular factors also interact and influence blood pressure to various extents. Most patients with primary hypertension show heightened vascular and cardiac responses to sympathetic stimulation. There is no evidence that excessive sodium intake, emotional stress, or obesity *causes* hypertension, although each of these factors may aggravate it or hasten its appearance in predisposed individuals.

Psychiatric investigation of hypertension has revealed difficulty in handling hostile feelings, subnormal assertiveness, and obsessive-compulsive traits. Hypertension may be considered a state of chronically inhibited rage (similar to Cannon's rage reactions in animals) arising from conflict between passive dependent longings and competitive feelings.

Antihypertensive medication remains the mainstay of treatment, although psychotherapy designed to promote better self-understanding and solution of conflicts and to encourage normal assertiveness may be helpful. Clinical studies report that biofeedback, meditation and other relaxation techniques can lower blood pressure; the results, however, seem temporary unless such relaxation becomes part of daily living.

ANGINA AND CORONARY OCCLUSION. It is a frequent observation that attacks of coronary insufficiency follow prolonged periods of fatigue and worry and may immediately follow a threat to vocational security. The effect of severe emotions such as loss of a spouse has been shown to increase the mortality from coronary artery disease by as much as 40%. As is well known, coronary insufficiency is a common disorder among men of high income, administrators, and physicians. Often they have a poor prognosis because of their need to deny emotional factors and their tendency to react to the illness itself as an intense frustration.

Friedman and Rosenman have described an overt behavior pattern important in the pathogenesis of coronary artery disease, particularly in younger Type A personalities, that is characterized by: (1) excessive competitive drive, (2) ambitious achievement orientation, (3) a chronic sense of urgency, (4) an inclination to multiple commitments, and (5) an immersion in deadlines.

VASODEPRESSOR SYNCOPE. Fainting occurs with a sudden drop in blood pressure. Emotional factors allow vasodilatation in muscles that are not contracting and hence blood can pool beyond a critical level. Fear or suppressed fear is an important factor, particularly in response to a real or fancied injury to the body, with the person in the erect posture. The phenomenon may be "contagious" in large groups.

OTHER CHANGES IN VASCULAR TONE. Reports of vasospasm or vasodilatation symptomatic of personality difficulty have appeared with reference to Raynaud's disease, migraine, and other conditions.

An illustration of this type of malady is *migraine*, an excruciating, pulsating, recurrent headache often presaged or accompanied by visual disturbances, vomiting, and transient sensorimotor changes. Migraine attacks lasting a few minutes to 2 or 3 days occur in 5% of the population (higher incidence in women than in men). Attacks are recurrent and there is often a positive family history. The discomfort arises from extreme dilatation of the external carotid artery branches and may localize and progress in a characteristic manner; transient neurological signs are thought to result from cerebral vasoconstriction. Personality studies of patients with migraine cover such a broad spectrum that at this time it is safe to say only that emotional stress may lead to an attack in vulnerable persons. The role of food and substance allergy seems of increasing importance.

Remedies are legion, with their effectiveness often depending upon the enthusiasm of the physician and the patient's confidence in him. Methysergide, 4 to 8 mg./day orally is effective but can cause retroperitoneal fibrosis. Acupuncture and biofeedback have been reported to be effective. Psychotherapy that aims at helping the patient to identify situations that stir resentment and to express himself more freely prevents further attacks.

Once commenced, the attack may be relieved in eight out of ten patients by parenteral administration of ergotamine tartrate. Caffeine, 0.5 mg., combined with ergotamine tartrate is available in tablet form; two tablets taken at the earliest premonition, one to four times as necessary, at half-hour intervals, may abort an attack. This medication is also available in suppository form for cases in which nausea and vomiting are severe.

SUDDEN DEATH. Emotional causes of sudden death seem to relate to the way the cardiovascular system responds to stress. The psychological setting is commonly one of hopelessness, powerlessness, and intense emotions. Collected histories usually reveal that such death occurs around losses, situations of personal danger, and occasionally some paradoxical situation of great relief, pleasure, or triumph. Surgical patients who are convinced that their death is inevitable and desirable have an increased surgical mortality rate. An increased score on the Social Readjustment Rating Scale (Table 6) has been found to correlate with an increased incidence of sudden death. The mechanism is most surely that of higher cortical influence upon cardiac function by way of the autonomic nervous system, with hypertension, arteriosclerosis, myocardial necrosis, and changes in cardiac rhythm being significant precedent conditions.

SUGGESTED READINGS

Appenzeller, O., editor: Pathogenesis and treatment of headache, New York, 1976, Spectrum Publications.

Blanchard, E. B., and Miller, S. T.: Psychological treatment of cardiovascular disease, Arch. Gen. Psychiatry 34:1402, 1977.

Blanchard, E. B., and Haynes, M. R.: Biofeedback treatment of a case of Raynaud's disease, J. Behav. Ther. Exp. Psychiatry 6:230, 1975.

Chambers, W. N., and Reiser, M. F.: Emotional stress in the precipitation of congestive heart failure, Psychosom. Med. 15:38, 1953.

Diamond S., and Dalessio, D.: The practicing physician's approach to headache, New York, 1973, Medcom Press.

Dimsdale, J.: Emotional causes of sudden death, Am. J. Psychiatry 134:12, 1977.

Fischer, H. K.: Hypertension and the psyche. In Brest, A. N., and Moyer, J. H., editors: Hypertension, Philadelphia, 1961, Lea & Febiger.

Gressel, G. C., and others: Personality factors in arterial hypertension, J.A.M.A. 140:265-271, 1949.

Jenkins, C. D.: Recent evidence supporting psychologic and social risk factors for coronary disease, N. Engl. J. Med. 294:984, 1976.

Millet, J. A. P., Lief, H., and Mittelman, B.: Raynaud's disease: psychogenic factors and psychotherapy, Psychosom. Med. 15:61, 1953.

Sacks, O.: Migraine: the evolution of a common disorder, New York, 1970, American University Press Services, Inc.

Stone, R. A., and DeLeo, J.: Psychotherapeutic control of hypertension, N. Engl. J. Med. 294:80, 1976.

Weiss, E.: Emotional factors in cardiovascular disease, Springfield, Ill., 1951, Charles C Thomas, Publisher.

Wolff, H. G.: Headache and other head pain, ed. 2, London, 1963, Oxford University Press.

Hemic and lymphatic disorders

A few studies and case reports have linked certain blood responses and blood dyscrasias with psychological stress. For example, men exposed to battle in Korea, but in whom no strictly organic explanation could be entertained, demonstrated a marked transitory fall in neutrophil count. Decrease in clotting time, rise in erythrocyte sedimentation, rise in relative blood viscosity, purpura, hemolytic crises, and changes in eosinophil and lymphocyte levels have been reported to follow emotional stress in certain cases. At the present time, however, the nature of these relationships remains speculative and controversial.

SUGGESTED READINGS

Benedict, R. B.: Psychosomatic correlations in certain blood dyscrasias. Psychosom. Med. **16**:41, 1954.

Bowne, W. J. Mally, M., and Kane, R. P.: Psychosocial aspects of hemophilia: a study of twenty-eight hemophiliac children and their families, Am. J. Orthopsychiatry **30**:730, 1960.

Miller, F. R., and Jones, H. W.: The possibility of precipitating the leukemic state by emotional factors, Blood **3**:880, 1948.

Gastrointestinal disorders

In early life, feeding activities are the all-important source of relief from physical discomfort. They provide security and emotional satisfaction. Early successes and failures of parents in meeting their infant's physical and psychological needs influence the first feelings a child develops about himself and about his own oral and anal activities. In later years as other sources of pleasure and relief from tension become available, these early patterns may persist and influence behavior in a wide variety of situations.

ANOREXIA. This symptom is common with both neurotic and psychotic disorders. Perhaps most frequently it is associated with depressive feelings.

Anorexia nervosa. Occurring particularly in fragile, immature girls, the triad of anorexia, emaciation, and amenorrhea may resemble initially an adolescent dietary fad. A developmental history of family overconcern with feeding problems and a confusion between sexual activities and feeding activities may be observed. In a few patients who find the demands of adulthood impossible to deal with, psychotic episodes, death by starvation, or suicide may take place. In cases where the patient shows little self-concern or desire for treatment, hospitalization on a closed ward, with psychotherapy, frequent small feedings, isolation from the family, and a planned daily program are required.

BULIMIA. An intense craving for food as a substitute for emotional drives is symptomatic of a wider personality disturbance; commonly, bulimia may be a defense against disappointment or depression. The syndrome of "binge" eating on a paroxysmal basis has been reported to respond to treatment with diphenylhydantoin sodium (Dilantin).

CARDIOSPASM. Constriction of the middle and lower portions of the esophagus in reaction to a situation the patient "cannot swallow" tends to be a conversion type of symptom. Diagnosis is confirmed by x-ray examination. Dilatations and surgical procedures should be a last resort since combined medicinal and psychotherapeutic efforts can usually bring complete relief.

NERVOUS VOMITING. This occurs in psychoneurotics and often during pregnancy. Where nausea and vomiting since infancy have habitually accompanied interpersonal conflict, these physiological reactions may become conditioned to a variety of life stimuli of which the patient may be only dimly aware. Symbolically, vomiting may express an unconscious desire (e.g., the wish to get rid of what is inside).

PEPTIC ULCER. Clinical experience indicates that ulceration with gastric hyperactivity, hypersecretion, engorgement of the mucosa, and hyperacidity is usually (about 80%) related to life situations. It tends to occur in a person who experiences frustration and resentment within the context of strong dependent attachments. Most psychiatric investigations have reported conflicts between passivity and aggressiveness, with reaction formation (the opposite type of behavior) a prominent defense mechanism which covers up a strong irrational need to achieve security from others. Studies by Mirsky found higher serum pepsinogen in subjects prone to ulcer formation. He found evidence of psychic conflict in these hypersecretors. Others have linked ulcer formation to excessive vagal discharge with oversecretion of HCl. Although long-term psychotherapy has been recommended, the advent of newer histamine H_2 antagonists such as cimetadine have provided the physician with an effective means to inhibit gastric acid secretions and quickly promote ulcer healing.

PROBLEMS OF ELIMINATION. Toilet training by those mothers who demand that the child "give to them" in terms of obedience, punctuality, excessive neatness, and regular production of feces may create strong functional associations between interpersonal giving-and-taking conflicts and bowel regulation. Thus feces may be viewed symbolically as something of value, a gift or a possession; in such cases constipation may express the wish to keep or retain, and diarrhea (irritable colon or mucous colitis) expresses resentful giving.

ULCERATIVE COLITIS. This physiological dysfunction apparently involves parasympathetic stimulation of the lower bowel with production of the mucolytic enzyme lysozyme, which deprives the bowel of its protective coating of mucin. In certain personalities this dysfunction may occur as a reaction to a variety of stresses, but it is reputed to occur particularly in situations which demand independent accomplishment or arouse fear of not being capable of doing something. There is little agreement among psychiatrists as to personality type, although ulcerative colitis as a suicide equivalent or as part of a grief reaction has been reported. Strong desires to be taken care of by others (oral dependent longings), reaction to frustration with bottled-up aggressive feelings, and attempted restitution through "anal giving" (diarrhea) have been formulated by some. It is generally agreed that many of these patients are immature and frequently do not permit successful psychotherapeutic intervention. When psychotherapy is attempted during a relapse, extreme care may have to be practiced around situations which may threaten the patient's infantile dependence on the therapist, to avoid worsening the disorder. At present there is no evidence demonstrating that in-depth psychotherapies are any more effective than simple supportive psychotherapuetic measures in conjunction with the medical treatment regimen.

SUGGESTED READINGS

Alexander, F., French, T. M., and Pollock, G.: Psychosomatic specificity, Chicago, 1968, University of Chicago Press, vol. 1.

Anthony, E. J.: An experimental approach to the psychopathology of childhood encopresis, Br. J. Med. Psychol. 30:146, 1957.

Beaumont, W.: Experiments and observations on the gastric juice and the physiology of digestion, Plattsburgh, N. Y., 1833, F. P. Allan.

Bliss, E. L., and Branch, C. H.: Anorexia nervosa, its history, psychology and biology, New York, 1960, Paul B. Hoeber, Inc., Medical Book Department of Harper & Bros.

Cannon, W. B.: The wisdom of the body, New York, 1939, W. W. Norton & Co., Inc.

Dally, P.: Anorexia nervosa, New York, 1969, Grune & Stratton, Inc.

Daniels, G. E.: Psychiatric factors in ulcerative colitis, Gastroenterology 10:59, 1948.

Daniels, G. E., O'Connor, J. F., Karush, A., Moses, L., Flood, C. A., and

Lepore, M.: Three decades in the observation and treatment of ulcerative colitis, Psychosom. Med. **24:**85, 1962.

Engel, J. L.: Studies of ulcerative colitis; V, Psychological aspects and their implications for treatment, Am. J. Dig. Dis. **3:**315, 1958.

Feinstein, A. R.: The treatment of obesity. An analysis of methods, results and factors which influence success, J. Chronic Dis. **11:**349, 1960.

Goldblatt, P. B., Moore, M. E., and Stunkard, A. J.: Social factors in obesity, J.A.M.A. **192:**1039, 1965.

Karush, A., and Daniels, G.: Ulcerative colitis, Psychosom. Med. **15:**140, 1953.

Liebman, R., Minuchin, S., and Baker, L.: An integrated treatment program for anorexia nervosa, Am. J. Psychiatry **131:**432, 1974.

Lucas, A. R., Duncan, J. W., and Piens, V.: The treatment of anorexia nervosa, Am. J. Psychiatry **133:**1034, 1976.

Mecklenburg, R. S., and others. Hypothalamic dysfunction in patients with anorexia nervosa, Medicine **53:**147, 1974.

Melzak, R.: The puzzle of pain, New York, 1973, Basic Books, Inc., Publishers.

Moore, M. E., Stunkard, A. J., and Srole, L.: Obesity, social class and mental illness, J.A.M.A. **181:**962, 1962.

Pilot, M. L., Muggia, A., and Spiro, H. M.: Duodenal ulcer in women, Psychosom. Med. **29:**586, 1967.

Sternbach, R. A.: Pain patients: traits and treatment, New York, 1974, Academic Press.

Sullivan, A. J., and McKell, T. E.: Personality in peptic ulcer, Springfield, Ill., 1950. Charles C Thomas, Publisher.

Taipale, V., and others: Anorexia nervosa in boys, Psychosomatics **13:**236, 1972.

Thoroughman, J. C., et al.: Psychological factors predictive of surgical success in patients with intractable duodenal ulcer: a study of male veterans, Psychosom. Med. **26:**618, 1964.

Ulett, G. A.: Control of chronic pain by acupuncture, Psych. J. Univ. Ottawa 3(3):Sept., 1977.

Wolf, S., and Wolff, H. G.: Human gastric function, New York, 1943, Oxford University Press, Inc.

Young, A. J. et al.: Psychiatric illness and the irritable bowel syndrome, Gastroenterology **70:**162, 1976.

Zigler, R., and Sours, J. A.: A naturalistic study of patients with anorexia nervosa admitted to a medical center, Comp. Psychiat. **9:**644, 1968.

Genitourinary disorders

Disturbances of genital and urinary functions may occur under stress in normal persons and also in a wide variety of psychopathological states. It is generally accepted that enuresis, amenorrhea, dyspareunia, frigidity, impotence, and premature ejaculation are, in most cases, strongly determined by psychological factors. Considerable evidence also exists that dysmenorrhea, infertility, chronic leukorrhea, urinary frequency, polyuria, oliguria, urinary retention, and urgency may, in certain persons, be produced or aggravated by life conflict. Individual case studies suggest that depressed or helpless feelings may lead more commonly to urinary retention, while feelings of fear may choose expression by urgency or frequency. Urgency as a response to stress is said to be experienced in the urethra, while urgency as a cue to bladder distention is sensed suprapubically.

Whereas menstrual disorders (amenorrhea, oligomenorrhea, and premenstrual tension) are generally recognized as occurring in response to endocrine imbalance, these may also often be aggravated by stressful emotional situations acting presumably through the hypothalamic-pituitary axis. Amenorrhea may also appear as part of the syndrome of false pregnancy (pseudocyesis) in which other signs of pregnancy such as abdominal distention, breast changes, and weight gain occur. This may be a covert expression of the wish for or fear of pregnancy.

Ten percent of pregnancies end in spontaneous abortion. Psychological stress is understandably a factor in many of these. Following the tragedy of a sudden infant death, 60% of mothers were found to have difficulty in conceiving and then had twice as many miscarriages as a control series.

SUGGESTED READINGS

Beach, F. A.: "Psychosomatic" phenomena in animals, Psychosom. Med. **14:**261, 1952.

Brown, E., and Barglow, P.: Pseudocyesis, Arch. Gen. Psychiatry **24:**221, 1971.

Ferenczi, S.: Sex in psychoanalysis, New York, 1952, Basic Books, Inc., Publishers.

Hastings, D. W.: Impotence and frigidity, Boston, 1963, Little, Brown & Co.

Life stress and genital disorders; part 12. In Wolff, H. G.: Life stress and bodily disease, Ass. Res. Nerv. Ment. Dis. Proc. **29:**1059, 1950.

Masters, W. H., and Johnson, D. E.: Human sexual response, Boston, 1966, Little, Brown & Co.

Schwartz, M. S., and Stanton, A. H.: A social psychological study of incontinence, Psychiatry 13:399, 1950.

Endocrine disorders

DIABETES MELLITUS. Long-term medical-psychiatric studies have shown close correlations between time of onset of diabetes mellitus or times of exacerbation of the disease (indicated by the appearance of ketonuria without changes in diet, activity, dosage of insulin, trauma, or infection) and times of life stress. The phenomenon of overeating in reaction to emotional conflict is also commonly reported in diabetics and provides a ready mechanism for metabolic decompensation. In addition in some cases a period of emotional tranquility may lead to a remission in diabetes. Certain investigators report a low marriage rate (47% of males between 25 and 55 years old are married), poor grading of all emotional responses, strong feelings of shyness, and a need to rely on others. Exacerbations are believed often to follow events which lead the patient further to devalue himself. Patients are said to react to the illness with exaggerated feelings of helplessness and may blame others for their condition.

HYPERTHYROIDISM. Apparently in this condition psychic dysfunctions are partly etiological and partly a result of metabolic disturbance. The behavioral symptoms that occur with hyperthyroidism are overactivity, emotional lability, anxiety, and overt fear. It has been stated that persons who are sensitive and impressionable and who react keenly to life, with marked feeling of insecurity and an unusual sense of responsibility, are those in whom an undue emotional stress may serve to precipitate hyperthyroidism. Counterphobic behavior (doing repetitively what one most fears) is reported to be frequent. Psychotic episodes are not uncommon and may take the form of a manic excitement, a depression, or a paranoid illness. The psychosis can disappear with correction of the thyroid disturbance but this is by no means the rule.

MYXEDEMA. In cases of myxedema the slowness and difficulty in thought and action may be confused with a depression. A small number of psychoses with varied symptomatology have been reported to accompany this condition. Disappearance of the mental disorder with administration of thyroid preparation has been demonstrated.

OBESITY. An increase in adipose tissue of 15% or more over the norm for a given height and physiological age has been called obesity. A morbid increase in hunger (bulimia), resulting from brain damage (rare), from cultural conditioning, or (most commonly) from an abnormal emotional dependence upon eating pleasures for security and self-esteem produces this positive energy balance. Endocrine and constitutional factors are usually important in determining metabolic efficiency as well as the distribution of fat in the body.

Therapy limited to drugs and reducing diets frequently fails in chronic cases. With such patients, too forceful or rapid reducing regimes have been known to be attended by psychiatric illness. Because of these patients' craving for love and esteem, their sensitivity to criticism, and underlying loneliness, they are often difficult to keep in individual therapy. Group therapy is believed by many to be particularly helpful. Successful weight loss programs, however, are those that aim at long-term modification of behavior such that permanent changes are made in food selection, eating habits, and, perhaps most important of all, the institution of a program of regular physical activity.

SUGGESTED READINGS

Bale, R. N.: Brain damage in diabetes mellitus, Br. J. Psychiatry **122**:337, 1973.

Bruch, H.: Physiologic and psychologic interrelationships in diabetes in children, Psychosom. Med. **11**:200, 1949.

Burdon, A. P., and Paul, L.: Obesity, Psychiatr. Q. **25**:568, 1951.

Crowley, R. M.: Psychoses with myxedema, Am. J. Psychiatry **96**:1105, 1940.

Dinko, J. D., and Kaebling, R.: The psychiatric aspects of hypoparathyroidism, Acta Psychiatr. Scand. **38**(Suppl.): 164, 1964.

Gatewood, J. W., Organ, C. H., Jr., and Mead, B. T.: Mental changes associated with hyperparathyroidism, Am. J. Psychiatry **132**:129, 1975.

Hinkle, L. E., Evans, F. M., and Wolf, S.: Studies in diabetes mellitus, Psychosom. Med. **13**:160, 1951.

Lindstedt, G., and others: On the prevalence, diagnosis and management of lithium induced hypothyroidism in psychiatric patients, Br. J. Psychiatry **130**:452, 1977.

Lidz, T., and Whitehorn, J. C.: Life situations, emotions and Graves' disease, Psychosom. Med. **12**:184, 1950.

Pitts, F. N., and Guze, S. B.: Psychiatric disorders and myxedema, Am. J. Psychiatry **118:**142, 1961.

Reilly, E. L., and Wilson, W. P.: Mental symptoms in hyperparathyroidism, Dis. Nerv. Syst. **26:**361, 1965.

Wyden, P.: The overweight society, New York, 1965, William Morrow & Co., Inc.

Disorder of an organ of special sense

The diagnosis of a disorder of a special sense organ is applied to any disturbance of any organs of special sense in which emotional factors play a role. Ordinarily such disturbances are seen as one symptom of hysterical neurosis (conversion reaction). On the other hand, there is some evidence, as with primary *atypical facial neuralgia,* that neurological disturbance may on occasion be related to the emotions.

Other disorders

ACCIDENT PRONENESS. Many writers have considered accident proneness as a psychosomatic disorder. Certainly in these patients psychological factors and somatic disease are associated. Studies have shown that persons prone to repeated accidents, who seem unable to learn caution despite numerous painful experiences, differ in personality make-up from their more prudent peers. These individuals have been described as impulsive, resentful, and less able to control their hostility. They are anxious, fearful, and less able to tolerate tension. Accident-prone children have been said to have depression with a strong inner sense of guilt and an unconscious need for punishment.

PSYCHOLOGICAL FACTORS IN MALIGNANCY. The importance of psychological factors in the growth of cancer has been long suspected but has remained controversial. Numerous studies have reported on the influences of emotional factors in leukemia. Precarious life events and feelings of hopelessness have shown a positive correlation with positive cervical smears. Viral production of mammary cancer in mice has been shown to increase under laboratory-induced stress. Also, the medical literature has reported cases of "spontaneous" healing of various neoplasms.

Such reports are given increasing credence with the demonstration that many patients suffering from advanced cancer of certain types have been shown to have decreased immune responses. This is significant in view of recent findings of the role of stress upon hypothalamic function and its association with dysfunction and hypofunction of the immune system and, particularly, macrophage activities. Current interest has focused upon the prediction of the development of cancer from life stress scores. Recently it has been demonstrated that a therapy program including relaxation and guided imagery can prolong life in terminal cancer victims.

PAIN. Pain is a common and unpleasant experience primarily associated with tissue damage. The intensity and degree of pain, however, are determined by psychological and cultural as well as physiological factors. Acute pain serves as a useful warning, while chronic pain often produces useless suffering and disability.

Psychological influences can both raise and lower the threshold and tolerance for the many varieties of chronic pain: post-traumatic (causalgia), musculoskeletal (disc, bursitis, myositis, arthritis), iatrogenic (postsurgical), peripheral (neuralgia), central, and phantom-limb pain. Anxiety both increases muscle spasm and through the reticular activating system adds to the pain sensation. Chronic repressed anger as well as depression are common accompaniments of chronic pain. The MMPI of patients with chronic pain shows coping styles characterized by increase in hypochondriacal, hysterical, and depressive scales. Conversely it has also been shown that long-term suffering can increase signs of neuroticism. Cognitive influences that control pain levels include the conditioning of previous experiences (childhood abuse, being raised with a suffering parent, etc.), how well such are remembered, and the ability to understand the cause of the pain and the amount of optimism or pessimism about the meaning and outcome of the painful illness.

Some cultures from childhood condition their young to "take it in their stride," while others (more extroverted) encourage the expression of pain. The latter is especially true of females, blacks, Mediterranean cultures, the very young, and the very old. The diversion of attention can have transient salutory effect upon pain sensation.

Emotional disturbances, depression, lability of affect, and

dysaesthesia are known accompaniments of lesions in the thalamus (central pain). Less well understood are cases of persistent pain which in the absence of demonstrable CNS lesions continues long after the peripheral injury has healed. Such may be explained by reverberating circuits in the brain, often amplified by anxiety, muscle tension, depression, and concern over unsettled insurance claims.

Symptoms associated with chronic pain include sleep and appetite disturbances, decreased libido, irritability, social withdrawal, weakening of interpersonal relationships, and increased somatic preoccupation. Such persons are often resentful of unsuccessful previous treatment and the lack of attention received from previous physicians. If referred for psychiatric care they resent the implication that their pain is "in the mind."

In *diagnosis* it is important that some organic illness is not overlooked. A careful history will discern the presence or absence of segmental or peripheral nerve distribution corresponding to the anatomic location of the lesion. Pains with organic substrate typically awaken the patient at night and may change in character.

Our pill-popping culture often demands immediate relief, though such may carry the danger of addiction. The proper management of chronic pain is increasingly seen in multidisciplinary pain clinics staffed by neurologists, neurosurgeons, internists, anesthesiologists, physiatrists, psychiatrists, psychologists, social workers, nurses, and others. Treatment modalities include surgery, nerve block, transcutaneous electrical stimulation, acupuncture, biofeedback, hypnosis, relaxation therapies, as well as massage, heat, and exercise. Medications include a wide range of analgesics and often tricyclic antidepressants, including the combination of amitriptyline and fluphenazine. Psychotherapy includes a variety of approaches: (1) psychodynamic, aimed at the relief of pain aggravated by guilt and hostility; (2) hypnocognitive, seeking to alter the pain experience; (3) group therapy, to improve the communication and interpersonal problems of the pain state; and (4) behavioral techniques, operating with the concept that pain is a behavior with significant operational components and with the goal of teaching new responses through social reinforcement.

SUGGESTED READINGS

Freese, A.: S. Pain, New York, 1974, G. P. Putnam's Sons.

Melzack, R.: The puzzle of pain, New York, 1973, Basic Books, Inc., Publishers.

Simonton, O. C., and Simonton, S.: Belief systems in management of the emotional aspects of malignancy, J. Transpersonal Psychol. 7(1):29-48, 1975.

18

Transient situational disturbances and conditions without manifest psychiatric disorder

TRANSIENT SITUATIONAL DISTURBANCES

The term "transient situational disturbance" is used to refer to a variety of behavioral-emotional disturbances which can occur as acute reactions (adjustment reactions) to overwhelming environmental stress. In daily life situations one faces frequently the problems of illness, accident, disappointments in interpersonal relationships, and failure to achieve hoped-for goals. Major disasters differ from the above only in degree, unexpectedness, longer duration, unfamiliarity, lack of opportunity for escape or for effective action, and the absence of important support by others. The sudden death, loss, or illness of another valued family member would be an example of life trauma often precipitating an *adjustment reaction*. Healthy persons have a variety of conscious and unconscious mechanisms for effectively coping with such situations. If the patient has good adaptive capacity, his symptoms usually recede as the stress diminishes.

The immediate symptoms of stress are fear, anxiety, grief, annoyance, or anger, which can result in more or less appropriate reaction or, at the height of the stress, in paralysis of all action or in purposeless hyperactivity. From prolonged stress (as in combat reaction) there may be a residuum of restlessness, tremor, anorexia, asthenia, fatigue, insomnia, reaction to startle, phobias, nightmares, etc., that can last for months. Physical symptoms from chronic stress include tachycardia, precipitation of coronary attacks, and aggravation of peptic ulcer. Irrational behavior, drinking, and promiscuity can also result. Later symptoms too can include shame, guilt, depression, and loss of self-esteem from memories of one's inefficiency at the time of crisis. Symptoms from reaction to stress are often contagious: panic can spread through an audience, an anxious mother upset her children, or the unhappy home life of the boss increase the consumption of headache pills by the office force. In fortunate, healthy individuals the period of recovery from symptoms of stress may be brief and for some a good night's sleep is the best tonic. After prolonged stress the rebound may be less complete and the patient's life may not be characterized by quite the same vigor.

In differential diagnosis and in assessment of the patient's ability to manage stress, one must weigh the magnitude of the stress in terms of how it would be seen by others; also in terms of the stress tolerance of the individual, his life style and current life situation, his preparation to meet stress through past experiences ("sheltered life, etc."), the number of other stresses at this time ("last straw"); and the possible solutions available to him.

In preparing for treatment one must decide whether it is possible to change the situation, to change the patient, or to permit escape from that which is intolerable. One must judge the coping mechanisms of the patient and decide whether he perseverates in using coping mechanisms that are inappropriate or unworkable or whether he may be guided to use of better coping mechanisms. Reassurance, encouragement, and involvement in constructive activity are essential with the early return to duty or work situation. Adequate nutrition, sleep, and mild sedation are useful.

The prevention of situational maladjustments begins in early home training for the gradual responsibilities of growing up through shared responsibilities at home, preparation through wholesome, adequate adult interpersonal relationships, with good support at times of crisis in childhood and adolescence. A knowledge of life's traumata and emotional interplay is readily learned from one's peers and the communications media. A proper preparation for dealing with strong emotions and health matters is a responsibility of home and school as is the development of a personal supporting life philosophy. The balance of adequate support without the development of too much protection and dependence is a difficult parental task. In an enlightened employment situation the prevention of situational maladjustment is aided by clear lines of authority, good channels of communication, assignment of tasks within the range of the worker's competence, and personnel policies that enhance employment security. Continuing support from family, friends, and peers is of great importance. The important role the church can play in the development of a good life plan is too often overlooked in today's high-pressure society.

Transient situational disturbances are classified as follows:

ADJUSTMENT REACTION OF INFANCY. Crying spells and appetite disturbance may occur at separation from the mother.

ADJUSTMENT REACTION OF CHILDHOOD. Attention-getting behavior and nocturnal enuresis may occur with jealousy over a new sibling. The first day at school with its presentation of new and strange relationships, tasks, and situations may create intense temporary anxiety.

ADJUSTMENT REACTION OF ADOLESCENCE. At puberty the incidence of psychosis rises sharply. It is held by many that schizophrenic and manic-depressive psychoses which have their onset after the age of 20 years actually begin in this period of life. Signs and symptoms of such incipient psychoses are difficult, however, to distinguish from the normal vicissitudes of adolescence. Conflicts involving urges of self-expression, attempts at emancipation from parental control, emotional hypersensitivities, exaggerated self-assertiveness or regressive timidity, and tendencies toward intense or dereistic fantasies lead at times to fleeting psychoneurotic or psychotic disorganization which has been characterized by the general term "adolescent turmoil."

The symptom pictures presented in these patients—frequently similar to those of a schizoaffective psychosis—may indicate the necessity for physical methods of therapy such as phenothiazine medication or electroshock therapy. One should apply such methods with caution because prognosis with hospitalization and brief psychotherapy alone is often good.

ADJUSTMENT REACTION OF ADULT LIFE. The adjustment reaction may revolve around difficulties of the marital relationship, stress or fear of military combat, pregnancy and child rearing, unwanted pregnancy, bereavement, and the like. If the symptoms are of sufficient gravity or tend to persist, the appropriate diagnosis of psychotic disturbance is used.

ADJUSTMENT REACTION OF LATER LIFE. In aging persons major adjustment reactions occur not only with awareness of the problems of the climacteric and an increasing number of physical disturbances but also as a result of retirement from work, attendant loss of goal drive and motivation, decreasing daily activity, and a reduction in financial income. Breakup of the family through separation or death and loss of old friends are additional factors. Attention must be given to orderly planning for retirement with proper scheduling of preventive physical examinations and medical procedures, attention to diet, physical exercise, and the involvement in group interaction (golden age clubs, etc.) together with emotional support from family and friends.

SUGGESTED READINGS

Ausubel, D. P.: Theory and problems of adolescent development, New York, 1958, Grune & Stratton, Inc.

Both, H. M., Modlin, H. C., and Orth, M. H.: Situational variables in the assessment of psychotherapeutic results, Bull. Menninger Clin. **26:**2, 1962.

Eaton, M. T., Jr.: Executive stresses do exist but they can be controlled, Personnel **8:**18, March-April, 1963.

Eaton, M. T., Jr., and Livingston, D.: Marriage counseling by the family doctor, New Zeal. Med. J. **61:**359, 1962.

Holmes, A. J.: The adolescent in psychotherapy, Boston, 1964, Little, Brown & Co.

Horney, K.: The neurotic personality of our time, New York, 1937, W. W. Norton & Co.

Raush, H. L., Goodrich, W., and Campbell, J. C.: Adaptation to the first years of marriage, Psychiatry **26:**4, 1963.

Reinhardt, R. F.: The flyer who failed, an adult situational reaction, Am. J. Psychiatry **6:**740, 1924.

SOCIAL MALADJUSTMENT WITHOUT MANIFEST PSYCHIATRIC DISORDER

Current psychiatric terminology permits the use of diagnostic classification for individuals who are without diagnosable psychosis, or other classic psychiatric illness, but who nevertheless have problems severe enough to warrant examination by a psychiatrist. For them the term "social maladjustment without manifest psychiatric disorder" has been suggested. Under this category would fall persons with *marital maladjustment,* who appear psychologically normal but who are unable to adapt to meaningful situations and demonstrate significant conflict and maladjustments therein, yet for whom life is otherwise normal. The term *social maladjustment* is used to describe persons unable to adjust when thrown into a new culture, whereas *occupational maladjustment* is used to describe persons with significant and handicapping conflicts within the work situation. *Dyssocial behavior* describes persons who are not classifiable as antisocial personalities yet who manifest disregard for the usual social codes and often come into conflict with them as a result of living their lives in an abnormal environment. Here we find persons who are predators and who follow more or less *criminal tendencies,* such as racketeers, gamblers, prostitutes, and dope peddlers. These persons may be capable of strong loyalties. They usually do not show significant personality deviations other than those implied by adherence to the values or codes of their own predatory, criminal, or other social group.

These categories clearly are of direct interest to psychiatrists, since preventive psychiatry depends largely upon interventions during normal life crises which assist the individual to master potentially disorganizing experiences and thus prevent them from becoming fixed as behavioral disorders. Potentially disruptive stresses tend to occur in relation to specific developmental stages or life situations. These include early changes in child adaptation which require new learning such as weaning, toilet training, the first experience of leaving the family to attend school, and in adolescence the experience of graduation and the first intense heterosexual commitment. Later in life marriage or parental relationships as well as certain job situations may provide intense stress. Marital and occupational stresses tend to arise when the original bases for initial marital or job choice have modified with time. A marriage which may have been satisfactory before the arrival of children may not be well-adapted to parenthood. Certain occupational roles develop new personality functions or interests which then lead to alteration in values which can affect marital or parental adaptation. In all of these situations the task of a psychiatrist is first of all to differentiate between chronic established disorder and transient social maladjustment. This can be done by examining the duration of the symptoms, the temporal proximity of symptoms to the particular social stress, and the appropriateness of the intensity to the stress. The nature of the symptoms occurring with social maladjustment are limited to anxiety, depression, insomnia, mild psychosomatic disturbances, and the like. More serious symptoms such as phobia, delusion formation, and obsessional symptoms are indications of psychiatric illness rather than an isolated problem of social maladjustment. Previous levels of intellectual, affective, and social functioning achieved by the patient also contribute to the differentiation.

TREATMENT. Brief psychotherapy carried on in close proximity to the stress involved, with a focus on the present situation, can be useful in instances of social maladjustment. Within several weeks a follow-up should be planned to be sure that the pathological responses to stress do not become fixed.

SUGGESTED READINGS

Ackerman, N. W., Beatman, S., and Sherman, S. N., editors: Exploring the base of family therapy, New York, 1961, Family Service Association of America.

Ackerman, W.: The psychodynamics of family life, New York, 1958, Basic Books, Inc., Publishers.

Birren, J. W.: The psychology of aging, Englewood Cliffs, N.J., 1964, Prentice-Hall, Inc.

Boszormeny-Nagy, I., and Framo, S., editors: Intensive family therapy, New York, 1965, Hoeber Medical Division, Harper & Row, Publishers.

Burgess, E. W., editor: Aging in Western societies, Chicago, 1960, University of Chicago Press.

Erikson, E.: Childhood and society, ed. 2, New York, 1964, W. W. Norton & Co., Inc.

Farber, S. M., et al., editors: Man and civilization: the family's search for survival; a symposium, New York, 1964, McGraw-Hill Book Co..

Group for the Advancement of Psychiatry: Death and dying: attitudes of patient and doctor, symposium no. 11, New York, 1965, The Group.

Group for the Advancement of Psychiatry: Psychiatry and the aged: an introductory approach, symposium no. 59, New York, 1965, The Group.

Lidz, T.: The family in human adaptation, New York, 1963, International Universities Press, Inc.

McCord, W., and McCord, J.: Psychopathy and delinquency, New York, 1956, Grune & Stratton, Inc.

Post, F.: The clinical psychiatry of late life, New York, 1965, Pergamon Press, Inc.,

Schneider, K.: Psychopathic personalities, Springfield, Ill., 1968, Charles C Thomas, Publisher.

19

Behavior disorders of childhood and adolescence

Interest in child psychiatry has developed rapidly during the past quarter of a century. Within this time the management of disturbed children has shifted from the juvenile courts, schools, and churches into the psychiatric setting of child guidance clinics. In 1909 William Healy initiated a 5-year study of juvenile delinquents, and in 1912 the Boston Psychopathic Hospital had the first mental hospital outpatient clinic to accept children as patients. Great inspiration has come from the mental hygiene movement wherein it has been hoped that early attention to the disorders of childhood would prevent major neuroses and psychoses in later adult life. For example, Melanie Klein taught that psychoanalysis at the age of 2 to 4 years may promote healthier adult ego integration and prevent later pathogenic defenses against disruptive aggressive drives. The verity of such an assumption as yet awaits conclusive data, but it is now recognized that the emotional disorders of childhood form, within their own right, a medical specialty in which the child psychiatrist devotes attention not only to the child patient but also to the child's family.

The general principles underlying etiology, diagnosis, and therapy of adult psychiatric disorders apply also in child psychiatry. A number of problems, however, assume special importance.

CASE FINDING. Although no easily administered screening tests exist for the early detection of child psychiatric disorders,

245

nevertheless certain general principles guide the pediatrician, the schoolteacher, or the parent in defining such problems. Only rarely is the behavior disorder identified as a clear-cut new entity. Usually the problem is more confusing, being an exaggeration of established behavior patterns in the child. For adequate evaluation such a shift in adaptation usually requires repeated observations of the child and family and must be carried out by a clinician with considerable experience.

In well-baby clinics, pediatricians' offices, and nursery schools the infant's slow development of walking, talking, or socialization requires a differential diagnosis between constitutional defect, prenatal brain damage, environmental understimulation, or early emotional trauma. It has been shown that mild brain damage is associated with poor prenatal and obstetrical care and is one cause contributing to some emotional disorders. This factor being present does not diminish the importance of a thorough study of the child's and the family's psychological processes, which often determine the outcome of treatment. After the child's problems have been clarified, special psychotherapeutic skill and tact are necessary to bring this unwelcome possibility to the parents' awareness without creating an avoidance of the problem but, instead, instilling a desire to cooperate in further diagnostic study. This is a particularly difficult situation when the child is a victim of parental rejection, overprotection, overstimulation, overpermissiveness, overindulgence, overcontrol, or physical abuse—situations in which the parent's own needs serve to blind her or him to the child's real nature.

The *diagnostic study* aims to assess psychopathology—a particularly difficult task because of the normal disturbances that attend growth—and also to evaluate the developmental state as compared to the development expected at a given age in the child's social milieu. The treatment plan depends upon an evaluation of the problems for further personality growth imposed (1) by the disorder itself and previous distorted development and (2) by socioenvironmental forces such as parental personalities, influence of other family members or people at school, cultural values held by adults about this particular symptomatic behavior, and the motivation of those responsible for the child to help the child and to face their own part in the disturbance. A complete diagnosis may include investigation of possible constitutional, medical, psychological, and social factors in etiology, a description of the child's methods of dealing with anxiety and of his capacities for interpersonal relatedness, as well as a prediction of potential assets within the child and within his psychological habitat. Obviously, gathering this information requires an extensive intake evaluation sometimes involving contacts with parents, teachers, family physician, neighbors, etc., as well as with the child. A trial period of case work with a parent and exploratory psychotherapy with the child are often required before the problem becomes clear.

The new classification by the A.P.A. refers to the behavior disorders of childhood and adolescence as being divided into six major categories: (1) hyperkinetic reaction, (2) withdrawal reaction, (3) overanxious reaction, (4) run away reaction, (5) unsocialized aggressive reaction, and (6) group delinquent reaction. The *hyperkinetic reaction* is one observed frequently in males and consists of restlessness in the classroom, impulsive action, and a difficulty in concentration and intellectual development. Frequently the referral is by the teacher who has difficulty in controlling the child's focus of attention and the child's tendency to distract others in the classroom. In some cases there is evidence of minimal organic brain damage, and this may occur in the absence of intellectual deficit. In these cases amphetamines as well as psychotherapy can be useful. In other instances such behavior may be an aspect of a childhood neurosis. Like the *withdrawal reaction*, the *overanxious reaction* and the *run away reaction* are symptomatic of either neurotic or transient situational personality disorders. The *unsocialized aggressive reaction* has been seen in children described by F. Redl and others and should be considered as a personality growth disturbance. These children have extremely poor control over their aggressive and sexual impulses, and usually they have been poorly socialized by their parents and even subtly encouraged by the pleasure of their parents in their expressions of aggression. Finally, the *group delinquent reaction* is a subculture-specific condition, found particularly in the slums of our large cities, where groups of late childhood or early adolescent children find security in anti-social acts supported by mutual peer identifications.

The present classification is behavioristic in orientation and does not fit with the classification used to describe adult disorders.

Therefore, we shall also present the more traditional categories of childhood syndromes here.

Transient situational personality disorders. Because of the almost unlimited variety of disorders, there seems to be even less unanimity about nomenclature among child psychiatrists than among those who work with adults. A child may be easily influenced by environmental changes of all kinds, and the behavior disorders of childhood have been classified as adjustment reactions of infancy and childhood under the general heading given above. This grouping includes (1) *habit disturbance* such as nail biting, thumb sucking, enuresis, soiling, masturbation, and tantrums; (2) *conduct disturbance* such as truancy, stealing, destructiveness, cruelty, sexual offenses, and use of alcohol; and (3) *neurotic traits*, including tics or habit spasms, somnambulism, stammering, overactivity, and phobias. Often underlying these symptoms are rather severely disturbed self-expectations and perceptions of others as having hostile, rejecting motives.

Personality growth disturbances. Somewhat analogous to adult personality pattern disturbances are those problems in personality growth which interfere with school or social adjustment. Here may be mentioned as illustrations the overconforming pseudomature child, who cannot relate childishly to other children, the child with a reading or other educational disability, and the pseudofeebleminded child.

Psychophysiological disorders. The commonly encountered disorders in the group include feeding difficulties (chronic anorexia, food faddism, recurrent vomiting, obesity), difficulties of coordination (writing dysfunctions), respiratory dysfunctions (asthma, rhinitis), neurodermatitis, enuresis, lower bowel dysfunctions (colitis, constipation), etc.

Since physical handicaps and diseases with their possibly frightening accompaniments (medical examinations, hospitalizations, temporary separation from home) involve particular emotional stress for the child, the psychological reactions and social retardations resulting therefrom are an important part of pediatric psychiatry. In managing such situations, as Pearson has stated, pediatric psychiatry may be only common sense, but it is surprising how little the average person knows about this kind of common sense.

Psychoneuroses. The classic psychoneuroses are diagnosed in children but not with the frequency that such disorders occur in adults. Phobias, anxiety states, hysterical symptoms, and depressive states are seen. In addition, neurotic symptoms unique to childhood occur. For example, Spitz has described "anaclitic depression" and chronic withdrawal states resulting from the institutional environment in infants, and Bowlby has described a similar withdrawal phenomenon in children $1^1/_2$ to 4 years old, following placement in a general hospital for brief periods.

Psychoses. Psychoses are comparatively rare in the period of childhood but increase as adolescence is approached. Marked disorganization of affect and thinking, bizarre, reversible sensory or motor dysfunctions, inhibitions of learning, and severe interpersonal difficulties are seen. Kanner has presented the concept of the "autistic child" as a contribution to the study of schizophrenia in childhood. Goldfarb has shown that about 50% of autistic children have "soft" neurological signs and less severe family psychopathology. These mildly organic types of autistic children can sometimes be helped with special education for the child and with family or individual psychotherapy for the parents, who may be withdrawn and confused about a child who can actually be handled more effectively if the parents are given understanding. It has been found that these children and some of their mothers have speech disorders; there is a disorder in perception of time, space, and causality. Most of the children with autism have severe language disorder and a significant group are mute. The disorder presumably arises during the first year of life as a failure of attachment to the mother and a failure, therefore, to develop a self-concept as a human being. These children tend to orient toward inanimate objects in a very stereotyped, repetitive way and to demonstrate active withdrawal from relationships which apparently make them quite anxious. Although Eisenberg reports a poor outcome with outpatient psychotherapy, Bettleheim has reported two-fifths of these patients as markedly improved when given intensive long-term residential treatment. Presumably the most effective approach to autism lies in the prevention of disturbed early mother-infant relationships and in the prevention of organic brain disorder in fetal or early infant development. The differential diagnosis between psychoses and neurological disorders is frequently difficult; in fact, some autistic children have been misdiagnosed as deaf or brain-damaged patients.

TREATMENT. Psychotherapy with children must be adapted to the communication skills of each developmental stage. Treatment of infants is in terms of substitute mothering. With young children, in play therapy, interchange occurs largely at a symbolic or purely emotional level. With somewhat older children, the therapist still communicates via play but can also make interpretations and encourage verbal understanding of important issues. With the young adolescent (perhaps the most challenging therapeutic relationship) at certain times an adult type of interview may be possible, and at other times communications may be smoother if supported by a card game or other recreation which does not prevent sensitive discussion of feelings; at still other times a pal type of companionship, perhaps taking a walk together, is what can be accepted. No matter what the child's age, the psychotherapist becomes more emotionally involved than is the case in work with most adult patients. For the child, the therapist usually becomes a supportive, identification figure, as well as one who uncovers, interprets, or confronts preconscious or unconscious elements. Because of the child's immaturity and great dependence, the therapist must take pains not to evoke more intense affect or guilt than can be borne without panic, withdrawal, or further regression.

In recent years clinicians have increasingly recognized that for many child disorders the focus of work should be the family rather than the child alone. The child's psychopathology in these cases is not simply an internalized structure but is rather an expression of an active family interaction process. For these cases the clinician must try to ascertain what relationships within the family represent the core conflict. Many times the child's symptoms serve to uncover a much more significant marital conflict; in these cases the treatment of choice may be group or individual therapy with the parents. In situations in which each member of the family seems to make a significant contribution to the conflicts, family therapy is indicated. Particularly with certain kinds of chronic handicaps such as infantile autism or mild brain damage in a child, it may be useful to form a group of parents, all of whom have the same type of problem child, to assist each other in managing the particular difficulties of that disorder and in accepting the child's limitations. With middle-class verbal families therapy tends to identify pathological types of communication and interaction, including the double bind, chronic power alignments as of mother and son against father and daughter, family myths which serve as rationalizations for disturbed behavior, and special family roles such as the "helpless one" or the "scapegoat." With poor disadvantaged families the therapist may initially have to visit the home and will be required to give more of himself emotionally and to face the practical survival problems of the family with them in order that a psychotherapeutically useful process can be initiated. These families tend to use violence rather than verbalized principles for influencing each other. This may be extreme, with the inflicting of multiple fractures and burns on the child, known as the "battered child syndrome" or the "child abuse syndrome." State agencies have been organized to offer services to the parents, and reporting is mandatory. This violence in the families of delinquent children has no predictability but fosters constant vigilance and a sense of helplessness. These families lack a sufficient sense of the past and the future and need models for identification. Often the parents, being occupationally and economically as well as psychologically helpless, abdicate parental responsibility to one of the older children so that family power is vested much more in the children than is true in middle-class families.

The problem of whether to provide institutional treatment, always a difficult one, is particularly so here. On the one hand, insitutional treatment is an especially powerful tool because of the child's psychological dependence upon the environment; on the other hand, removal from the family may do violence to normal identifications and the development of a "me-feeling" based upon family tradition. Institutional treatment is indicated where the family and social circumstances are unusually malignant and where the child's disorder is severe and chronic. In addition to psychotherapy and other medical treatment where indicated, the institution provides a therapeutic group-living milieu designed to encourage his interpersonal adaptiveness and also provides parental surrogates, usually by the device of "cottage parents," who sleep and eat with a fixed group of children.

In conclusion, then, the specialty of child psychiatry is a multidisciplinary one. While the rationale for treatment grows out of the child's problem, most frequently the child is treated in conjunction with the family or larger social group. The psychiatric team approach is particularly indicated. Therefore, the basic clinical staff of a children's clinic is made up of pediatrician, psychiatrist, clinical psychologist, and psychiatric social worker.

SUGGESTED READINGS

Bakwin, H., and Bakwin, R. M.: Clinical management of behavior disorders in children, ed. 3, Philadelphia, 1966, W. B. Saunders Co.

Beller, E. K.: Clinical process, New York, 1962, The Free Press of Glencoe, Inc.

Burks, H. I.: Effects of amphetamine therapy on hyperkinetic children, Arch. Gen. Psychiatry **11**:604, 1964.

Chess, S.: Diagnosis and treatment of hyperactive child, New York J. Med. **60**:2379, 1960.

Conners, C. K., and Eisenberg, L.: The effects of methylphenidate on symptomatology and learning in disturbed children, Am. J. Psychiatry **120**:458, 1963.

Curran, W. J.: Failure to diagnose battered child syndrome, N. Engl. J. Med. **294**:795, 1977.

Eisenberg, L.: The management of the hyperkinetic child, Develop. Med. Child Neurol. **8**:593, 1966.

Erikson, E. H.: Childhood and society, ed. 2, New York, 1963, W. W. Norton & Co., Inc.

Fish, B.: Drug use in psychiatric disorders of children, Am. J. Psychiatry **124**:31, 1968.

Freud, A.: Concept of developmental lines, Psychoanal. Stud. Child **18**:245, 1963.

Freud, A.: Psychoanalytical treatment of children, London, 1946, Imago Publishing Co., Ltd.

Gamer, E., Gallant, D., Greenbaum, H. V., and Cohler, B. J.: Children of psychotic mothers, Arch. Gen. Psychiatry **34**:592, 1977.

Graham, P.: Management in child psychiatry: recent trends, Br. J. Psychiatry **129**:97, 1976.

Jenkins, R. L.: Classification of behavior problems of children, Am. J. Psychiatry **125**:68, 1969.

Kanner, L.: Child psychiatry, ed. 4, Springfield, Ill., 1971, Charles C Thomas, Publisher.

Kerr, W. C.: Lithium salts in the management of a child batterer, Med. J. Aust. **2**:414, 1976.

Kraft, I. A.: The use of psychoactive drugs in the out-patient treatment of psychiatric disorders of children, Am. J. Psychiatry **124**:1401, 1968.

Macht, L. B., and Mack, J. E.: The firesetter syndrome, Psychiatry **31**:277, 1968.

O'Neal, P., and Robins, L. N.: The relation of childhood behavior problems to adult psychiatric status: a thirty-year follow-up study of 150 subjects, Am. J. Psychiatry **114**:961, 1958.

Panter, B. M.: Lithium in the treatment of a child abuser, Am. J. Psychiatry **134**:1436, 1977.

Pincus, J. H., and Glaser, G. H.: The syndrome of minimal brain damage in childhood, N. Engl. J. Med. **275**:27, 1966.

Reichard, C. C., and Elder, S. T.: The effects of caffeine on reaction time in hyperkinetic and normal children, Am. J. Psychiatry **134**:144, 1977.

Rexford, E. N.: A developmental approach to problems of acting out, a symposium, New York, 1966, International Universities Press, Inc.

Robins, L. N.: Deviant children grow up; a sociological and psychiatric study of sociopathic personality, Baltimore, 1966, The Williams & Wilkins Co.

Sanders, R. W.: Systematic desensitization in the treatment of child abuse, Am. J. Psychiatry **135**:483, 1978.

Shaw, C. R.: Psychiatric disorders of childhood, ed. 2, New York, 1970. Appleton-Century-Crofts.

Shirley, H. F.: Pediatric psychiatry, Cambridge, Mass., 1963, Harvard University Press.

Werry, J. S., Weiss, G., Douglas, V., and Martin, J.: Studies on the hyperactive child. III. The effect of chlorpromazine upon behavior and learning ability, J. Am. Acad. Child Psychiatry **5**:292, 1966.

20

Mental retardation

Mental retardation is a disorder defined by incomplete maturation of attention, perception, and cognition as well as of social adaptability. Psychological tests are particularly important in establishing the diagnosis, whereas neurological, psychiatric, and social service studies help to evaluate and form an appropriate treatment plan. About 3% of school-age children are sufficiently retarded to require special classes or other services to promote their development.

Since 1961, patients with mental retardation have been classified into eight etiological patterns, and the degree of deficiency in adaptive behavior is specified as part of the diagnosis.* Their classification and recommended coding as given at the end of this chapter clearly demonstrates that there are many different kinds of mentally retarded patients. Only a few of the classic varieties will be discussed here.

Patients with milder cases of mental retardation may not be diagnosed before reaching school, where they manifest difficulty in learning but may attain sixth-grade performance level toward the end of adolescence. Although they are not capable of a high-school education, with special help those patients with mild impairment can become self-supporting. They require supervision as adults only in serious stress situations. Moderately severe retardates can talk but lack social awareness and usually can accomplish only a fourth-grade level in school. Under careful super-

---

*See A Manual on Terminology and Classification in Mental Retardation, Willimantic, Conn., 1961, American Association on Mental Deficiency.

254

vision and with special adult help, many of these patients can eventually undertake an unskilled or semiskilled occupation. Severe retardates, so-called levels III and IV in degree of retardation, require hospitals or other special care environments throughout their lives. Various degrees of guidance, support, and control are indicated, depending upon whether the patient has learned speech, mastery of bodily functions, and ways to protect himself. With those who do learn to communicate one tries to inculcate simple health habits.

The psychiatrist's job in diagnosis is a complex one and places special emphasis upon the maturation level of the patient's motor, auditory, visual, and speech functions. Educability depends on the patient's potentials for conforming to his culture and for responsive interpersonal relationships. Such a complex diagnosis is necessary in order to make a prognosis and proceed with a treatment plan.

The etiology of mental deficiency is varied. Some 30% of patients show no other symptoms but may have a family history of mental defect. Prenatal infections (especially viral) or childhood encephalitides apparently cause about 20% of cases. Asphyxia, anoxia, and cerebral hemorrhage resulting from prolonged labor or from brain damage associated with prematurity account for perhaps another 20% (cerebral palsy, cerebral diplegia, choreoathetosis). In mild form in children, the syndrome may be difficult to distinguish from incipient schizophrenia.

An undetermined number of patients show a mild or moderately severe retardation apparently associated with loss of interest and curiosity about the world around them which begins within the first year or year and a half of life as a result of parental neglect. Commonly this syndrome occurs in large cities in very poor families who leave their infants and young children to be cared for in situations in which there is very little activity, social stimulation, or contact of any kind with other adults or children. The child's interest in learning becomes so muted that the developmental process is disrupted.

Mongolism. Less than 10% of defectives suffer from mongolism. In one study such children occurred once in every 688 births. This form of amentia is said to occur more frequently when mothers are past 40 years of age. Although first described by Down in 1860, it was not until 100 years later (1960) that cytologists succeeded in numbering the chromosomes of afflicted patients, thus permitting a major breakthrough toward understanding etiology. A chromosomal abnormality (trisomy) was found as an extra forty-seventh chromosome in the twenty-first and twenty-second pair of chromosomes. Such chromosomal nondysjunction was present, particularly when the patient was the offspring of an older mother. The defect appeared as a deformed chromosome, because of translocation, in one of a pair of 46 chromosomes in the offspring of younger mothers, and here there appears to be some hereditary predisposition. Defects occur in the skull, eyes, tongue, hands, and feet. A narrow, sloped palpebral fold and frequent epicanthus give the patient an oriental appearance. Usually these patients are placid and inert and show considerable variation in the degree of mental defect.

Cretinism. Cretinism occurs sporadically as a result of congenital aplasia of the thyroid gland. It is endemic to some areas of the world. The child appears normal at birth but by the sixth month shows signs of the illness. There are retardation of growth and bone development and a general lethargy. The skin is often yellowish in color, loose, and wrinkled. There may be puffiness of the features with thickening of the eyelids, nostrils, and lips. Myxedematous swelling of the hands, feet, and back of the neck is common. The abdomen may be prominent, with umbilical hernia. Hair on scalp and eyebrows is scanty, temperature subnormal. Breathing may be sonorous and the child has a dry, "leathery" cry.

All degrees of mental impairment are found, but usually the patient is an imbecile. Usually he is weak and often placid, good tempered, and affectionate.

Treatment should be begun immediately with whole thyroid (dried gland). Begin in children 3 to 6 months of age with ¼ grain daily. This may be increased with age. Tredgold recommends ½ grain per day for each year of the child's age. Maximum dose is 5 grains daily. Treatment must be continued after the symptoms have disappeared or they will return. Maintenance medication one to two times weekly is often sufficient. If treatment is delayed until the patient is an adult, little or no improvement will be seen.

• • •

There exist also in any large hospital for the mentally deficient a number of patients whose conditions are hereditary in nature and are associated with signs and symptoms apart from those of mental deficiency. The following conditions are included.

Phenylpyruvic oligophrenia. Phenylketonuria characterizes this rare, recessive, inherited biochemical defect. Clinical imbecility may be accompanied by dwarfing, seizures, dermatitis, kyphosis, and accentuated reflexes. Fair hair and blue eyes are common features. These patients excrete phenylpyruvic acid in the urine, which may be detected by the development of a transient, deep bluish green color upon the addition of a few drops of 5% ferric chloride solution.

Treatment of these patients by phenylalanine-restricted diets has produced definite improvement in the EEG's and some promising clinical results. Hemocysteinuria is a similar syndrome recently defined, and it would appear likely that additional defects specific to the metabolism of single essential amines may yet explain other cases of retardation.

Huntington's chorea. In the majority of cases this has its onset in middle life as a chronic, progressive psychosis with dementia, and it is accompanied by chronic movements, wasting, and rigidity. In a number of cases, however, the onset occurs in childhood and so this illness is then classified as a mental deficiency.

Epiloia. This is a syndrome of tuberous sclerosis, sebaceous adenoma, and epilepsy. The mental symptoms range from idiocy to the level of a high-grade moron.

Neurofibromatosis. In this condition, also known as von Recklinghausen's disease, multiple nerve tumors are found covering the whole body. Pigmented patches of skin and mental defect are variable accompaniments.

Oxycephaly. Oxycephaly, or acrocephaly. is an anomaly in which a high or pointed head is accompanied by mental defect. A similar defect is also found with *hypertelorism,* in which the head is too wide, or with *microcephaly,* in which the skull is smaller than normal size, both conditions being due to premature synostosis of the cranium.

Arachnodactyly. This is a condition in which long spidery fingers and toes, combined with long limbs, occur with mental defect and often with coloboma, dislocation of the lens of the eye, and cardiac defect.

Nevoid amentia. This condition, known also as Sturge's or

Weber's or Kalischer's disease, shows a combination of mental impairment and meningeal and facial angioma.

Friedreich's ataxia, Laurence-Moon-Biedl syndrome, retinitis pigmentosa, polydactyly, and **pituitary dystrophy** are found among the mentally deficient.

Amaurotic idiocy. Both the juvenile type and the infantile type (Tay-Sachs disease) show progressive cerebromacular degeneration with severe mental deficiency.

TREATMENT. In the treatment of conditions of limited brain capacity, the patient's actual performance will depend to a considerable extent upon his motivation to train himself and upon the skill and persistence of those who are helping him to develop. Initially, it is the physician's responsibility to assess the severity of presumed cortical deficiency. With level III or IV patients the parents need to recognize the real situation and to consider institutional placement. Involved in this decision are not only the availability of special schools and clinics but also an evaluation of how much emotional and physical strain the parents and siblings could withstand were the child to remain in the family. With children who score over 20 to 30 I.Q. points, more serious consideration may be given to the possibility of maintaining the child in the home, provided the parents have the energy and personal resources to work intensively, under professional guidance, to train the child. Many communities now have special educational counselors and clinics to advise parents about special home training techniques and to evaluate at regular intervals the child's readiness for more complex tasks. Public schools often maintain special classes for the retarded. During his childhood years, daily routines should avoid complexity and stress personal hygiene, social amenities, punctuality, and understandable speech. As the child grows older, vocational guidance becomes important and the social worker acts as interpreter of the illness to the family or to the employer. The rate of development, although much slower than in normal persons, need not be inconsequential. Recently psychologists skilled in conditioning and reinforcement learning schedules have developed new methods of programmed education which break down learning to read and learning to count skills into smaller units more manageable by the patient. By skillful repetitive use of principles of reinforcement and associative learning, some formerly uneducable retardates have been able to obtain simple schooling. With an adequate educational program, it may be that even level II and level III patients could become more self-sufficient in the future than has been true in the past. Hospital programs not infrequently discharge such patients in their twenties or thirties to begin a semi-independent life.

The psychiatrist can assist in evaluating attitudes and symptoms which interfere with attainable educational or job achievements. Commonly, for example, these patients experience conflict around dependence-independence problems and may react by either exaggerating or denying their handicaps. Parents of these patients, as with parents of any chronically helpless child, commonly show intrusiveness and an overcontrolling attitude because of their deep concern to be helpful and push the child to accomplishments beyond his capacity. This common parental syndrome often leads to a lack of self-confidence and various types of neurotic responses.

SUGGESTED READINGS

Bowman, T. W., and Mautner, H., editors: Mental retardation, New York, 1966, Basic Books, Inc., Publishers.

Brown, E. S., and Warner, R.: Mental development of phenylketonuric children on or off diet after the age of six, Psychol. Med. **6:**287, 1976.

Clarke, A. M., and Clark, A. D., editors: Mental deficiency. The changing outlook, ed. 2, New York 1966, The Free Press.

David, O., and others: Low lead levels and mental retardation, Lancet **II:**1376, 1976.

Ellis, N. R., editor: Handbook of mental deficiency, New York, 1963, McGraw-Hill Book Co.

Franks, C. M., editor: Annual review of behavior therapy: theory and practice, New York, 1976, Brunner/Mazel.

Hanson, J. W., and others: Risks to the offspring of women treated with hydantoin anticonvulsants with emphasis on the fetal hydantoin syndrome, J. Pediat. **89:**662, 1976.

Kanner, L. A.: A history of the care and study of the mentally retarded, Springfield, Ill., 1964, Charles C Thomas, Publisher.

Leitenberg, H., editor: Handbook of behavior modification and behavior therapy, Englewood Cliffs, N. J., 1976, Prentice-Hall, Inc.

Lilienfeld, A. M.: Epidemiology of mongolism, Baltimore, 1969, The Johns Hopkins University Press.

Luria, A. R.: The mentally retarded, New York, 1963, The Macmillan Co.

A manual on terminology and classification in mental retardation, Willimantic, Conn., 1961, American Association on Mental Deficiency.

Menolascino, F. J., editor: Psychiatric approaches to mental retardation, New York, 1970, Basic Books, Inc., Publishers.

Noland, R. L.: Counseling parents of the mentally retarded: a sourcebook, Springfield, Ill., 1970, Charles C Thomas, Publisher.

Penrose, L. S.: The biology of mental defect, ed. 2, New York, 1963, Grune & Stratton, Inc.

Phillips, T., editor: Prevention and treatment of mental retardation, New York, 1960, Basic Books, Inc., Publishers.

Piaget, J.: The origins of intelligence in the child, London, 1953, Routledge & Kegan Paul, Ltd.

Robinson, H. B., and Robinson, N. M.: The mentally retarded child, New York, 1964, McGraw-Hill Book Co.

Tarjan, G.: Research and clinical advances in mental retardation, J.A.M.A. **182:**617, 1962.

Thompson, T., and Grabowski, J., editor: Behavior modification of the mentally retarded, ed. 2, New York, 1977, Oxford University Press.

Tredgold, R. F., and Soddy, K.: A textbook of mental deficiency, ed. 10. Baltimore, 1964, The Williams & Wilkins Co.

III

THERAPEUTIC MEASURES

21

The psychiatric treatment team

As the multidimensional nature of many illnesses has become clearer, the focus of medical concern has begun to move from treating the illness to treating interacting dysfunctions of related systems which either exist within the patient (biological or physiological) or impinge upon the patient from without (environmental or social). To employ this complex concept of disease often requires a harmoniously effective team of specialists. This is particularly true in psychiatry, where disabling disorders may, in a sense, reside as much within the disturbed relationships surrounding the patient as within the patient himself. Here, therefore, the therapeutic task may involve working in a coordinated manner with several "patients"—for example, with the patient and his family or with the patient and his employer.

Depending upon the setting for treatment, whether state hospital, general hospital, clinic, school, or juvenile court, the professional identity of members of the treatment team varies considerably. Thus in a hospital, under supervision of the occupational therapist, a person trained primarily as a muscian, artist, or teacher may perform a variety of socializing and ego supportive functions. Within the juvenile court, the probation officer or lawyer may be called upon to perform functions the aims of which do not differ, substantially, from the goals of supportive psychiatric treatment. In medical settings, the primary members of the team may commonly include the psychiatrist, internist, surgeon, pediatrician, social worker, psychologist, and nurse. For special problems the resources available from a mental health-oriented clergyman, dietitian, vocational guidance specialist, marriage counselor, physical therapist, library assistant, or volunteer aide should be kept in mind.

THE PSYCHIATRIST

Because of the complex nature of psychiatric disorders, the psychiatrist, more than most physicians, tends to become involved in administrative, educative, and professional leadership functions. The psychiatrist's approach both to patients and to colleagues must be in some respects more collaborative and less authoritative than the approach of his brother physicians.

For example, when psychiatrist and social worker collaborate in the psychotherapy of a disturbed parent-child pair, the emotional relationship and communication pattern worked out between the two therapists is a dynamic factor powerfully affecting the new balance to be achieved within the family of the two patients. Energies spent in improving the individual self-awareness and group effectiveness of psychiatric team members will directly benefit patients. Traits of competitiveness, dominance over others, excessive need for approval, or indecisiveness in the team director should be courageously self-scrutinized.

THE COLLABORATING PHYSICIAN

Commonly an internist, surgeon, pediatrician, or general practitioner may be involved at the time of referral, of disposition after the treatment, or when physical diseases accompany psychiatric disorders. The art of referring to a psychiatrist a patient who may be attached to "his" doctor and who believes his illness to be primarily somatic is indeed a difficult one. Later success in relating positively to the psychotherapist is much more likely if the outside physician consults with the psychiatrist before planning the timing and the rationale for the referral. For it is true that if the patient arrives on the psychiatrist's doorstep feeling rejected or insulted, or perhaps confused by a rather hurried explanation from his physician, the initial stages of forming constructive rapport are made more difficult than usual, if not impossible. When the patient in psychotherapy is being attended regularly by another physician, it may occur that the latter's attitudes affect the patient's involvement in, and benefit from, psychotherapy. Some type of regular consultation is desirable between the two physicians to clarify the changing problems in the relationship each maintains with the patient.

THE SOCIAL WORKER

The psychiatric case worker is trained to undertake care of a great variety of social or emotional problems which are not so threatening to the organism as to require a physician's guidance. In addition, under supervision, experienced social workers may, on occasion, carry psychotherapeutic tasks. As a result of thorough training, the social worker contributes to the team an alert awareness for family and cultural pressures which may be aggravating to the patient's symptoms. The social worker is prepared to go into the patient's house or to meet the patient's employer at the latter's office in order to evaluate at first hand and report back upon the realities which face the patient. In the patient's efforts to make concrete changes in job or living arrangements, the social worker may function actively to encourage or to support the patient in defined directions.

In recent years a new type of social worker—the group worker—has been trained to function as an active participant with patients in group situations. These persons work to produce changes through sensitive environmental planning, group leadership, and intuitive on-the-spot guidance. In institutions and community organizations they have played vital roles in creating a therapeutic milieu.

THE PSYCHOLOGIST

Nurtured by an academic tradition rooted partly in philosophy and partly in the laboratory, the clinical psychologist is best prepared to represent behavioral science. Although psychological test instruments are still fairly crude and accurate predictions of important variables still difficult, it is the psychologist who is ready to aid the team in evaluating treatment results and in using the therapeutic setting for research purposes. Besides diagnostic and research functions, the clinical psychologist is also trained in psychotherapy (under medical supervision). In clinic practice it often happens that psychologist, social worker, and psychiatrist may among themselves carry three members of a family in treatment and then meet weekly in order collaboratively to evaluate progress.

THE NURSE

The nurse on the psychiatric ward combines a bewildering variety of functions. These include being responsible for the patient's immediate physical needs, mediating patients' requests for attention or special privileges, using her own intimacy with patients as a medium for behavior modification, supervising and training students and volunteers, participating with the occupational therapist or group worker in planning activities for patients, and assisting the physician in physical modes of treatment. When intensive psychotherapy is being done within the hospital, a regular meeting between therapist and nursing staff is usually valuable both to the nurse, in providing insight into disturbed behavior, and to the psychotherapist, in understanding transference reactions and other disturbed behaviors both in and outside the interview. In some therapeutic wards an administrative separation is made between the personnel who are responsible for the patient (aide, nurse, and clinical director) and the psychotherapist; with responsibility taken off the psychotherapist for any decisions about the patient, it is hoped that the patient will feel free to trust the therapist, to express hostile or anxiety-laden impulses, and to work them through. Like the attendant or the activity therapist, the nurse becomes deeply involved in a patient's disturbed attitudes and actions and in some ways is in a unique position to observe and record for the physician subtleties of improvement or relapse.

ADJUNCTIVE THERAPISTS

Occupational therapy came to be regarded as a new profession, particularly from its important role in the rehabilitation of physically ill patients during World War I. Various forms of art (painting, sculpture), handicraft (wood, metal, leather, ceramics), dancing, music, and certain recreational therapies require specially trained personnel. Attempts to fit the activity to the patient's needs have taken the form of "occupational therapy prescriptions." Some hospitals prefer to give the patients a free choice in an unstructured workshop setting.

Industrial therapy is a most meaningful step toward returning the patient to community living. Such experience can lead to discharge for patients who need training in some marketable skill or vocation. Often mentally retarded patients who would otherwise spend an institutionalized lifetime can, through industrial training, graduate to a sheltered community workshop and special living arrangements apart from an institution. Hospitals may contract with local industries for piece work that can be performed in a hospital workshop and for which patients can earn wages even while still hospitalized.

Pastoral counseling attempts to meet the spirtual needs of patients through religious services for patients of several religious persuasions while they are hospitalized; the pastoral counselor also serves as an important link to the community and arranges for patients during the process of rehabilitation to attend community churches of their own choice. Very often the engagement in social activities with community religious groups can serve as an important step toward recovery. Increasingly, the clergy of community churches are seeking to gain psychiatric knowledge and counseling skills in order to better recognize incipent mental disorders and to learn proper management and referral techniques. In the mental hospital the pastoral counselor with special training participates in group therapy, counseling with special groups such as alcoholics, and learns to listen with a psychological as well as ecumenical religious ear to the problems of each client.

SUGGESTED READINGS

Aguilera, D. C.: Review of psychiatric nursing, St. Louis, 1977, The C. V. Mosby Co.

Barker, R. L.: Trends in the utilization of social work personnel, New York, 1966, National Association of Social Workers, Inc.

Caplan, G.: The theory and practice of mental health consultation, New York, 1970, Basic Books, Inc., Publishers.

Clark, D. H.: Principles of administrative therapy, Am. J. Psychiatry **117:**506, 1960.

DePaul, A. V.: The nurse as a central figure in a mental health center, Perspect. Psychiat, Care **6:**17, 1968.

Deschin, C. S.: Future direction of social work. I. From concern with problems to emphasis on prevention, Am. J. Orthopsychiatry **38:**9, 1968.

Fairweather, G.: Social psychology in treating mental illness, New York, 1964, John Wiley & Sons, Inc.

Freger, H.: The police-social work team: a new model for interprofessional cooperation: a university demonstration project in manpower training and development, Jane Addams School of Social Work, University of Illinois at Chicago Circle, Springfield, Ill., 1975, Charles C Thomas, Publisher.

Peplau, H. E.: Principles of psychiatric nursing. In Arieti, S., editor: American handbook of psychiatry, New York, 1952, Basic Books, Inc., Publishers, vol. 2.

Schwartz, M. S., and Shockley E. L.: The nurse and the mental patient, New York, 1956, Russell Sage Foundation.

Stanton, A., and Schwartz, M.: The mental hospital, New York, 1954, Basic Books, Inc., Publishers.

Stein, S. P., and Charles, E.: Emotional factors in juvenile diabetes mellitus. Study of early life experiences of adolescent diabetics, Am. J. Psychiatry **128:**700, 1971.

Tudbury, M. A.: The psychiatric nurse in the general hospital, Springfield, Ill., 1958, Charles C Thomas, Publisher.

Weiss, J. M. A., editor: Nurses, patients and social systems, Columbia, Mo., 1968, University of Missouri Press.

West, W. L.: Changing concepts and practices in psychiatric occupational therapy, New York, 1959, American Occupational Therapy Association.

Zaslove, M. O., Ungerleider, J. T., and Fuller, M.: The importance of the psychiatric nurse: views of physicians, patients, and nurses, Amer. J. Psychiat. **125:**482, 1968.

22

Individual psychotherapy

Of the many qualities of different psychotherapeutic relationships, we will present only those common aspects which seem to lend themselves to brief verbal description. The variety of experiences—whether from the physician's point of view or from the patient's—depends upon a multitude of factors, including differences in the participants' capacities for a continuing, intimate, creative relatedness, differences in their ideas concerning the goals of psychotherapy, and differences in their beliefs about the process of psychotherapy. Differences between settings for psychotherapy are relevant also although it cannot always be predicted how a given patient will be affected by whether he is seen in his hospital bed on the ward, sits in a bare, somewhat noisy clinic cubicle, lies down in a well-appointed private office, or receives psychotherapy in a soundproofed room with a listening tape recorder.

At the outset it is well to recognize that the interview as a form of communication need not be therapeutic. Many interviews are conducted for other purposes: social research, childhood education, moral suasion, authoritarian intimidation, selling merchandise, and so on. Whether an interview, or a series of interviews, has a therapeutic influence depends upon the motivations and psychological capacities of the participants, the structuring of communication, the subjective experiences fostered by the interviews, and the resulting encouragement or inner permission for the patient to experiment with new patterns of action. When the interview is therapeutic in intent and is successful, such an experience leads to increased mastery by the patient of his everyday social interactions and is accompanied by relief from symptoms.

The interview room should be quiet, comfortable, and conducive to inner contemplation without disturbance by telephone or street noises. Complete privacy of communication should be assured. Brief notes may be taken if they do not interfere with the therapist's attention. No furniture should intervene between the patient and physician (the stage should not be set for authoritative looks across a desk). A slight divergence of chairs in the face-to-face interview allows both doctor and patient a natural and easy avoidance of direct embarrassed stare.

Physician-patient contacts of whatever length, including the initial, history-taking interview, can be psychotherapeutic. It is recommended, however, that therapeutic interviews be scheduled regularly and that each last a definite period of time. Thirty-five to fifty minutes has been found, by experience, to be sufficiently long to permit the divulgence of worthwhile material, and yet not be too emotionally tiring for the patient. Shorter interviews may be indicated when the longer time produces too much anxiety. On the other hand, at the time of an acute emotional crisis, it may occasionally be valuable to stay with a patient for a prolonged period, until the storm has somewhat subsided. For intensive analysis of personality problems, interviews are held daily, 4 to 6 days a week. Less intensive psychotherapy is commonly carried on with interviews one to two times a week and, for supportive psychotherapy, as often as financial and geographical difficulties conveniently permit. When treatment is being terminated, even longer spacing of interviews may be used. Both therapist and patient should be punctual, as tardiness may indicate resistance to treatment. A brief interval of time should be left between patients. This is helpful for relaxation and for organization of notes.

The doctor is more than just a listener; he is an active participant whose attentive attitude, encouraging mood, and occasional words are calculated to help the patient uncover and clarify his feelings and behavior. Early, a question-and-answer technique may be necessary—particularly with passive, dependent patients. Gradually, however, the patient is encouraged to take more initiative and to discuss whatever topic comes into his mind. Initially, a brief explanation of therapy may be helpful and the patient can be given the following types of explanation:

"We seek to find an explanation for, and means to alter, repetitive ways of behavior in meeting conflict situations that make you uncomfortable and produce your symptoms."

"It will be necessary to review your life in considerable detail, emphasizing not only what you have done but also how you feel and have felt about what you have done and about important persons in your life."

"It is best for you to talk about whatever comes to your mind. As time goes on, you will be able to discuss matters that at first seem too personal or too emotionally painful to mention. It is very important that you learn to do this, because such areas of thought are usually the most important to study to help you get well. Our basic rule will be to say whatever pops into your mind, even if it does not always seem to make good sense at the time."

When the patient blocks, a period of silence may occur as the result of a thought that is important and so the therapist may, after a few moments of silence, inquire, "What is on your mind now?" or "What thought caused you to stop talking?" Yet, in helping the patient achieve greater spontaneity and insight, at times—for fear of mobilizing too much anxiety—care must be exercised not to press the patient into revealing too much too soon. The therapeutic sessions will never run short of material, for we are reviewing the patient's whole life; therapy could therefore occupy years. Practically, however, the subjects covered include all areas of life which are meaningful in terms of currently disturbed interpersonal relationships.

The therapist may obtain insight into facets of the patient's behavior of which he (the patient) is totally unaware. It is not so helpful to point this out to the patient directly as it is to lead him by means of carefully worded questions and directed associations to discover meaningful relationships for himself. Occasionally interpretations are given by the therapist in the form of "Could it perhaps be that this feeling toward your employer is like what you felt toward somebody else, you father, for example?" A "yes" answer from the patient, however, does not always imply emotional acceptance of the idea. Consequently his total (verbal and nonverbal) reaction to such interpretations should serve as clues to direct further exploration. At other times the patient may be confronted with some characteristic interview behavior or speech pattern that he is using to avoid emotional pain or to avoid serious contemplation of a central life issue.

The golden rule of therapy states, "It is more rewarding to listen than to speak." It is the patient who is being helped by verbalizing, confessing, and analysis—not the physician. Insofar as possible, considering the practical realities of living, it is well that patients not make major decisions while they are in treatment. One important goal of therapy is to help them mature so that they can make such decisions on their own. Even though it is obvious to the therapist what path should be followed, the patient is *not* the therapist; he has different goals, wishes, plans, etc.; hence, what would be a good solution for the therapist could well lead to further unhappiness for the patient. In this regard, remember that therapy is intended to preserve the individuality of the patient and is not a process of fashioning personalities in the likeness of the therapist. It follows from this that moral, religious, or ethical judgments must not be implied by the therapist.

The content includes all mental production of the patient and especially such topics as the following:

1. Subjective and somatic symptomatology
2. Family constellation and the complex emotional forces sensed within relationships to members of the family, in both the present and the past
3. Affects of fear, dread, loneliness, helplessness, confusion, anger, bitterness, depression, guilt, lust, hope, joy, and humor
4. Fantasy, dream material, and free association—with attention to recurrent or dramatic themes
5. Habitual interpersonal attitudes of clinging, isolation, defiance, accusation, complaint, domination, submission, provocation, rejection, inquiry, cooperation, helpfulness, or hero worship—as expressed to the psychotherapist or in other relationships
6. Recurrent patterns of action at work or at play, whether constructive or self-defeating

All psychotherapy is an elaboration and continuation of the original history-taking session. As time goes on, similar insights into similar problems begin to repeat themselves. This process, which follows the initial correction of distorted perceptions and which consists of numerous trial-and-error attempts at healthier solutions, is called *working through*. It may extend for weeks, months, or years. Indeed, after termination of psychotherapy this process can continue to operate. Psychotherapeutic alleviation of symptoms can occur soon after the first few interviews, during the middle of the working-through process, or not until close to termination.

THE DOCTOR-PATIENT RELATIONSHIP

The relationship between psychotherapist and patient occurs within certain broad psychosocial *structures* and utilizes a variety of interpersonal and intrapsychic *processes*. The societal position of the physician, a role defined through the ages as the healer, is a structure which fosters attitudes of dependence, trust, passivity, and suggestibility in all patients—without regard to personality or disease. As has been demonstrated in studies of the placebo effect, the popularity and public acceptance of any therapeutic agent contribute powerfully to its valuation by patients and staff and thereby to its objective influence. Another structural element in any doctor-patient relationship is the basic fit of their personalities. Does the physician have enough basic communality of personal experience with the patient to be able to establish a sensitive and genuine rapport? The beliefs and values held by the physician about matters of interpersonal influence, too, are important structural elements in the relationship, since they contribute to the goals and limits of the process. The nature of the patient's central conflicts, whether primitive and highly disorganizing to effective communication or less primitive and less disorganizing, contributes to the relationship. Similarly, the psychiatrist's own areas of continued immaturity, selective inattention, or latent anxiety will determine in a regular fashion those aspects of the patient's communication to which he can respond usefully.

Within the structure of a given doctor-patient relationship, many processes may be openly recognized and consciously utilized or, on the other hand, remain implicit or even relatively unimportant. The element of *hope,* the opportunity for the patient's hidden potentials for change and growth to be realized, remains implicit in many therapies and is utilized with greatest explicitness by the existential therapists. In nearly all psychotherapies, the therapist fosters some degree of *ambiguity* in the patient's knowledge of the therapeutic process and of the therapist as a person. In the organismic approach of K. Goldstein, this is thought to be analogous to social isolation and sensory deprivation experiments which permit awareness of experiences bound to the less peripheral brain structures. Psychoanalytically oriented therapists also foster ambiguity as a way of *clarifying transference manifestations* and of *maximizing regression in the service of the ego.* On the other hand, in the client-centered approach of Carl Rogers, as well as in the psychobiological approach, the accent is more upon *acceptance of the patient as he is* and *clarification* of the patient's self-defeating, symptom-connected interpersonal operations. Most psychotherapists utilize *abreaction* or *catharsis,* the relief from tension obtained by simple impulse expression in a permissive setting. In all psychotherapies the therapist reinforces through repeated, nonverbal patterns of response in the interview certain behaviors and tends to extinguish others. Learning-theory therapists tend to utilize the *operant conditioning processes* explicitly as a means of influence. The *educative* or psychopedagogical aspects of psychotherapy, in which the therapist acts as a parent or teacher in protecting or leading the patient, are recognized by all schools of therapy.

The psychobiologists particularly stress the value of *systematic rational review* of the patient's life history and symptom development. The *psychobiological point of view* is particularly adapted to psychotherapy within the traditional medical context and can be readily combined with physical examinations, drugs, or other physical therapies. It is based upon the principle of *negotiation.* The patient is encouraged to spell out his view of the nature of his symptom pattern and the physician then presents his or her view. Certain empirical attempts at trying this or that remedial behavior or attitude may serve to convince the patient or physician of the correct formulation or may bring to light new information. No rigid limits or requirements are placed upon the patient and any or all of the principles and processes described in this section may come into play at one time or another in this approach.

When patients displace upon the therapist irrational or infantile attitudes, originally developed in relation to early familial figures, the behavior is referred to as parataxic or prototaxic (by the Sullivanian therapists) or as a *transference manifestation.* Such inappropriate expressions often evoke emotional feelings or behaviors in the therapist. When consciously sensed and controlled, these *countertransference manifestations* are among the most informative psychotherapeutic phenomena. They may be further classified as to whether they are the outcome of a momentary *complementary identification* with the patient (in which the therapist's feeling of anger, for example, would complement the patient's provocativeness) or the outcome of a momentary *concordant identification* (in which the therapist's feeling of helplessness, say, agreed with the patient's experience). In the psychoanalytic frame of refence, constructive changes in patients are considered a result of *transference cures* or of the *release of conflicted portions of the ego* to grow and make fresh identifications. The process of *identification,* unlike conditioning or rational learning, refers to the total shift in inner psychological forces rather than to changes in specific behaviors or feelings. While no therapist encourages his patients to emulate him, it is nevertheless true that patients can sense more useful ways of thinking, feeling, or reacting by relying on the therapist's understanding as a kind of borrowed ego. In instances in which the usual *nonjudgmental* and *nondirective* attitudes have been tried without effect over a long period of time or in which the patient seems on the verge of foolish, precipitous action the therapist can become quite active, giving *advice* or even exhorting. Such a direct approach, to be effective and scientifically based, must be eschewed on most occasions.

SUPERVISION AND CONSULTATION

Whether the psychiatrist is a beginner or an expert in psychotherapy, there will be cases in which regular sharing of personal experiences and problems with a skilled outside therapist will serve to remove areas of selective inattention by the therapist and to clarify further the patient's problems. A collaborative atmosphere should be fostered in which the supervisor or consultant seeks to sense vicariously how the patient presents himself and his difficulties. Reporting by the psychotherapist may be by playing a tape recording, by reading from detailed notes, or by depending on memory of the patient's communications to summarize and formulate the latter's behavior. By presenting the interplay between patient and psychiatrist and focusing equally upon the experiences of both persons in the relationship, or by emphasizing heavily the psychotherapist's own subjective fantasies, feelings, and behavior while in the patient's presence, the consultant can clarify otherwise obscure facets of the treatment interaction. Each of these aspects may shed a somewhat different light upon the case. Perhaps in most successful supervision a mixture of all these processes takes place. The beginning psychotherapist would do well to avoid either too great a dependence upon or too great a competitiveness with the mentor.

TERMINATION OF PSYCHOTHERAPY

The question of when to end the relationship depends upon the needs and capacities of the patient and the goals set at the beginning. Symptomatic relief with some modifications in behavior can—in some patients—apparently be achieved in a very few interviews. With most patients, however, regardless of the frequency of interviews, it is well to plan on a period of several months to several years before closing the door. Even then it is well to leave with the patient the knowledge of a continued interest and of his freedom to return if necessary for further work. The neophyte psychotherapist would do well to regard any unexpected sudden desire, either on the patient's part or on his own, to end the relationship as a possible manifestation of transference or countertransference anxiety. Decision to terminate may take into consideration such factors as the current severity of symptoms, the current directions of change in the patient, the degree of stress or support in the patient's environment, the patient's latent potentiality for further constructive changes, and his motivation to undertake further psychotherapy.

SUGGESTED READINGS

Fenichel, O.: Problems of psychoanalytic technique, Albany, N.Y., 1941, The Psychoanalytic Quarterly, Inc.

Frank, J. D.: Recent American research in psychotherapy, Br. J. Med. Pscyhol. **41:**5, March, 1968.

Karasu, T. B.: Psychotherapies: an overview, Am. J. Psychiatry **134:**851, 1977.

Luborsky, L., Singer, B., and Luborsky, L.: Comparative studies of psychotherapies, Arch. Gen. Psychiatry **32:**995, 1975.

Sloane, R. B.: Psychotherapy versus behavior therapy, Cambridge, 1975, Harvard University Press.

VARIETIES OF PSYCHOTHERAPEUTIC APPROACHES
Psychoanalysis

The most elaborate conceptual frame of reference for psychotherapy is that developed by Sigmund Freud. Classic pyschoanalysis rests upon five points of view, each of them tied to rather extensive theoretical speculations and observations about human experience. While most psychotherapies draw upon various of Freud's discoveries, only psychoanalysis utilizes all five points of view. The *topographical* approach assumes that the mind contains three regions, the unconscious, the preconscious, and the conscious. The *genetic principle* states that present patterns of functioning shall be understood in terms of past experience and that neurotic phenomena are essentially manifestations of fixation at or regression to earlier developmental levels. Here lies the importance to the theory of the three stages of pregenital development: it provides a basis for classifying psychopathology according to whether the conflicts and defenses seem more to be oral, anal, or phallic. According to the *dynamic point of view* overt behavior and conscious experience are seen as outcomes of a struggle between the *instinctual impulses* to find expression and the counter forces *(countercathexes)* which operate to maintain self-control and self-esteem. The *economic viewpoint* states that the question of whether a patient is sick or well or whether he permits expression of impulses is a question of distribution of energies between the portions of the mind. If too large a proportion of energies is locked in unconscious conflict, fatigue and decreasing capacity for dealing with external stimuli *(reality)* result. The *structural point of view* is a working formulation which refers to the inner reservoir of basic aggressive and sexual energies (all unconscious) as the *id;* to the apparatus of control and mediation between action, sensation, and inner need as the *ego;* and to the internalized parental and guiding social models as the *superego* and *ego-ideal.* The psychic processes of the id are dominated by the *pleasure principle* and are referred to as *primary processes* (association by contiguity, displacement, condensation, and similarity). The functions of the ego are *perception, logical thought, memory, judgment, synthesis of experience,* and *control of motility* and are characterized as the *secondary processes* (association by logical, temporospatial, and causal relations).

The goal of psychoanalysis is to produce structural changes in the patient's ego by re-creating and resolving the *infantile neurosis.* The re-creation of the early pathogenic situation within the therapeutic relationship is called the *transference neurosis.* It is permitted to emerge by the use of the couch, with analyst sitting behind or out of the patient's line of vision, by meeting three to six times a week, and by encouraging the patient to follow the *basic rule of free association*. The patient is instructed to say everything which occurs to him, without censorship. As he listens the analyst adopts an *attitude of freefloating attention* in which he vacillates between vicarious emotional participation and objective evaluation and review. Classically the transference neurosis is resolved only through insight; that is, the analyst's *interpretations* are the instrument of cure. Early in the analysis interpretations are directed only at *resistances* to progress; later, basic conflicts are interpreted, as well. Following a prolonged period of *working through* in which the patient attempts to shift to new ways of handling life experience, and following resolution of the transference and countertransference distortions, the analysis is terminated.

SUGGESTED READINGS

Alexander, F., and French, T.: Psychoanalytic therapy, New York, 1946, The Ronald Press Co.

Brill, A. A.: Lectures on psychoanalytic psychiatry, New York, 1946, Alfred A. Knopf, Inc.

Dewald, P. A.: The process of change in psychoanalytic psychotherapy, Arch. Gen. Psychiatry **35**:535, 1978.

Dewald, P. A.: Toward a general concept of the therapeutic process, Int. J. Psychoanal. Psychother. **5**:283, 1976.

Fenichel, O.: Problems of psychonanalytic technique, Albany, N.Y., 1941, The Psychoanalytic Quarterly, Inc.

Freud, S.: The dynamics of the transference. In Collected papers, New York, 1959, Hogarth Press, Ltd., vol. 2.

Fromm-Reichmann, F.: Principles of intensive psychotherapy, Chicago, 1951, University of Chicago Press.

Glover, E.: The technique of psychoanalysis, New York, 1955, International Universities Press, Inc.

Schafer, R.: The termination of brief psychoanalytic psychotherapy, Int. J. Psychoanal. Psychother. **2**:135, 1973.

Jungian psychotherapy

Carl Jung early split off from Sigmund Freud in his theory of personality. A basic difference arose between them as to the sources of psychic energy. While Freud viewed the libido as arising from some chemical substrate in the brain, Jung felt that the nature of psychic energy derived from evolutionary and primitive social myths and archetypes. He found evidence that in all peoples there are common symbols such as the mandala, the symbol of wholeness or the symbol of the whole self. He also pointed out the universality of phallic and other sexual symbols and the common content of fairy tales and religious rituals across different cultures. Jung's theory states that there are these universal unconscious sources of energy. Jung also differentiates within the unconscious specific personality tendencies referred to as "the shadow" and "animus" and "anima." The latter two refer to innate male and female character tendencies which are somewhat universal for all humanity but have a unique form in each individual.

Within this frame of reference the goal of Jungian psychotherapy is self-discovery and rebirth. By this, Jung means that psychotherapy should attempt to identify latent psychological tendencies arising from inner fantasies and feelings. The Jungian therapist tries to assist the individual to find means of expression for these repressed potentials leading to a revision of roles and functions in life. Thus the end result of Jungian psychotherapy is a new life style and a process referred to as individuation.

Underlying the Jungian psychotherapy process is a philosophy of time, space, and matter which differs from the prevalent empirical position of most scientists today. Jung believes that there are certain forces in people and in the universe which are not recognized by modern science but which find expression in extrasensory perception and in the expression of human purposes. He believes in a "synchronistic" or interactive relationship of psychological experience with the brain. Most psychologists today believe that psychological experience is based on neuronal events and on the functioning of the central nervous system. Jung, on the other hand, believes that there are independent psychological energies which interact with the brain within the person but are not dependent upon the nervous system.

In practice there are many competent Jungian therapists whose concern with individuation does not differ substantially from interests of other schools of psychotherapy except with regard to a greater concern for positive potentials arising from the unconscious.

SUGGESTED READINGS

Jacobi, J., and Hull, R. F. C., editors: C. G. Jung's psychological reflections: a new anthology of his writings 1905-1961, Princeton, 1970, Princeton University Press.

Jung, O. G.: Collected works, New York, 1953, Pantheon Books, Inc.

Jung, C. G.: Man and his symbols, Garden City, N. Y., 1964, Doubleday & Co., Inc.

The psychology of Alfred Adler

Alfred Adler, an early disciple of Freud, diverged to found his own school of individual psychology. Its approach differs from that of Freud in stressing goal-directed behavior and social adaptation.

Although emphasizing that persons differ in physical stature, predisposition to illness, etc., he believed it was less the actual inferiority itself than the *feelings of inferiority* in reaction to stresses, frustrations, and failures that shaped the *life style*. He felt that the human was neither a passive recipient of events from without nor of forces from within but rather that he had *innate capabilities* and a *creative power* to fashion his own life course.

Adler's psychology was not that of the individual alone. Innately friendly and cooperative, humans develop a trend to neurotic behavior if parents and teachers are overindulgent or overprotective or if they show the child hatred and rejection. He stressed the importance of birth order: the oldest being displaced by later siblings, the second having to cope with a stronger sibling, the youngest often being petted and indulged, and the only child suffering from lack of social interaction. Females, he felt, developed a *masculine protest* by reason of a world that puts greater premium on male status.

Adler felt that deep inferiority feelings were universal and normal, that they resulted from self-evaluation and led to a striving for superiority. Whereas the world initially appears chaotic to the child, he soon stabilizes it by the building of apperceptual schema (ideas about the world).

Each person develops a *life style* (self, ego, general methods of problem solving, total attitude) which is fixed by the time he is 5 years old. It affects the manner in which he strives to fulfill his goals and wishes in life's constant struggle to become superior. The very effort of striving makes a person seem more adequate. As much of it develops before the child can speak, it is unconscious; i.e., it cannot be verbalized.

Disturbed behavior is due to a maladaptive life style, with feelings of inadequacy and faulty compensatory responses. The same underlying principle exists for all failures or abnormalities, psychotic, neurotic, or whatever psychopathological entities.

The neurotic lives in fear that his exaggerated self-evaluation of superiority will be exposed, and he therefore develops self-guarding tendencies—"neurotic safeguards"—which include both aggressive acts and the seeking of distance by escape and avoidance (suicide, phobia, refusal to act, indecision, etc.); he further guards himself through limiting the sphere of action to that which he can control. Symptoms are formed at the point and time of crisis; hence, the onset of neurosis is seen as failure with life's major tasks (marriage, career, etc.).

To Adler, psychotherapy was essentially a social relationship applicable to all disorders in which the patient directed toward the therapist his habitual modes of reaction to significant persons in his life. By means of this relationship, the therapist could bring about a reduction in the feelings of inferiority and increase the patient's ability to meaningfully interact with others.

The therapist learns about the subjective responses of the patient by empathy and intuitive guessing, by eliciting reports from the patient, and by observing the interrelationships among situational events and the responses that occur in the presence of the therapist. The goals of treatment are (a) to reduce feelings of inferiority, (b) to correct erroneous perceptions and thinking, (c) to develop greater concern for the welfare of others with more affection and skills in interpersonal relations, (d) to reappraise goals, and (e) to increase initiative and courage to act in social situations.

Adler focused treatment on better understanding and felt that, when understanding was complete, improvement automatically followed. It was only necessary that the patient accept the need for change and for collaboration with a therapist whom he liked and trusted.

The therapist is required to remain attentive, sympathetic, and tactful and must maintain patience and tolerance in the face of hostility and resistance. The series of topics explored in therapy include childhood memories, childhood disorders, aggravating life conditions (including "organ inferiority"), family pressures, pampering, rivalry, neurotic patterns within the family, events that precipitate an aggravation of symptoms, birth order, dreams and fantasy, and expressive movements. Initial partial improvement is anticipated to occur within 3 months.

Unfortunately, Adler's writings were poorly systematized; and although much of what he said presaged current interest in ego psychology and has been widely accepted in clinical practice, even in everyday language, yet as a system it has many deficiencies and has now been considerably outdated.

SUGGESTED READINGS

Adler, A.: What life should mean to you, New York, 1958, G. P. Putnam's Sons.

Adler, A.: Problems of neurosis, New York, 1964, Harper & Row, Publishers.

Ansbacher, A. L., and Ansbacher, R. R.: The individual psychology of Alfred Adler, New York, 1956, Basic Books, Inc., Publishers.

Otto Rank's psychotherapeutic approach

Otto Rank, onetime personal secretary to Freud, developed his own separate psychological system. Although his clinical experience was limited mainly to patients with compulsive neurosis and hysteria, he displayed considerable insight into human behavior and his writings have been widely read. Although his theories were loose and poorly organized, he became known for his concepts of *will, counter-will, life-fear, death-fear, birth trauma,* and *end-setting.* He believed that, although situational events played an important role in behavior, man had control over his own destiny. Rank postulated that, although individuals from birth had basic impulses (hunger, sex, thirst), the kinds of responses each showed were individualized and varied with learning. He postulated an original "trauma of birth," which represented a basic conflict and struggle, experienced by all people, between complete dependency and autonomous action. The individual, through exercise of his will, achieves a typical mode of adjustment so that he may live with his conflict in reasonable comfort. In this way Rank's approach was a precursor of more recent interests in existentialism in psychotherapy.

Rank conceptionalized humans as purposive, self-determining individuals with power to control primary physiological responses (drives) and affects (fear, guilt) and to select constructive, creative responses. Rank believed that neurotic behavior developed when fear and guilt became chronic or strong and when self-directing patterns were inadequate to control. The nature of the behavior disorder is determined by the nature of the patient's fear—either assertive-independent (life-fear) or submissive-helpless (death-fear). In this philosophy neurotics are considered not to be persons of action; they are thought to substitute thinking instead, and their self-evaluations are negative. Rank believed that an individual could stop his affective thoughts, could suppress them, and thereby reduce his discomfort. He rejected Freud's "psychology of the unconscious" as only furthering the neurotic attempt to avoid assuming responsibility for his own behavior.

The goals of treatment are (a) to change the patient's thoughts about himself from being critical and rejecting to approving and accepting and (b) to change the affective responses from negative to positive. With fear and guilt thus reduced and with self-confidence thus established, overt behavior could become constructive rather than avoidant. Man needs some kind of belief to be happy, and Rank's therapeutic attempts were directed toward giving him that belief in the form of faith in himself.

Rank outlined few techniques of therapy but felt that the therapist, from personal knowledge and experience, would develop a new technique tailored for each patient. After reducing his fears to a controllable level, the patient is encouraged to take the initiative in the treatment process. The therapy period focuses on discussing the here-and-now as an experience in living rather than as a mere discussion. Little attention is paid to content, but the therapist gets the patient to experience the full range of emotional expressions in the treatment situation and to learn to control and accept his emotional reactions toward others. The therapist makes no moral evaluation; he or she does not punish the patient through criticism, evaluation, or derogatory remarks. Past history is explored only if it leads to a clearer understanding of the current situation. The patient is encouraged to express openly all behaviors and connected emotions (fear, pride, shame, etc.). Dreams are discussed only in a symbolic way by discussing responses which were already conscious in another form. Free association is not used, as it would weaken the patient's control of directing his thoughts.

The patient is encouraged to react to the therapist emotionally as to human beings in general. The therapist guards against too strong a dependent emotional attachment through early establishment of a date the treatment process will terminate (*end-setting*) and manipulating the length of time of the therapy session as a reality factor. This planned ending of psychotherapy is believed to assist the patient to reexperience with greater mastery earlier separation and birth traumas.

SUGGESTED READINGS

Rank, O.: Will therapy and truth and reality, New York, 1950, Alfred A. Knopf, Inc.

Rank, O.: Otto Rank, New York, 1958, Julian Press, Inc.

Taft, J.: The trauma of birth, New York, 1952, Robert Brunner.

Psychotherapy in the mode of Karen Horney

Dr. Horney was one of the first of the early psychoanalytic group to join with Harry Stack Sullivan and to emphasize the importance of the social environment and the cultural stresses in accounting for neurotic phenomena. She fully accepts the basic concepts of psychoanalysis such as repression, the unconscious, and the use of defense mechanisms but emphasizes much more in her dealing with patients a careful analysis of actual, present-day life stress. Thus, Horney has contributed to a reorientation of psychiatry toward current conflicts (marital, job, and cross-cultural) as now expressed in the recent A.P.A. classification under the heading of "Social Maladjustment."

Horney, like Jung, has felt that the task of psychotherapy lies in the direction of clarification of the individual's identity and preferred social mode of functioning. Unlike Jung and Freud, however, she places less emphasis on working to understand innate or inner conflicting tendencies, such as conflicts between the drives, and places greater emphasis on the psychological tasks of resolving pressures from current and past social relationships. For example, in relation to understanding dream content she would be somewhat more likely to interpret dream material as expressions of actual life choices and alternatives rather than simply as expressions of primitive biologically based conflicts.

Horney's view of anxiety has depended somewhat less on the structural theory of the personality and more upon unresolved social conflicts.

SUGGESTED READINGS

Horney, K.: The neurotic personality of our time, New York, 1937, W. W. Norton & Co., Inc.

Horney, K.: Self-analysis, New York, 1942, W. W. Norton & Co., Inc.

Horney, K.: Neurosis and human growth, New York, 1950, W. W. Norton & Co., Inc.

Client-centered psychotherapy

Client-centered psychotherapy was developed by Rogers and his school in the period from 1938 to 1950. The use of the word *client* was intended to underscore a focus on the internal phenomenological world of the client, indicating that the individual seeking help was perceived as a self-responsible person rather than as an object (patient) for treatment. The distinctive characteristics of this therapy include (a) the hypothesis that certain attitudes in the therapist constitute the necessary and sufficient conditions for treatment, (b) the concept that the therapist is immediately accessible to the client in the experiencing of the treatment relationship, (c) a continuing focus on the phenomenological world of the client, (d) the theory that therapeutic process is marked by a change in the client's manner of experiencing, along with an increased ability to live more fully, (e) a continuing emphasis on the self-actualizing quality of a human organism as the motivational force in therapy, (f) a focus on the process of personality change rather than upon the structure of the personality, (g) an emphasis on the need for continued research upon the method of psychotherapy, (h) the belief that the same principles of psychotherapy apply to psychotic, neurotic, and normal individuals, and (i) the opinion that psychotherapy is but one specialized example of all constructive interpersonal relationships.

In client-centered psychotherapy it is stressed that success in treatment is not so much dependent upon the technical training or skills of the therapist as it is upon the presence of certain attitudes in the therapist. Therapeutic progress and personality change depend upon the communication of these attitudes and their perception by the client. These important attitudes include (a) the therapist's genuineness or congruence, (b) the therapist's complete acceptance and unconditional positive regard for the client, and (c) a sensitive emphathic understanding of the client. Throughout the treatment process the therapist openly reflects the feelings and attitudes being experienced via self-awareness. Genuine positive regard for the client is communicated in a warm acceptance of the client's expressions regardless of their nature. It is important not to imply disapproval of painful, hostile, defensive, or abnormal feelings but to accept them in the same manner as good, positive, and mature feelings without the necessity of making judgment. Thus the therapist creates a "safe" environment in which the client is motivated to explore his own deepest thoughts and feelings and to share them with another human being. The therapist develops an empathy in which he or she is completely at home in the client's world, sensing and understanding the client's inner world of personal private meanings as if it were his or her own world.

It is important for therapeutic success that the client reciprocate the therapist's attitudes, that, in an atmosphere of complete acceptance, he express his thoughts and feelings little by little, and that he become increasingly able to listen to communications from within himself. He realizes best at a time when he is angry, frightened, or experiencing feelings of love that he can reveal these hidden and "awful" aspects of himself without changing the therapist's regard for him, and slowly he moves toward adopting this same attitude toward himself, i.e., accepting himself as he is. Finally, he is free to change and grow in the directions which are natural to the maturing organism. From a position of remoteness he moves toward an immediacy of experiencing to discover its current meaning. There is no time limit on the therapy, and, indeed, it is felt that even in a relatively limited number of hours significant changes in personality attitudes and behavior can be produced.

SUGGESTED READINGS

Rogers, C. R.: Client-centered therapy, Boston, 1951, Houghton Mifflin Co.

Rogers, C. R.: On becoming a person, Boston, 1961, Houghton Mifflin Co.

Rogers, C. R., Gendlin, E. T., Kelser, D. J., and Truax, C. B.: The therapeutic relationship and its impact: a study of psychotherapy with schizophrenics, Madison, 1967, University of Wisconsin Press.

The learning theory approach to psychotherapy

The learning theory approach to psychotherapy leans heavily on the assumption that individual behavior is shaped by patterns of response from the social environment. As with behavior in animals, human behavior is considered to be learned in an automatic fashion; man's freedom to direct his own behavior is more apparent than real. In the course of growth and development, each person is taught by others ways of handling and reducing the intensity of such drives as hunger, thirst, curiosity, and sex. External events connected with these satisfactions acquire for him an individual and motivating significance. Fear is a normal response which initiates protective behavior. It may, however, become intense, inappropriate, and too generalized; such a fearful person must learn to reduce the intensity of the fear so that other functionally important behavior is not disrupted. The richness of behavior in man, as compared with animals, is made possible by thoughts which can stand in the place of action.

The kinds of habit patterns, both of action and of thought, learned in dealing with drives and emotions, are characteristic for each individual. The acquisition of disordered behavior follows these same principles of learning as does normal behavior. Neurosis is thus seen as the result of faulty child-rearing practices and the pressures of unhealthy social customs. Thus the environment may have taught the child a conflict between the sex drive and the need to reduce fear. Besides conflict based upon incompatible drives, there can be conflict stemming from incompatible rewards and punishments presented simultaneously from the environment.

The learning theorists speak of *avoidance conflicts* (of which fear is the most important) and *approach conflicts* (in which incompatible goals exist). The gradient concept relates to increase of intensity with either a spatial or temporal proximity to the conflict. Conflict may be solved temporarily by running away for a time, by the suspension of all activity, by suppression, or by repression. Repression places a conflict beyond conscious awareness and thus renders neurosis inaccessible to ready verbal examination, as is also true of conflicts formed in the child before speech patterns were developed.

Factors predisposing to a neurosis include poor childhood training and inconsistent behavior on the part of teachers and parents, particularly when children are small and helpless and easily influenced due to a limited choice of behavioral action. Society often provides a matrix with built-in conflicts, relating especially to patterns associated with eating, elimination, sexual responses, and aggressive behavior. In some cases a chance exposure to some emotion-provoking event triggers the neurosis.

The symptoms that develop from fear and anxiety are both physiological—cardiac, gastrointestinal, etc.—and learned—phobias, compulsions, etc. Thus the patient appears both miserable and, due to his maladaptive behavior, somewhat stupid.

The learning theorists believe that removal of symptoms is not a sufficient goal of treatment but rather that the underlying conflict must be searched out and relieved. Therapeutic goals are designed to help the patient acquire a conscious control over his thoughts, to help him unlearn the consequences of inhibition and inadequate responses, and to help him learn to consciously delay responses and substitute more adequate and discriminative responses by the use of higher mental process.

The therapist seeks to discover the kinds of events that elicit anxiety and the kinds of responses involved. The patient is taught through free association to reveal his full train of thoughts and emotional sensations. The therapist demonstrates this art through an ability to observe carefully and to accurately identify crucial behavior sequences. In judging which events can be manipulated, intended behavior modification is achieved by helping the patient *extinguish* (get rid of) old, inadequate responses and *learn* new, adaptive ones. In the interview situation the therapist must give the appearance of a nice kind of person with whom the patient can identify, yet must be sufficiently neutral so that the patient can generalize, in his interaction with the therapist, patterns and responses he uses with others. It is not enough that new behavior patterns are discussed; they must also be tried out in real life; and if failure occurs, they can be discarded or tried differently anew.

The therapist must remain free from emotional involvement and unaffected by the acts and emotions of the patient. He or she must show restraint and must have sufficient sensitivity to the feelings of others to empathize with the patient, to maintain a positive attitude, and to instill sufficient motivation to continue treatment.

The actual work in the treatment hour consists of maintaining a verbal productivity, keeping the patient focused on productive themes, and overcoming hesitance and blocking by explanations or interpretations of any resistance to speak and to explore. The therapist points out responses that are occurring but should not occur, and initiates responses that are not occurring but should occur; unmasks the true meaning of acts and thoughts that are but repetitive or symbolic; points out ways to modify the fear response; helps the patient identify and appropriately label attitudes and emotions, and leads the patient toward satisfying episodes of behavior; uses the therapeutic interaction as a real-life model—movies, videotape, or specially designed group experiences may be presented regularly so that, in graded fashion, the appropriate responses may be seen in others and learned by imitation of these others in action.

SUGGESTED READINGS

Dollard, J., and Miller, N. E.: Personality and psychotherapy: an analysis in terms of learning, thinking and culture, New York, 1952, McGraw-Hill Book Co.

Hilgard, E. R.: Theories of learning, New York, 1956, Appleton-Century-Crofts.

Mowrer, O. H.: Learning theory and the symbolic process, New York, 1960, John Wiley & Sons, Inc.

Hypnotherapy

The history of hypnosis has been characterized by periods of great interest and of rejection. Beginning with Franz Mesmer (1734-1815), its proponents have included James Esdaile (1808-1859), a Scottish surgeon; James Braid (1795-1860), a Manchester physician; A. A. Liebeault (1823-1904), a French country physician in Nancy; Hippolyte Bernheim (1837-1919), a professor of medicine who worked with Liebeault; Jean Charcot (1825-1893), of the Salpêtrière in Paris; Joseph Breuer (1841-1925), a Viennese physician; Sigmund Freud (1856-1939); Morton Prince (1854-1929), founder of the Harvard Psychological Clinic; Clark Hull, Professor of Psychology at Yale; and, more recently, Grinker,

Spiegel, Brenman, Gill, Erikson, Wolberg, Hilgard, Barber, Orne, and others. Recent experimental work has suggested a physiological predictor (EEG) of hypnotizability and has shown that changes in brain electrical activity with hypnosis differ from the EEG patterns of moderate or deep sleep and rather suggest a state of increased vigilance.

Hypnosis has been widely used in obstetrics, dentistry, and surgery and has found many applications in medicine, including psychiatry, where its appropriate use in selected cases can expedite and shorten the process of psychotherapy. The concept of the "hypnotist" is to be rejected. Rather hypnosis should be considered a useful tool, an extension of the doctor-patient relationship which can affect the ease and speed of communication. Hypnotizability is the ability to accept uncritically and to act upon a verbal or nonverbal suggestion, given either directly or indirectly, either deliberately or inadvertently. It is an intrinsic characteristic of the human mind, present in all individuals to a variable degree, and operative more or less all of the time. It is our experience that the great majority of patients can achieve a degree of hypnosis that is helpful to treatment.

There is probably in all of medicine no technique in which the doctor plays so active, directive, and authoritative a role and in which, on occasion, his ministrations can gain such prompt and dramatic results as with hypnosis. It should be remembered, however, that behavior and mood alteration or even symptom removal during the trace state is no substitute for an understanding of the dynamics, nor is an abreaction alone so valuable as the integration of acquired insights into conscious awareness.

A good doctor-patient relationship, rapport, and positive suggestion blend imperceptibly into hypnosis. Patients vary greatly in the extent to which they show signs of deep hypnosis (amnesia, somnambulism, and posthypnotic suggestion). About 20% of all persons can achieve a deep hypnotic trance on the first attempt, and practically all can be helped by light hypnoidal states or simply positive suggestion.

Hypnosis is readily accomplished. Many elaborate induction methods and rituals are described in readily available texts. Most of these, however, simply involve principles of restricting the perceptual field/visual fixation), monotonous suggestion ("sle-e-e-e-p, relax, sle-e-e-e-p, relax," etc.), visualization ("TV screens"), and confusing verbalization ("When you are sure you can't open your eyes, try to open them to make sure you can't."). A simple method is to have the subject gaze upward at a pencil until the eyes feel tired and close. "You feel so relaxed and sleepy—relax, relax, let yourself go—away-y-y in-n-n." "When you are sure your eyes won't open, try to open them." "Let your head fall." Words are repeated in a low voice and monotonous manner. Successful suggestions tested by successful challenges deepen the trance. (Suggest and test for anesthesia, suggest arm levitation, etc.)

The skillful hypnotist tailors this technique to the needs of the patient (i.e., uses visual techniques with those who visualize well, arm levitation with tense, poor visualizers, etc.). The trance should be structured so that something useful can be accomplished. The ultimate purpose should be a more traditional psychiatric approach in which hypnosis is merely one tool. In exploring the patient's past life, it may be important to relive earlier life periods. This can be helped by *age regression* accomplished by hypnosis. The patient may play-act events of earlier years. Other useful techniques include *hypnotic dream induction, automatic writing, visualization under hypnosis, role playing of hypnotically induced conflicts,* and *abreaction.* The therapeutic process can continue after the treatment hour by means of *posthypnotic suggestions.* Here by the setting of a predicted, neutral, and nonembarrassing time for their appearance, significant memories may be brought to consciousness.

In summary: (1) People are suggestible and may be helped by positive suggestion, given deliberately or under hypnosis. (2) Formal hypnotic techniques may be used as a part of, but not as a substitute for, the psychotherapeutic approach. (3) Properly used, hypnosis is a useful adjunct to psychotherapeutic methods and may greatly shorten the time needed to reach the desired therapeutic goal.

SUGGESTED READINGS

Barber, T. X.: Hypnotizability, suggestibility and personality; part V, a critical review of research findings, Psychol. Rep. **14**:229, 1964.

Brenman, H., and Gill, M.: Hypnotherapy, New York, 1947, International Universities Press, Inc.

Kline, M. V.: Clinical correlations of experimental hypnosis, Springfield, Ill., 1963, Charles C Thomas, Publisher.

Meares, A.: A system of medical hypnosis, Philadelphia, 1960, W. B. Saunders Co.

Orne, M. T.: Hypnosis, motivation and compliance, Am. J. Psychiatry **122:**721, 1966.

Ulett, G. A., Akpinar, S., and Itil, T. M.: Hypnosis—physiological, pharmacological reality, Am. J. Psychiatry **128:**7, 1971.

Ulett, G. A., and Peterson, D. B.: Applied hypnosis and positive suggestion, St. Louis, 1965, The C. V. Mosby Co.

Winn, R. B.: Dictionary of hypnosis, New York, 1965, Philosophical Library, Inc.

Wolberg, L. R.: Medical hypnosis, New York, 1948, Grune & Stratton, Inc., vols. 1 and 2.

Psychotherapy through reciprocal inhibition

The *reciprocal inhibition* approach to psychotherapy represents a serious alternative to the repression theory approach. It is based upon the assumption that neurotic habits are learned and can best be eliminated through unlearning. It is only necessary that the therapist arrange for the proper sequence of events.

The therapeutic model is based upon the *drive reduction* conditioning theories of Clark Hull.

Habits result as a recurring response to a given stimulus. Such a response may be generalized to other situations which are similar or contain an element in common even though inappropriate. Habits become stronger when rewarded and tend to become inhibited when reward is lacking. Other stimuli occurring simultaneously interfere with a habit's recurrence on future occasions.

A special case of conditioned inhibition occurs when a response antagonistic to the response to be extinguished is associated with it, as both responses cannot occur simultaneously. Thus, through proper association, one can be strengthened and the other extinguished. Wolpe, with whose name this approach is commonly associated, states that neuroses are learned behavior patterns, basically unadaptive, conditioned anxiety reactions. The resultant anxiety disrupts major aspects of an individual's life or restricts or limits his behavior. Predisposing conditions are physiological differences in reactivity to anxiety-provoking situations. Some persons, through previous learning, have already acquired many inappropriate anxiety responses. Other predisposing factors are fatigue, drugs, hormones, etc.

Precipitating events produce severe anxiety. Fear may be associated with any of a number of events that were present at the time of the major fear stimulus. Previously conditioned childhood emotions may serve as a focus of restriction of the number of responses in a person's repertoire and may result in inadequate responses as may also a misinterpretation of the situation. Not only events but also thoughts can become anxiety elicitors. Associated events that have occurred at the same time as anxiety is produced may also elicit anxiety—shadows, odors, noises, etc.; it only demands that they make an impression on the central nervous system. Associated with the anxiety may be physiological changes, such as increased pulse rate or respiration, and these in turn may also become elicitors. Once anxiety becomes a habitual occurrence, it may impair other aspects of a person's behavior. Muscle tension may produce headaches, thinking may be disrupted, and psychosomatic symptoms, stomach reactions, etc., may occur. These symptoms produce more anxiety, and a vicious circle results.

The patient himself may learn to control anxiety by (a) physical avoidance, (b) displacing his attention, (c) the use of drugs, alcohol, etc., (d) the development of excessive and compulsive behavior which exerts control, or (e) amnesia—forgetting the content of the emotional response.

The goals of therapy are (a) to alter to extinguish the symptoms and (b) to help the patient unlearn the anxiety response to inappropriate events.

In order to effect behavioral change, anxiety-eliciting situations must be presented to the patient under circumstances in which responses other than anxiety will occur. The first step is to identify the troublesome anxiety sequences and to select the appropriate treatment procedures. The patient is presented with events, situations or responses, or symbolic representations of such events which inappropriately elicit anxiety and symptoms, and these learned conditions are then weakened. A sufficient number of repetitions must occur so that the troublesome connections will be abolished and more adaptive behavior will take place.

Among techniques used by the therapist are (a) assertive responses, including anger or friendly responses, (b) sexual responses, (c) muscular relaxation, (d) respiratory responses using CO_2, (e) competitively conditioned motor responses, (f) anxiety relief responses, (g) pleasant responses in life situations, e.g., with drug enhancement, and (h) interview-induced emotional response and abreactions.

The therapist collects data on which to judge events: the patient's behavior, present life situation, etc.; determines what stimuli do or can evoke symptoms at the present time; and collects data on developmental history with emphasis on habitual emotional responses in each setting. Such tests as the Bernreuter Self Sufficiency questionnaire and the Willoughby Personality Schedule (a kind of systematic interview) are employed.

The goals of therapy include symptom improvement, increased productiveness, increased adjustment to and pleasure in sex, improved interpersonal relationships, and improved ability to handle and to change psychological conflicts and reality stresses. Improvements is judged by the patient's report, the reports of others, clinical assessments, and changes in the Willoughby scale. The first step to changing neurotic behavior is by acting, not by thinking.

Therapy relationship as a general procedure is a human interaction which provokes emotions, friendly sympathetic experiences. Assertive responses are used in life situations—aggressive, relaxing, affectionate, sexual—only when anxieties are provoked by interpersonal situations. The therapist sells the patient on the idea of trying it in a real-life situation and then discusses and corrects the patient's performance. Behavior is shaped by consequences—systematic desensitization occurs during interviews. The therapist establishes a list of circumstances eliciting anxiety, from the strongest to the weakest. He trains the patient to muscle relaxation with hypnosis, he forces the patient's attention on anxiety-provoking circumstances, and he then helps him relax. Progress is made from the simplest to the more difficult visualized scenes. CO_2 respiratory responses may be used for freefloating anxiety. CO_2 produces muscle relaxation and is antagonistic to anxiety. Competitive motor responses are produced in the presence of conflict situations—through the patient's imagery in the treatment situation. Mild shocks may elicit other motor responses than those usually associated with anxieties. Real life behavior is the most effective therapeutic tool, and the patient is urged to experience success in the community.

Proponents of this theory believe that the majority of candidates for psychotherapy can be significantly helped, with a relatively small number of sessions.

SUGGESTED READINGS

Bugenthal, J. F. T.: Search for authenticity, New York, 1965, Holt, Rinehart & Winston, Inc.

Eysenck, H. J.: Behavior therapy and the neurosis, New York, 1960, Pergamon Press, Inc.

Eysenck, H. J., and Rachman, S.: The causes and cures of neurosis, San Diego, Calif., 1965, R. R. Knapp.

Franks, C. M., editor: Conditioning techniques in clinical practice and research, New York, 1964, Springer Publishing Co., Inc.

Parker, B.: My language is me, New York, 1962, Basic Books, Inc., Publishers.

Strupp, H. H.: Psychotherapists in action, New York, 1960, Grune & Stratton, Inc.

Ulman, L. P., and Krasner, L., editors: Case studies in behavior modification, New York, 1965, Holt, Rinehart & Winston, Inc.

Wolpe, J.: Psychotherapy by reciprocal inhibition, Stanford, Calif., 1958, Stanford University Press.

Wolpe, J.: The experimental foundations of some new psychotherapeutic methods. In Bachrach, A. J., editor: Experimental frontiers of clinical psychology, New York, 1962, Basic Books, Inc., Publishers.

Transactional analysis

Transactional analysis (T.A.) was developed from the attempts of Dr. Eric Berne to create a unified system of individual and social psychiatry, both comprehensive at the theoretical level and effective at the applied level. Although similar in some concepts, T.A. opposes the use of the elaborate language and definitions of psychoanalysis. Instead it substitutes the vocabulary of the man in the street. T.A. is operationally a method of examining the stimulus-response patterns of an individual with the goal of personality growth through an understanding of how one's habitual manner of responding developed and by substituting more mature response patterns. Thus T.A. begins by analyzing, "I do something to you and you do something back."

Three active elements are distinguished in each person: Parent, Adult, and Child. The Parent describes the "don't's" and a few "do's" implanted in one's earliest years and hence accepted as gospel. The Child represents spontaneous emotion. Both Parent and Child must be kept in proper relation to the Adult, whose function is seen as that of a reality-oriented computer that formulates decisions based upon the data of experience. The goal of T.A. is the strengthening and emancipation of the Adult from the archaic recordings in Parent and Child to make possible the freedom of choice and creation of new options.

Four life positions are assumed: (1) I'm not OK—you're OK (immature). (2) I'm not OK—you're not OK (despair). (3) I'm OK—you're not OK (criminal). (4) I'm OK—you're OK (mature adult at peace with himself and others). T.A. is well suited to group treatment where there is an abundance of transactions to analyze.

SUGGESTED READINGS

Berne, E.: Games people play, New York, 1964, Grove Press.

Berne, E.: Transactional analysis in psychotherapy, New York, 1961, Grove Press.

Harris, T.: I'm OK—you're OK, New York, 1967, Harper & Row, Publishers.

Relaxation and biofeedback techniques

Relaxation is an old technique. Healing temples for rites of relaxation and meditation, spas, and baths abound in the early history of civilization. Stress has long been with mankind. Relaxation through hypnosis was recorded in Egypt 4000 years ago and is still used today. In a modern adaptation, Johannes Schultz's Autogenic Training uses rote repetition of relaxing phrases: "my right foot is heavy, both feet are heavy," "heartbeat calm and regular," etc., with phrases repeated daily until both outer and inner parts of the body are relaxed.

Ancient meditation techniques from the Far East, yoga, and Zen Buddhism have all had a recent rebirth in the form of transcendental meditation (T.M.). These have long been acceptable means for controlling body physiology. Posture and breathing exercises are commonly used together with repetition of some verbal formula, such as a mantra (two-syllable Indian word) so that concentration is focused on a nonemotional act and worries are hence blocked out. In 1929 Edmund Jacobson wrote of progressive relaxation. He recommended a process in which each limb and body part (legs, arms, trunk, eyelids, eyes, etc.) were the center of relaxation practice for days at a time. Finally after weeks, or longer in some cases, visual imagery was accomplished and improved.

The most modern and highly publicized of these techniques is biofeedback. Using electronic circuitry, muscle tension (EMG), heart rate, blood pressure, EEG, skin temperature, galvanic skin response, and any other physiological function whose changes are accessible to electronic recording, are monitored. The change (improvement) in body function is converted into a signal (sound or light), whose variation is then "fed back" to the patient. The latter (listening through earphones or watching the monitor light but otherwise relaxed) is thus made aware of his progress in controlling blood pressure, etc. Although high claims for specificity have been made for this technique it is often apparent that achieving the relaxation of one part of the autonomic nervous system also requires relaxation of voluntary muscles, mental functioning, and other bodily functions controlled by the autonomic nervous system as well. The American public's love of gadgetry and competition for sales among equipment manufacturers have popularized this method beyond others despite inadequate evidence of any superiority.

Because much attention is given to stress as a cause of psychophysiological disorder, these techniques are all being used for the treatment of a host of psychosomatic conditions. It has been demonstrated that relaxation techniques can produce a deeper state of relaxation of some body responses than are seen in natural sleep and that they occur much more quickly. Thus it is usual to prescribe one or two 20-minute periods of relaxation daily. Significant changes in lowered blood pressure and relief from tension, vascular headaches, GI disturbances, etc., have been achieved by these methods. It is necessary to carry out the relaxation practice daily and indefinitely, however, as cessation of relaxation leads in many cases to the prompt return of symptoms.

Acupuncture

A related technique that often promotes relaxation, may assist in healing of psychosomatic illness, and is of considerable assistance in pain control is acupuncture. This is perhaps the most controversial of treatments in contemporary American medicine. A traditional form of Chinese medicine, this treatment modality originated some 5000 years ago and has been of interest in the United States for less than a decade, although it has been widely used in Europe since early in this century and universally acclaimed for its pain-relieving qualities. Despite abundant clinical documentation, careful research work is only now beginning to appear. American physicians have failed to embrace acupuncture because it has lacked documented scientific validity and has been taught as a practice based upon ancient Taoist philosophy passed down through the centuries with relatively little change. In acupuncture theory man is thought to be a "microreflection" of the cosmos, with two major forces (Yin and Yang) affecting his energy balance (Chi). Diagnosis is derived from a ritualistic palpation and interpretation of twelve different radial pulses. Therapeutic decisions are based upon formulae involving the relationship of five basic elements (fire, earth, metal, water, wood). Treatment is instituted by the insertion of needles into several of more than 400 carefully described acupuncture points. These latter are located on twelve paired and two unpaired major meridian, hypothetical, lines of force, which traverse the body from head to toe.

Work from many laboratories around the world has recently suggested alternative explanations for the action of acupuncture that are based upon acceptable scientific principles. Foremost among these explanations is Melzack and Wall's gate theory, which postulates a segmental interaction between large and small diameter afferent fibers. Activity in small (A-delta and C) fibers mediating the sensation of pain would open the gate to the afferent pain pathway, whereas activity in large afferent fibers (A-alpha, beta, gamma) would close the gate. This hypothesized mechanism of inhibition and facilitation lies within the substantia gelatinosa of the spinal cord, modifies the ability for cephalad transmission by the T cells, and in turn is modified by descending impulses from higher centers. Other higher level gating mechanisms have been postulated. Chang has demonstrated that stimulation of acupuncture points can interfere directly with the reception of pain impulses in cells of the medial thalamic nuclei. Pertinent findings include recent work identifying some acupuncture points as classic motor points. Some acupuncture points are identified as the trigger areas described in the 1950's by Dr. Travel. Felix Mann has suggested that these points are areas of stimulation for cutaneocutaneous reflexes. Other workers have postulated that the acupuncture message may be carried by chemical mediators resulting from local tissue injury produced by the acupuncture needles. Recent evidence of the role of the hypothalamus in the regulation of immune processes broadens the support for reports of the effectiveness of acupuncture in some allergic and psychosomatic illnesses.

Perhaps the most exciting evidence in support of the effectiveness of acupuncture lies in the recent discovery of the endorphins. These endogenous endokinins, polypeptide substances produced by the pars intermedia of the pituitary, brain, and GI tract, when released block pain receptor sites in the periaqueductal gray matter. They produce a variety of effects on behavior as well through stimulation and inhibition of basal brain structures. Pomeranz has reported that removing the pituitary gland, the probable source of endorphin release, blocks the pain-relieving action of acupuncture. Goldstein and co-workers have shown that electrical stimulation of the brain releases endorphins and completely blocks pain. They have described endorphins as a ". . . built-in tranquilizer for reducing anger and tension" as well as for modifying chronic pain.

From a review of these data it would appear that there are several mechanisms by which acupuncture needles inserted into the skin may produce physiological effects in the body, including attenuation of pain. Different points and different methods of stimulation may well account for the different types of therapeutic results. While, as seen in the foregoing, much emphasis on acupuncture research has dealt with the problem of pain, with less documented rationale acupuncture is widely used for psychosomatic illness and in the Orient particularly for the treatment of psychiatric and emotional disorders. At the 1000-bed Shanghai Institute of Psychiatry one of the authors has seen the routine use of electrically stimulated needles in the scalp, temples, and suboccipital areas as a major therapy for schizophrenia. Instructions prepared for Chinese Health Department personnel as well as manuals on acupuncture currently available in the United States chart the points on the skin where needles are placed for the treatment of various psychiatric diseases. In China acupuncture treatment for mental illness is usually not given alone but is combined with the use of selected herbs in accordance with traditional Chinese medicine, Western psychotropic medications, and milieu therapy, including group treatment and physical activity.

SUGGESTED READINGS

Andersson, S. A., and Holmgten, E.: On acupuncture analgesia and the mechanism of pain, Am. J. Chin, Med. 3:311-334, 1975.

An Outline of Chinese Acupuncture; The academy of Traditional Chinese Medicine, Peking, 1975, Foreign Language Press.

Bellis, J.: Emotional flooding and bioenergetic analysis. In Olsen, P., editor: New directions in psychotherapy: emotional flooding, 1976, New York, Human Sciences Press.

Benson, H.: The relaxation response, New York, 1976, Avon Books.

Blanchard, E. B., and Young, L. D.: Clinical application of biofeedback training, Am. J. Psychiatry 30:573, 1973.

Brown, M. L., Ulett, G. A., and Stern, J. A.: Acupuncture loci: techniques for location, Am. J. Chin. Med. 2(1):67-74, 1974.

Chang, H. T.: Integrative action of thalamus in the process of acupuncture for analgesia, Scientia Sinica 16:26-60, 1973.

Chen, J. V. P.: Acupuncture anesthesia in the People's Republic of China, National Institutes of Health Publication, 75-769, 1973.

Gersten, D. J.: Meditation as an adjunct to medical and psychiatric treatment, Am. J. Psychiatry 135:598, 1987.

Jacobson, E.: Progressive relaxation, Chicago, 1929, University of Chicago Press.

Kim, S. S.: Mediators of acupuncture, Am. J. Acupuncture, 4:28-32, 1976.

Lavenschuss, O.: Electroacupuncture progress and effectiveness, Am. J. Acupuncture 3:347-351, 1975.

Liu, Y. K., Varela, M., and Oswald, R.: The correspondence between some motor points and acupuncture loci, Am. J. Chin. Med. 3(4):347-358, 1975.

Mayer, D. J., Price, D. D., and Rafii, A.: Antagonism of acupuncture analgesia in man by the narcotic antagonist Naloxone, 121:368, 1977.

Mann, F.: Acupuncture. The ancient Chinese art of healing and how it works scientifically, New York, 1973, Vintage Books.

Neurology—Psychiatry in the People's Republic of China, National Institutes of Health Publication, 74-56, 1973.

Nicholas, T.: How to teach yourself meditation, Wilmington, Del., 1975, Enterprise Publishing Co.

Ping, W. W.: Chinese acupuncture. Translated by J. Lavier. Rustington, Sussex, England, 1962, Health Science Press.

Schultz, J., and Luthe, W.: Autogenic training, New York, 1959, Grune & Stratton, Inc.

Yogi, M. M.: Transcendental meditation, New York, 1968, New American
Library.

Brief therapy

Most commonly patients come for relief of symptoms of less
than 6 months' duration or symptoms referable to a recent life situation which has led to intensification of a chronic set of difficulties.
In many such cases it is possible to set rather limited goals and yet
provide the patient with substantial symptomatic relief as well as
some opportunity for psychological growth. The initial *ventilation
of feelings* and *uncovering of major current sources of anxiety* can
most effectively be done in the first or second interview while the
patient is suffering and highly motivated to receive help. Such an
initial contact may extend for 2 hours in order to obtain a full account and demonstrate the physician's concern. The work of
psychotherapy in such situations tries the observational and intuitive capacities of the therapist, who needs to thresh out the wheat
of the precipitating life crisis from the chaff of accumulated but
generally manageable dissatisfactions. This can sometimes be
done through a focus on the situation surrounding the development of the most recent or acute symptom. Once the nidus of current stress has been defined, a confrontation of the patient with the
nature of the situation may give considerable relief through insight, provided the patient's personality is sufficiently resilient. In
patients who exhibit diffuse symptomatology, panic, confusion,
social withdrawal, or bizarre attitudes, an underlying severe personality defect may be suspected, and a more gentle *supportive
approach* be employed. Here the therapist may utilize personal
understanding as a basis for *giving advice* or *clarifying certain assets* in the patient which the latter may be overlooking. At any rate,
in brief therapy one must take special pains to present material to
the patient in ways consistent with the later's self-esteem, since
time has not permitted much testing out of the therapist or development of a deep rapport.

SUGGESTED READING

Small, L.: The briefer psychotherapies, New York, 1971, Brunner/Mazel,
Inc.

23

Group therapy

Since ancient times many leaders, particularly state or religious leaders, have recognized the power of a unified group in producing certain psychological changes within individual members of the group. Wherever individuals form such a stable group for the purpose of relieving symptoms or of strengthening certain personality functions, group therapy may be said to exist. Although some of the qualities of a group and part of the direction in which it proceeds depend upon the personality of the group leader, it is important to recognize that any group has the latent power of self-direction; it may, in one way or another, resist a leader who tries to produce changes which are too divergent from the standards, beliefs, or defenses of the members. The effects a group has upon participants' personality or social adjustments seem to be influenced by the tolerance developed within the group for emotional expression, for self-scrutiny without loss of self-esteem, for attempting corrective emotional experiences, and for identifying or empathizing with each other.

In the United States, group therapy was originated by Pratt in 1905 when groups of patients suffering from tuberculosis were brought together to discuss their reality problems, to help each other solve these problems through discussion, and to receive emotional support. In Vienna, Moreno used this technique in 1910 with a group of prostitutes and later in dealing with children's emotional problems. In 1929 Wender began experimenting with group therapy with psychoneurotics and became convinced that for certain patients it was a more powerful tool than individual therapy. Since then, with Marsch's report in 1931 of group therapy with psychotics, with Schilder's and Slavson's use of psychoanalytic concepts in group therapy during the 1930's, and with Moreno's development of psychodrama during the same period, group techniques have had increasing application. Group therapy permits treatment of more patients by a single therapist and therefore has economic advantages. Partly because the military psychiatrist needed to treat many patients at once and partly because of the communality of soldiers' problems, the use of group therapy was greatly increased during World War II.

Very recently there has been a movement toward group experience as the "in thing," a popular way to help people learn by experience how to relate more easily and happily to other people. Such "sensitivity groups" are also known as T-groups, intensive group encounters, personal growth groups, and marathons. That such groups can have a beneficial effect upon a person's day-to-day relationships is attested to by the wide use of this technique by industry in management training. The best of such groups are run by trained professional leaders. Without trained leadership, danger exists that unstable personalities will be overstimulated and stressed to the point of acute emotional disturbances.

No matter what the type of group therapy, special problems arise which make the experience quite different from individual psychotherapy. At the outset it is desirable to plan to group patients together who are sufficiently similar so that sharing of attitudes and experiences will not be made too difficult without, however, having patients so similar that they will rigidly reinforce each other's perceptual distortions or anxieties. In fitting patients together the leader may consider how aggressive or inhibited a candidate seems compared to other members, how anxious he will be made by anticipated behaviors of others, and whether his cultural background and value system have enough in common with the others. If both sexes are included in the group, special problems arise which make a rough balance in numbers of men and women desirable. In a group of rather conforming or inhibited patients it is valuable to consider adding one or two individuals who have greater capacity for open expression of primitive impulses. While the usual size of a psychotherapeutic group is a workable 5 to 8 members, in dealing with psychotics a larger group of 12 to 15 members has been found to have advantages. It is usually important that those in the group not have outside obligations to one another. Some experiences indicate that after the first dozen or so sessions of a coherent group it becomes increasingly difficult to add new members.

Like individual psychotherapy with children or psychotics, group psychotherapy tends to put the therapist much more "on the spot" and to bring into operation his own neurotic tendencies. Since patients have tended to attack the leader quite freely at times and may not spare the leader's own sources of anxiety, it is well for the therapist to have some type of supervision. Members of the group will react sensitively to whether the therapist genuinely is able to accept their hostility and anxiety without being too disturbed.

It is possible to describe roughly a number of phases of this process. Particularly with passive leadership, initial anxious silences are common. Soon thereafter one or two members may impulsively "confess" a great deal; this may frighten the more isolated, inhibited patients, particularly if pressure is put on them to do likewise. Before long, rivalries appear and the formation of shifting subgroup allegiances occurs. At times a member may attempt to usurp leadership through incessant talking. Throughout the experience the therapist works to help the group clarify the meaning of individual behavior and to establish reality.

At the present stage of our knowledge, group therapy cannot be said to have any specific indications. Recent experiences suggest that the following disorders may sometimes be handled better in groups than by individual psychotherapy: alcoholism, severe psychosomatic disorders, ambulatory psychoses, transient situational neuroses, student counseling, vocational guidance problems, and adjustment problems such as new patients' adapting to a hospital ward situation. In addition, group therapy has been found of value as a preparation for individual therapy in persons who are not sure of their own motivation for individual therapy and as an adjunctive therapy providing social contacts and emotional support for severely disturbed immature characters, chronic psychotics, or psychopaths.

To the extent that human beings change their behavior through corrective action and identification with others rather than through detailed personal insight, group therapy may be potentially more effective than individual therapy. There is less time for each individual member to discuss his problems; on the other hand, inappropriate reactions, when expressed in the group, may be more visibly pathological than in individual therapy. Thus, if a patient on various occasions expresses a neurotic attitude, in relation to first one and then another member of the group, it soon becomes evident to all that this is a problem of the patient rather than of the other members. Group therapy may be arbitrarily divided into several types, each determined by the goals of the group and the leader's behavior.

Psychoanalytic group psychotherapy

In the psychoanalytic group type of therapy the group aims at considerable insight and personality modification and the leader assumes a rather passive role. This form mobilizes the most anxiety and the most acting-out behavior within the group. Concepts of transference and countertransference are utilized in analyzing members' perceptual distortions and in understanding the outbursts of affect.

Social group work

At the opposite pole from the first type named is social group work, a way of modifying individual and group behavior through skillfully designed patterns of group action. The goal here is to employ unused personal assets and to encourage their further growth. Analysis of symptomatic behavior is usually attempted only as required to remove obstacles to growth. The curative effects of settlement houses, clubs, political organizations, activity groups, religious orders, and schools may be said to fall within this general category. The active community group leader utilizes the energies of persons so that they receive emotional satisfaction from the action and the emotional interplay and so that healthy behavior patterns become stabilized.

The *life-space interview* or *marginal interview* is a psychotherapeutic approach appropriate in the group activity setting. It provides a well-timed opportunity to bypass defenses against discussion of interpersonal conflicts in a more formal interview. Disturbed behavior has been demonstrated before the eyes of the participant therapist and is thus more accessible to exploration.

Psychodrama

An elaborate theory and set of techniques for psychodrama have been worked out over the years since 1914 by J. L. Moreno. Many of the basic psychodynamic postulates are similar to those underlying psychoanalysis, but benefit is sought through action expression, reliving on the therapeutic stage, and working through in action. Moreno refers to *resistance* and employs special techniques (*warming up* the group, having the patient's role taken by a *double,* assisting dramatic expression of conflict through *auxiliary egos*) to overcome resistance. The patient is referred to as the *protagonist* and may portray on the stage either his own inner problems or a central problem of concern to the therapeutic group.

Flexible group psychotherapy

The term "flexible group psychotherapy" designates a variety of forms of therapy which aim at sufficient insight and personality change to achieve relief of symptoms or improved social adaptation. Patients are encouraged to express their problems in a permissive family atmosphere. Behavior patterns are discussed in historical terms but interpretation of transference feelings may be avoided. The patient learns new ways of meeting specific life situations through discussion, redefining his conflicts, and corrective emotional experiences. The leader may vary his behavior considerably from time to time and, where desirable, may introduce psychodrama, role-playing, or play therapy techniques to assist the group's progress.

SUGGESTED READINGS

Barber, T. X., editor: Advances in altered states of consciousness and human potentialities, New York, 1976, Psychological Dimensions, Inc.

Frank, J. D.: Group therapy in the mental hospital, monograph series no. 1, Washington, D.C., Dec., 1955, American Psychiatric Association.

Friedman, A. S., and others: Psychotherapy for the whole family, New York, 1965, Springer Publishing Co., Inc.

Gans, R.: Group co-therapists in the therapeutic situation, Int. J. Group Psychother. **12:**82, 1962.

Howells, J. G.: Theory and practice of family psychiatry, New York, 1963, Brunner/Mazel, Inc.

Jones, M.: Beyond the therapeutic community: social learning and social psychiatry, New Haven, Conn., 1968, Yale University Press.

Laqueur, H. P., Wells, C. F., and Agresti, M.: Multiple family therapy in a state hospital, Hosp. Community Psychiatry **20:**13, 1969.

MacLennan, B. W.: Group approaches to problems of socially deprived youth: the classical psychotherapeutic model, Int. J. Group Psychother. **18:**481, 1968.

Moreno, J. L.: Psychodrama. In Arieti, S., editor: American handbook of psychiatry, New York, 1959, Basic Books, Inc., Publishers, vol. 2.

Powdermaker, F., and Frank, J.: Group psychotherapy, Cambridge, Mass., 1953, Harvard University Press.

Rogers, C.: On encounter groups, New York, 1970, Brunner/Mazel, Inc.

Slavson, S.: Analytic group psychotherapy with children, adolescents and adults, New York, 1950, Columbia University Press.

Wolberg, L. R., editor: Group therapy, 1975: an overview, New York, 1975, Intercontinental Medical Book Corp.

Yalom, I.: The theory and practice of group psychotherapy, New York, 1969, Basic Books, Inc., Publishers.

24

The physical therapies (ECT, insulin, sleep therapy, psychosurgery)

ELECTROCONVULSIVE THERAPY

The production of convulsive seizures by pharmacological means was introduced by von Meduna as a treatment for schizophrenia. Later (1937) Cerletti and Bini introduced the simpler method of electroshock or electroconvulsive therapy (EST, ECT). The manner in which treatments of this type produce remission from emotional disorder is not understood, but their ability to relieve the symptoms of psychotic depression is universally accepted. Their effectiveness in other psychiatric disorders, however, is still open to question. Although early observations suggested that the use of antidepressant drugs might ultimately replace ECT, it is now apparent that ECT still remains the treatment of choice for severe suicidal depressions that require hospitalization. Because of the slow onset of action of these drugs, there exists a delay of 3 to 21 days in treatment results, during which period suicide may occur. To cope with this problem the antidepressant drug can be given concurrently with and following the administration of ECT, with the goal of earlier termination of the course of electroshock and a reduction in the number of ECT treatments that are required.

INDICATIONS. The best results with ECT have been obtained in patients with involutional psychotic reaction (depressed type) or manic-depressive reaction (depressed type). The duration of the depression is shortened and the incidence of suicide is decreased, resulting in a higher recovery rate. There is no evidence that a course of ECT prevents subsequent attacks or alters the frequency of recurrences. In manic-depressive reaction, manic type, the manic attacks may be shortened, but treatments may have to be given intensively (once daily or oftener). In schizophrenia, those patients in whom prognosis is judged to be good regardless of treatment (young patients with short duration of illness, with acute onset, and with pronounced affective component) seem to have remission within 2 to 6 weeks when ECT is used. There is much debate regarding the use of ECT for patients with psychoneurosis and other disorders. In such cases where the depressive element is marked, ECT may be of some help in a combined therapeutic approach. Maintenance ECT given every 4 weeks is used prophylactically in patients with recurrent psychotic depressions.

TECHNIQUE. Prior to ECT, the patient should be given a thorough physical examination with special attention to cardiac and pulmonary status. Chest x-ray films, an electrocardiogram, and a signed permit from relatives should be obtained. Lateral x-ray views of the spine and an electroencephalogram are advisable.

Preparation of patient. Before the patient receives an electroconvulsive treatment, the following steps should be taken.

1. Allow only clear fluid after midnight and give no breakfast.

2. It is important to prepare the patient psychologically for the treatment, with understanding reassurance. Apprehensive patients may receive a sedative the night before or intravenously prior to treatment. This also tends to lessen the postshock excitement, and its effect on raising the convulsive threshold is usually not sufficient to interfere with the treatment.

3. Nauseated patients and those who have a tendency to vagal crises may be given 1/200 grain atropine. This is a routine precaution in many hospitals. Larger doses, 1 to 2 mg., are given I.V. 3 to 5 minutes prior to the treatment as a preventive for cardiac complications.

4. Instruct patient to void bladder and bowels just before treatment.

5. Remove dentures and hairpins. Search for chewing gum or other loose bodies in the mouth.

6. Loosen tight clothing.

7. Succinylcholine chloride (Anectine) may be used to soften

the convulsion in patients with orthopedic or cardiac complications, but it must be used with great caution and with full realization that the muscles of respiration may be completely paralyzed and that artificial respiration is often necessary. Such muscle relaxants are used routinely by many psychiatrists, with a variety of techniques for administration. Combination with Pentothal sodium or Brevital is used to suppress the apprehension that may occur. When adequate relaxing doses of such drugs are given, positive-pressure oxygen is often necessary. The objection to the use of muscle relaxants is that, although decreasing the rate of fracture complication, they unquestionably increase the chance of fatal accident. Some hospitals require the presence of a trained anesthetist during this procedure.

Position of patient. Hyperextend the back with a pillow.

Treat on a hard stretcher or with a bedboard under the mattress and use a mouth gag.

Hold lightly to prevent extreme motions and immediately after shock watch the patient, during the confusional period that may follow treatment, to avoid his rolling from the stretcher or bed.

Electrode placement. Usually electrodes are placed approximately over the lower motor area (bitemporal). It has been proposed that posterior placement (i.e., hypothalamic, so-called) is better for the relief of anxiety whereas anterior placement is better for treating depression. A midvertex lead is sometimes substituted for one of the lateral leads, thus permitting stimulation of one hemisphere only. Other special techniques have been described for use primarily with unidirectional currents: One uses multiple leads; another is the so-called monopolar stimulation, in which a large indifferent lead is placed on the right arm and the stimulating lead is moved over the scalp to the approximate region of the brain to be stimulated. Placement of a small electrode in the nasopharynx and a large electrode on the scalp is said to concentrate stimulation upon basal brain structures. The advantages of these several methods of electrode placement over the conventional bitemporal application are still matters of individual opinion.

Number of treatments. Usually treatments are given three times a week. For psychotic depressions, 8 to 14 in a series are often used although, with concurrent administration of antidepressant drugs, this number can be reduced to as few as 3 or 4 treatments; 15 to 25 are usually considered necessary for schizophrenics. Patients have been given hundreds of treatments administered over many months without clinically obvious psychological or neurological deficit. The administration of several treatments per day over a period of several days produces the picture of a severe organic psychosis with confusion and loss of control over body functions. This so-called regressive shock therapy (REST, RECT) has found little acceptance.

COMPLICATIONS. Potential complications in the use of ECT are suggested briefly below.

Death rate. The overall death rate is usually given as about 0.08%. This varies from as much as 0.5% in patients over 60 years of age to as little as 0.02% in patients under 30 years of age.

Fractures and dislocations. These are estimated to occur in 25% of cases. The number reported varies considerably from series to series and with the care in which x-ray films of the spine are taken and read. Fractures are detected much less frequently if one relies only upon the patient's complaints and clinical findings than if the dorsal vertebrae are studied carefully with x-ray films before and after treatment.

Respiratory arrest. In case of such arrest, give artificial respiration. A rebreathing bag and oxygen tank should be available for emergency use.

Cardiovascular difficulty. Cardiac arrest can occur. Atropine may be given prophylactically.

Psychiatric complications. Blurring of memory is the most common complication. In some patients the dramatic symptoms of a Korsakoff type psychosis may develop. It is important to recognize this organic syndrome so as not to give more shock, because it will clear spontaneously and symptoms are only prolonged by more electroshock. It is believed by some that in older persons with confusion, niacin, 400 mg. per day, should be given a trial prior to shock, as ECT may aggravate the organic picture.

EEG changes. Changes in EEG occur almost universally. Slowing is seen in all leads, progressing maximally by 10 or 12 treatments and disappearing in most cases within a few weeks. Such induced cerebral dysfunction has been reported to be a necessary but not sufficient cause for the induced behavioral alterations, in that it may provide the means for a change in adaptation of the subject to his environment.

MODE OF ACTION. Although many theories exist as to the mechanism by which improvement occurs with ECT, we still lack a definitive answer to this problem. There is evidence that repeated convulsions are necessary to obtain therapeutic results and that the method by which the seizure is produced is of little importance. Confusion and memory loss are apparently not necessary for therapeutic success. Fink has presented his conclusions in a neurophysiological-adaptive hypothesis which states that the changes in brain function that follow repeated convulsions produce a necessary substrate which facilitates mechanisms for behavioral change and improvement. The induced biochemical changes, which may be reflected in EEG or spinal fluid studies, permit changes in thinking, mood, and affect, which in turn depend upon the subject's personality for their expression and duration. This theoretical view thus combines both the physiological and psychological data of electroshock research. The demonstration that ECT increases the permeability of the blood brain barrier may well be of importance.

CONTRAINDICATIONS. There are few absolute contraindications to the use of ECT, inasmuch as it in itself is frequently a treatment of emergency nature or desperation. All ages have been treated, from 3 to 80 years, and patients in all stages of pregnancy. In patients with tuberculosis electroshock can activate a lesion. Insulin (IST), however, is more dangerous in this regard. Patients with bone and joint disease are treated after medication with succinylcholine. Patients with aortic aneurysm, once thought to be an absolute contraindication to ECT, have now been successfully treated with SCG-Pentothal-modified convulsive therapy. Coronary disease makes one reluctant to give shock. With disease of the myocardium one would sedate and otherwise avoid exhausting the patient. A contraindication to ECT is the presence of brain tumor. In patients with hypertension, ECT may lower the blood pressure. Serious and even fatal complications have been reported from giving electroconvulsive therapy to patients receiving reserpine. However, combined chlorpromazine-ECT has been reported as a safe procedure and of help in those patients who fail to respond to either treatment alone. The daily dose of chlorpromazine should be kept under 750 mg. and probably should not be administered in the period just preceding treatment.

EQUIPMENT. In principle, no complex apparatus is required to induce a therapeutic convulsion electrically. Any electrical stimulus capable of irritating the cerebrum sufficiently to produce excitation of the motor cortex can induce a seizure. A patient of ours once treated himself by tearing a lamp cord apart and holding the frayed ends to his temples.

The shock machines in current use have controls to permit the administration of measured amounts of current for controlled periods of time, as most psychiatrists seek to produce the seizure with a minimal stimulus. In some equipment the voltage is held constant and the milliamperage of current delivered is varied, although in most equipment the voltage can also be altered. The electrical stimulus usually employed is the commercially available alternating current at 60 cycles per second.

Attempts to produce a gentler onset of the seizure resulted in the glissando control, which permits an initial build-up or rise of current during a second or more, rather than the instantaneous application of the full stimulus. Unfortunately, if the rise is slow enough to effectively alter the severity of seizure onset, the patient is uncomfortably aware of the treatment, and intravenous barbiturates must be administered before a course of such treatments.

Other attempts to improve upon conventional ECT resulted in the so-called unidirectional current stimulators (Reiter, Liberson-Offner B.S.T., etc.), which use forms of rectified current interrupted and modulated variously by different manufacturers. These modifications have not satisfactorily eliminated the complications of ECT, although they in general seem to induce milder seizures with less confusion and less alteration of the brain wave pattern than seen with conventional ECT. Unfortunately, however, it is often necessary to give a greater number of these milder treatments to achieve the desired therapeutic result.

OTHER TECHNIQUES

In an attempt to broaden the usefulness of ECT a number of cerebrostimulation procedures have been developed. Much careful work utilizing matched control groups must be done before the effectiveness of such methods can be known.

Subconvulsive and stimulative electrocerebral therapy

Subconvulsive (ESnc) and high-frequency stimulative electrocerebral therapy (Sedac) are produced by means of unidirectional stimulating equipment. In these techniques only sufficient current is used to induce clonic movements and autonomic effects. Since the patient remains conscious and has an unpleasant memory of this procedure, it is usually given only after the prior intravenous administration of sodium Amytal, Brevital, or Pentothal. Following this, the stimulation is given until the anesthetic wears off. Recent work seems to indicate that at least part of the effect of this treatment comes about through stimulation of the peripheral sensory nerves of the head; therefore, similar effect may be achieved by a method of peripheral stimulation in which the electrodes are applied against the legs and the small of the back, with the treatment otherwise given similarly.

Recent controlled studies of subconvulsive treatment using both electrical and photoshock methods seem to indicate that this method is without significant effect either in patients with psychotic depressions or in patients with anxiety states. Nonconvulsive electrostimulation immediately following a grand mal seizure (countershock) has been shown to have no value in alleviating the amnesia that may follow ECT.

Electrosleep

For many years Russian scientists have been investigating the properties of electrosleep as a therapeutic tool. More recently, considerable interest has been shown by American investigators. The term "electrosleep" has been considered inappropriate due to the fact that sleep is not induced in all subjects. It has been suggested that the term be replaced by "transcerebral electrotherapy."

Such transcerebral stimulation is today widely used to procure not sleep but relaxation. It is reputed to be beneficial in a variety of psychosomatic conditions and tension states as well as in minor forms of mental illness. An element of suggestibility is definitely present and is considered an important factor in the results obtained. Considerable research is necessary in this field.

In electrosleep therapy negative electrodes are applied over the eyes, and postive electrodes are placed over the mastoid processes. A weak, pulsed current (up to 1.5 mA and up to 50 V) for a total period of 1 hour per treatment session is used. Treatments may be given daily.

Pharmacological treatments

Generalized seizures can be produced pharmacologically by a variety of substances. Therapeutic convulsions induced by Metrazol were early abandoned for a number of reasons, which included undependability of seizure production, severity of seizures, unwanted multiple seizures, and production of marked apprehension in the patient during the period of induction. Other convulsant drugs for intravenous administration are now available which seems to obviate at least some of the above drawbacks.

Some workers have reported using currents of high voltage—but of brief duration—in conjunction with analeptics and anticonvulsants in an attempt to produce maximal stimulation of deeper structures in the brain.

Indoklon (hexafluorodiethyl ether), a convulsant ether, has been utilized for the production of generalized seizures. It is inhaled by the patient during a procedure of administration that is similar to that utilized with any gas anesthetic. Indoklon may also be given intravenously.

Photoshock

Photoshock is a treatment in which the intravenous injection of an analeptic such as hexazole (4-cyclohexyl-3-ethyl-1,2,4-trizole) is given in conjunction with intermittent photic stimulation of a stroboscope set to give 15 flashes per second. The resulting treatment is at least as effective as electroshock and appears to be gentler and produces less confusion in the patient.

Insulin therapy

The use of insulin (IST) to induce severe hypoglycemic states for the treatment of psychoses was reported by Manfred Sakel of Vienna in 1933. This treatment has shown a marked decline since World War II. The term "insulin shock" refers to the state of vasomotor collapse induced by this method.

INDICATIONS. Schizophrenia of recent onset.

CONTRAINDICATIONS. This treatment is time-consuming and not without danger. It requires careful attention to technique. Specific contraindications are cardiovascular disease, especially coronary disease or pulmonary tuberculosis, febrile illness, diabetes, acute or chronic diseases of liver, kidney, pancreas, thyroid, or adrenals.

PREPARATION. Complete physical examination, posteroanterior x-ray films of chest, and an electrocardiogram. Give preliminary test for insulin sensitivity (use 5 to 10 units regular insulin subcutaneously, examine in 6 hours for wheal, and watch for hypoglycemia the first hour).

TECHNIQUE. Insulin therapy may be used for either subcoma or coma.

Subcoma. Regular insulin (not crystalline or PZI) is given subcutaneously at 6:00 A.M. to patients fasting and in bed. An initial dose of 15 U. is increased by 10 U. until desired effect is achieved. From time to time it may be necessary to decrease or increase the dose by 5 to 10 U. to hold the patient at the required level.

Goal. The goal is to produce hypoglycemic reactions of drowsiness or sleep for $1/2$ to 1 hour.

Termination. Oral adminstration or gavage of 400 ml. orange juice with glucose, 2 Gm. per unit of insulin, or 10 to 50 ml. 50% glucose intravenously.

Course. Depending upon the clinical course of the patient, 20 to 100 treatments.

Coma. Give regular insulin, 15 U., subcutaneously; increase by 10 U. each day until brief periods of coma occur (usually around 100 U.); then proceed with greater caution until goal of 1 hour's coma is reached. Alter to maintain; usually can decrease by 5 U. per day. If no coma occurs with 400 U., increase by 25 to 50 U. At 500 U., try zigzag reduction (350, 150, 300, 75, etc).

Alternatively, use a multiple-injection technique, with increasing daily dosages to 20-20-20 or 30-20-20 U. of insulin given 15 minutes apart.

Goal. Comatose reactions of 60 minutes' duration. Watch for a dangerous stage in which contracted pupils fail to respond to light, corneal reflexes are absent, pulse rate runs between 50 and 60, and respiratory difficulties and muscular hypotonia occur. This deep coma is reputedly therapeutic but should not be maintained for over 20 minutes. Immediate termination is indicated if systolic blood pressure drops below 100 mm. Hg and pulse below 55.

Termination. Give 50 ml. 50% glucose intravenously (or 500 ml. by stomach tube) followed by oral orange juice with 2 to 400

Gm. glucose (i.e., 2 Gm. per insulin unit given) or glucagon injected intramuscularly in 1 to 5 mg. doses. Patient is then encouraged to eat breakfast and all meals during the day. Sugar-fortified orange juice in midafternoon is a precaution against delayed insulin reactions, which are not uncommon.

Course. Coma is produced 6 days a week for 2 weeks to 3 months if necessary.

Combined IST and ECT. Both electroconvulsive therapy (ECT) and Metrazol convulsions have been used in combination with and to terminate insulin coma treatments in cases refractory to insulin alone. The increased possibility of lasting organic brain alteration makes this combination a treatment of desperation.

COMPLICATIONS. Prolonged irreversible coma, respiratory and circulatory complications, intracranial hemorrhage, and death sometimes follow insulin therapy.

Prompt recognition of prolonged coma is essential. If comatose patient does not begin to revive in 10 to 15 minutes following normal gavage, administer 30 to 50 ml. 50% glucose intravenously. If no signs of arousal appear in 5 minutes, suspect prolonged coma.

Treatment of prolonged stupor is by use of intravenous glucose and dehydrating agents such as 50 ml. 50% sorbitol solution intravenously. Fifty milliliters 50% concentrated lyophilized human serum solution may also be given. Adrenocortical hormones should be used and are said by some, if given prophylactically, to prevent prolonged coma. Thiamine and blood plasma may be repeated every 2 or 3 hours until recovery. If the stupor continues for longer than 12 hours, adequate provision must be made for parenteral fluids, proteins, and carbohydrates to maintain an optimal state of nutrition. The therapist must be prepared for a long wait. It should be kept in mind that episodes of prolonged stupor often serve to sensitize the patient to the effects of insulin, so that if treatment is continued the dose of insulin may be decreased as much as nine-tenths of the previous amount and irreversible stupors still can result.

Convulsions may be avoided by the administration of phenobarbital or Dilantin at the time insulin is given. If subcoma is employed in patients over 45 years old and those with cardiovascular complications, special care must be taken to avoid coma.

RESULTS. Results obtained with insulin therapy depend

upon the factors included in case selection. Studies of patients followed for 5 to 10 years after treatment reveal remission rates from 13% to 84%. As in all treatment of schizophrenia, good prognosis is augured by youth, short duration of disease, precipitation of attack by external events, pyknic or athletic habitus, and good premorbid personality adjustment. A weight gain of 30 pounds or more during treatment is a favorable sign.

Insulin hypoglycemia produces marked slowing in the EEG, and there remains the question of permanent localized damage. Although insulin coma treatment has been largely replaced by psychopharmacology and ECT, there are some who believe it still has a role in the therapy of treatment-resistant patients.

Other coma-inducing techniques that have been used include acetylcholine (Fiamberti, 1937) and atropine (Forrer, 1951).

Carbon dioxide therapy

Carbon dioxide therapy was introduced by Meduna in 1945 as a treatment for psychoneurosis. A mixture of 30% CO_2 and 70% O_2 is used with an ordinary anesthesia mask, rubber bag, and reducing valve arrangement, with the patient in a supine position. Usually from 15 to 50 inspirations are needed to induce narcosis. The patient may abreact or report dreams.

Continuous sleep therapy

One of the oldest treatment methods in psychiatry is prolonged sleep therapy. This received considerable attention during World War II and is widely used in Russia today but is little used in civilian psychiatry in the United States. The once popular Cloetta's mixture (paraldehyde, 0.4864 Gm.; amylene hydrate, 0.1593 Gm.; chloral hydrate 0.1157 Gm.; alcohol, 92%, 0.1747 Gm.; isopropyl-allyl-barbituric acid, 0.0409 Gm.; Digalen, 0.0330 mg.; and ephedrine hydrochloride, 2.4600 mg.) rectally administered has more recently been replaced by mixtures of tranquilizers and barbiturates given orally. One such mixture that has been used consists of Seconal (short-acting), 100 mg.; Nembutal (moderate-acting), 100 mg.; sodium Amytal (long-acting), 150 mg.; and chlorpromazine, 50 mg.

In this treatment the nursing care and the adjustment of drug schedule and periods of awakening for elimination and food intake are critical. Pneumonia is a complication requiring cessation of sleep treatment and administration of antibiotic medication. The course of continuous sleep may be from 2 weeks to 2 months. Some excellent results reported from combat fatigue cases in wartime have not been duplicated in civilian medicine. Patients treated by this method range from those with psychoneurosis to those with chronic psychotic illness. More commonly used is the induction of sleep for brief periods of 2 to 8 hours by the slow, intravenous injection of 0.5 to 1.0 gm of sodium amobarbital (Amytal Sodium).

Hydrotherapy

The remedial use of water for mental ills had its origin in the baths of ancient times, and today swimming pools (group hydrotherapy) still play a role in the activities therapy programs of a number of mental hospitals. Individual hydrotherapy, however, is today rarely used in the hospital management of psychiatric patients. Prior to the advent of psychotropic drugs, it was widely applied in the form of continuous tub baths, showers, sprays, douches, and wet sheet packs.

Psychosurgery

Techniques of operating upon the human brain for the relief of psychiatric disorder originated from pioneer work of the Swiss psychiatrist Burkhardt (1888), that of Moniz and Lima of Portugal (1936), and subsequent popularization of the procedure in the United States by Freeman and Watts.

Psychosurgery was most commonly used for schizophrenics who had been chronic institutional problems, for severe chronic obsessive-compulsive neuroses, chronic anxiety neuroses, and severe chronic depressive states. With the widespread use of tranquilizing medications, psychosurgery is now rarely used. The most common indication today is for the relief of intractable pain, as in the case of terminal malignancy or severe hypochondriasis. Depth electrode stimulation methods have shown promising results for patients with chronic anxiety states and compulsive and phobic neuroses, but such techniques are today used mostly in research settings.

Literally, lobotomy is a cutting into the lobe, whereas *leukotomy* is a severance of white matter. Open lobotomy is performed under direct vision through large superior trephine openings. In closed lobotomy lateral small burr holes are used. Operation is blind, but with careful measurement from external land-marks the surgeon can limit section to superior or, more usually, inferior quadrants. Transorbital lobotomy was also called the "ice-pick" operation. A leukotome is plunged through the con-junctival sac and orbital plate into the orbital surface of the frontal lobe, where an arc swing of the instrument cuts the inferior quad-rant of the lobe.

A technique of some promise is the destruction of the deep white matter with ultrasonic vibrations.

The term lobectomy refers to the radical removal of all frontal areas as well as orbital surface. Gyrectomy is an open operative removal of cortical tissue (gyri) and was termed "topectomy" by the Columbia-Greystone Project Group who removed areas 9, 10, and 46 by subpial dissection. Cingulectomy is the removal of the cingulate gyrus. Thalamotomy (Spiegel and Wycis) uses a stereotaxic apparatus to produce lesions deep in the thalamus.

COMPLICATIONS. Estimated morbidity is about 1%. Neuro-logical complications are 10% to 20%, including operative hemor-rhages, parasurgical cysts and necrosis, epileptic seizures (rates vary with the type of operative procedure), and a persistent uri-nary incontinence. Postoperatively, there may be apathy, a lack of creative drive, little foresight, and in general an attitude of not caring. Impulsive, aggressive behavior can at times result.

RESULTS. By conservative estimate, over one third of chronic, hospitalized psychiatric patients treated by lobotomy are returned to the community; another third remain unchanged. Some op-timistic studies boost the number recovered to well over 50% and compare this to control groups (in which permission for the opera-tion was refused by the relatives) where over 90% remained un-changed. Obviously such figures are not too meaningful without careful description of the types of cases selected and without a matched control series given an equal amount of hospital atten-tion. Studies of 1000 patients of all types followed for 1 to 16 years after lobotomy (Freeman) reveal satisfactory adjustment out of the hospital. Results are better in those cases in which the duration of the illness is short, and results become progressively worse with increasing chronicity. Results in obsessive neurotics and in pa-tients with involutional psychosis are, on the whole, better than in those with schizophrenia.

Psychological studies reveal no significant change in I. Q. Self-reference, self-consciousness, and concern over poor performance are alleviated—with a frequent shift from tension to apathy. Impairment of abstract thinking, concept formation, and planning is seen, along with perseveration and stereotypy.

Sociological studies of postlobotomy patients have indicated a trend toward improved work and family adjustment, but in neither of these areas were pre-illness achievements attained. The degree of acceptance by members of the family of the postoperative patient and lapses of judgment and of modesty have been observed to be important factors in determining whether the patient can make a community adjustment. In recent years the number of lobotomies performed has steadily decreased. At present the more mutilating types of procedure are rarely seen and the emphasis currently is on smaller lesions following exploratory brain stimulation done in centers where elaborate research investigations are possible.

SUGGESTED READINGS

Asnis, G. M., Fink, M., and Saferstein, S.: ECT in metropolitan New York hospitals: a survey of practice, 1975-1976, Am. J. Psychiatry **135:**479, 1978.

Azima, H.: Prolonged sleep treatment in mental disorder, J. Ment. Sci. **101:**593, 1955.

Fink, M.: The mode of action of convulsive therapy: the neurophysiologic-adaptive view, J. Neuropsychiatry **3:**231, 1962.

Fink, M., and others: Inhalant-induced convulsions: significance for the theory of the convulsive therapy process, Arch. Gen. Psychiatry **4:**259, 1961.

Forrer, G., and Miller, J.: Atropine coma: a somatic therapy in psychiatry, Am. J. Psychiatry **115:**455, 1958.

Freeman, W., and Watts, J. W.: Psychosurgery, ed. 2, Springfield, Ill., 1950, Charles C Thomas, Publisher.

Fulton, J. F.: Frontal lobotomy and affective behavior, New York, 1951, W. W. Norton & Co., Inc.

Geller, M. R.: The treatment of psychiatric disorders with insulin, 1936-1960, a selected annotated bibliography, Washington, D.C., 1962, U.S. Department of Health, Education, and Welfare, Public Health Service.

Goldman, D.: Brief stimulus electric shock therapy, J. Nerv. Ment. Dis. **110:**36, 1949.

Gordon, H.: Fifty shock therapy theories, Milit. Surg. **103**:397, 1948.

Grantham, E. C.: Prefrontal lobotomy for relief of pain, J. Neurosurg. **8**:405, 1951.

Greenblatt, M., and Solomon, H. C.: Studies of lobotomy, Res. Pub. Ass. Res. Nerv. Ment. Dis. **35**:15, 1958.

Itil, T. M., Gannon P., Akpinar, S., and Hsu, W.: Quantitative EEG analysis of electro-sleep using frequency analyzer and digital computer methods, Dis. Nerv. Syst., 1972.

Johnson, L. C., Ulett, G. A., Johnson, M., Smith, K., and Sines, J. O.: Electroconvulsive therapy (with and without atropine), Arch. Gen. Psychiatry **2**:324, 1960.

Kalinowsky, L. B., and Hoch, P. H.: Somatic treatments in psychiatry; pharmaco-therapy; convulsive, insulin, surgical and other methods, New York, 1969, Grune & Stratton, Inc.

Lewis, W., Richardson, D., and Gahagan, L.: Cardiovascular disturbances and their management in modified electrotherapy for psychiatric illness, N. Engl. J. Med. **252**:1016, 1955.

Lindstrom, P.: Prefrontal ultrasonic irradiation—a substitute for lobotomy, Arch. Neurol. Psychiat. **72**:399, 1954.

Martin, D. J., and Kaelbling, R.: Diazepam-modified electroconvulsive therapy, Biol. Psychiatry **3**:129, 1971.

Meduna, L. J., editor: Carbon dioxide therapy, ed. 2, Springfield Ill., 1958, Charles C Thomas, Publisher.

Mettler, F. A.: Selective partial ablation of the frontal cortex, New York, 1949, Paul B. Hoeber, Inc.

Moniz, E.: Tentatives opératoires dans le traitement de certaines psychoses, Paris, 1936, Masson et Cie.

Nussbaum, K., and Kurland, A.: Bis (2,2,2-trifluorethyl) ether (Indoklon) modified with succinylcholine (Anectime) as a convulsant in psychiatric treatment, J. Neuropsychiatry **5**:143, 1963.

Oltman, J. E., and Friedman, S.: Long-term results of frontal lobotomy in schizophrenic patients, Amer. J. Psychiat. **118**:70, 1961.

Ottoson, J.: Experimental studies of the mode of action of electro-convulsive therapy, Acta Psychiat. Scand. **35**(supp. 145):5, 1960.

Putnam, T. J.: Procaine base in iodized oil introduced transorbitally as a test for the effects of lobotomy, Trans. Amer. Neurol. Ass. **75**:125, 1950.

Reynolds, D. V., and Sjoberg, A. E.: Neuroelectric research: electro-neuroprosthesis, electroanesthesia and nonconvulsive electrotherapy, Springfield, Ill., 1971, Charles C Thomas, Publisher.

Rylander, G.: Personality analysis before and after frontal lobotomy, Proc. Ass. Res. Nerv. Ment. Dis. **27**:691, 1948.

Sargant, W. W., and Slater, E. T.: An introduction to physical methods of treatment in psychiatry, ed. 4, Baltimore, 1963, The Williams & Wilkins Co.

Sem-Jacobsen, C. W.: Depth-electrographic stimulation of the human brain and behavior: from fourteen years of studies and treatment of Parkinson's disease and mental disorders with implanted electrodes, Springfield, Ill., 1968, Charles C Thomas, Publisher.

Shobe, F. O., and Gildea, M.: Long-term follow-up of selected lobotomized private patients, J.A.M.A. **206:**327, 1968.

Sykes, M. K., and Tredgold, R. F.: Restricted orbital undercutting: a study of effects on 350 patients over the 10 years 1951-1960, Brit. J. Psychiat. **110:**609, 1964.

Ulett, G. A., Gleser, G., Caldwell, B., and Smith, K.: The use of matched groups in the evaluation of convulsive and subconvulsive photoshock, Bull. Menninger Clin. **13:**138, 1954.

Ulett, G. A., Smith, K., and Gleser, F.: Evaluation of convulsive and subconvulsive shock therapies utilizing a control group, Am. J. Psychiatry **112:**795, 1956.

Wayne, G. J.: Use of succinylcholine chloride in electroconvulsive therapy, Dis. Nerv. Syst. **21:**149, 1960.

Wagender, E. M., and Schuy, S.: Electrotherapeutic sleep and electroanaesthesia, International Congress Series No. 136, New York, 1967. Excerpta Medical Foundation.

Wittenborn, J. R., and Mettler, F. A.: Some psychological changes following psychosurgery, J. Abnorm. Soc. Psychol. **14:**548, 1952.

Wood, M. W., and Rowland, J. P.: Bilateral anterior thalamotomy for the hyperactive child, Southern Med. J. **61:**36, 1968.

Wright, R.: Hydrotherapy in psychiatric hospitals, Boston, 1940, The Tudor Press.

25

Chemotherapy in mental illness

The treatment of the mentally ill by means of drugs is not new, but certainly it has been the focus of a renewed interest in the past few years. Unlike the antibiotics, whose action is against known etiological agents, drugs in psychiatry are, for the most part, used to alleviate undesirable symptoms. Initally, therefore, states of mania, delirium, and anxiety were treated with morphine, with chloral hydrate, and with paraldehyde. Such drugs often had the desired quieting effect on motor behavior but produced in addition an undesirable somnolence and lethargy which prohibited the patient's participation in other therapeutic activities. The newer ataractics produce tranquilization of behavior without lethargy, and recently introduced antidepressants relieve mood disturbances with fewer side effects than the earlier stimulating drugs.

The field of psychopharmacology is exciting and active, with an ever-increasing number of new agents being made available to the psychiatrist. The final chapter has not yet been written on the mechanism of action of these agents, but research in this field may well offer important insights into the etiology of psychiatric illness. The tables in this chapter itemize various drugs and doses which the psychiatrist may wish to use in the treatment of patients.

ANTIPSYCHOTIC AGENTS (NEUROLEPTICS—MAJOR TRANQUILIZERS)

Often called "tranquilizers," these drugs have produced a considerable change in the management of disturbed psychotic patients. Like the barbiturates, these have a quieting or calming effect; but, unlike the older hypnotic agents, these new ataractics accomplish the desired result without producing marked drowsiness. The tranquilizers have become one of the most frequently used drugs in medicine. The literature in this field is vast and confusing. These agents are probably neither specific nor "curative"; yet when they are properly selected for the individual patient and administered in a high dosage over a sufficiently long period of time, social restitution has occurred in cases in which the prognosis otherwise seemed to be extremely poor.

Extracts of plants of the rauwolfia variety were used for centuries in Asia for many illnesses, including hypertension and insanity. Introduction of the alkaloid reserpine into medical practice some two decades ago ushered in the new era of psychopharmacology. These compounds (Serpasil, etc.) are now rarely used in psychiatry, having been supplanted by the phenothiazines, butyrophenones, and related compounds. These latter drugs cause accumulation of the O-methylated metabolites of dopamine and noradrenaline within the brain, suggesting that they also block dopamine and noradrenaline receptors, thus causing compensatory activity of central neurones with monoamine transmitter release. There appears to be a selective distribution of these compounds in the brain with highest concentrations in the hypothalamus, basal ganglia, thalamus, and hippocampus. Some authors feel that action in the septal area is of particular importance.

Apart from strong antipsychotic and neuroleptic activity these drugs produce antiemetic effects. Extrapyramidal symptoms (pseudo-Parkinsonism, akathisia, dyskinesia, torsion spasms and oculogyric crises) are often seen and may cause the dose that is given to be limited. Such side effects may be controlled with appropriate doses of synthetic anticholinergic agents. Tardive dyskinesia is the term applied to Parkinson-type activity, particularly of a choreiform character involving especially the mouth and tongue, occurring after prolonged administration, and that is frequently exaggerated when the drug is no longer given.

Other adverse effects of some of these compounds include abnormal pigmentation of exposed areas of the skin, corneal and lenticular deposits, and, especially with thioridazine, retinal pigmen-

Text continued on p. 330.

Table 7. Neuroleptics (*major tranquilizers*)

Drug and how supplied	Dose range	Equivalent dose	Sedation	Extrapyramidal reaction
PHENOTHIAZINES				
Aliphatic				
Chlorpromazine HCl	50-1,000 mg.	100 mg.	++++	++
Thorazine				
Oral: 10, 25, 30, 100, 200 mg. tabs.; 30, 75, 150, 200, 300 mg. time-release caps				
Chlor-PZ				
Oral: 30 mg. and 100 mg./ml. concentrate				
Promatar and generic				
Rectal: 25, 100 mg. supp.				
I.M.: 25 mg./ml. in 1, 2, 10 ml. containers				
Triflupromazine HCl	25-150 mg.	25 mg.	++++	++
Vesprin				
Oral: 10, 25, 50 mg. tabs.; 50 mg./5 ml. suspension				
I.M.: 10 mg./ml. in 1.10 ml. container; 20 mg./ml. in 1 ml. container				
Piperidine				
Thioridazine HCl	50-800 mg.	100 mg.	++++	+
Mellaril				
Oral: 10, 15, 25, 50, 100, 200 mg. tabs.; 30, 100 mg./ml. concentrate				
Mesoridazine HCl	50-400 mg.	50 mg.	++++	+

Oral: 10, 25, 50, 100 mg. tabs.; 25 mg./ml.
concentrate

Drug	Dose range	Single dose		
Piperacetazine	10-160 mg.	10 mg.	++	++
Quide				
Oral: 10, 25 mg. tabs.				
I.M.: 2 mg./ml. in 10 ml. container				
Piperazine				
Trifluoperizine HCl	5-80 mg.	5 mg.	++	++++
Stelazine				
Oral: 1, 2, 5, 10 mg. tabs.; 10 mg./ml. concentrate				
I.M.: 2 mg./ml. 10 ml. vial				
Acetophenazine maleate	40-120 mg.	20 mg.	++	+++
Tindal				
Oral: 20 mg. tabs.				
Butaperazine maleate	15-100 mg.	10 mg.	++	++++
Repoise maleate				
Oral: 5, 10, 25 mg. tabs.				
Carphenazine maleate	25-400 mg.	25 mg.	++	++++
Proketazine				
Oral: 12.5, 25, 50 mg.; 50 mg./ml. concentrate				
Fluphenazine	1-20 mg.	2 mg.	+	++++
Fluphenazine HCL				
Prolixin				
Oral: 1, 2.5, 5, 10 tabs; 2.5 mg./5 ml. elixir				
I.M.: 2.5 mg./ml. solution				

Continued.

Table 7. Neuroleptics *(major tranquilizers)* —cont'd

Drug and how supplied	Dose range	Equivalent dose	Sedation	Extrapyramidal reaction
PHENOTHIAZINES—cont'd				
Piperazine—cont'd				
Fluphenazine decanoate–fluphenazine enanthate	Initial, 5 ml., then 1 ml.			
Prolixin decanoate	every 2 weeks			
I.M.: 25 mg./ml.	to 2-4 ml.			
Prolixin enanthate	every 2-6			
I.M.: 25 mg./ml.	weeks			
Permatil				
Oral: 0.25, 2.5, 5, 10 mg. tabs.; 5 mg./ml. concentrate				
Perphenazine				
Trilafon	12-64 mg.	8 mg.	+	++++
Oral: 2, 4, 8, 10 mg. tabs.; 8 mg. time release tabs; 16 mg./5 ml. concentrate				
I.M.: 5 mg./ml.				
Prochlorperazine	To 50 mg., divided	15 mg.	++	++++
Compazine				
Rectal: 2.5, 5, 25 mg. supp.				
Compazine (edisylate)	10-150 mg.			
Oral: 10 mg./ml. concentrate; 5 mg./ml. syrup				
Compazine (maleate)				
Oral: 5, 10, 25 mg. tabs; 10, 15, 30, 75 time caps				

Drug	Dose range		Sedative	Extrapyramidal
Chlorprothixene Taractan Oral: 10, 25, 50, 100 mg. tabs.; 100 mg./5 ml. concentrate I.M.: 12.5 mg./ml. sol.	25-600 mg.	100 mg.	+++	+
Thiothixene Navane Oral: 1, 2, 5, 10, 20 mg. tabs. Navane HCl Oral: 5 mg./ml. concentrate I.M.: 2 mg./ml. sol.	5-60 mg.	4 mg.	+	++++
BUTYROPHENONE COMPOUND				
Haloperidol Haldol Oral: 0.5, 1, 2, 5, 10 mg. tabs.; 2 mg./ml. concentrate I.M.: 5 mg./ml. sol.	1-100 mg.	2 mg.	+	++++
DIHYDROINDOLONE COMPOUND				
Molindone Moban Oral: 5, 10, 25 mg. tabs.	15-225 mg.	15-20 mg.	++	++
DIBENZOXAZEPINE COMPOUND				
Loxapine succinate Loxitane Oral: 10, 25, 50 mg.	20-250 mg.	15-20 mg.	++++	++++

tation. Jaundice of the cholestatic type is sometimes seen and, less commonly, dermatitis and blood dyscrasias. These drugs enhance the effects of other central depressants such as barbiturates, alcohol, and the narcotic analgesics. They are markedly cumulative —metabolic products have been detected up to 18 months after discontinuation of long-term treatment.

The use of these drugs is not curative but rather for the control of symptoms, and although some patients appear to respond better to one agent than another, claims of superiority must be carefully weighed against comparability of dose given with each agent and the frequency of side effects at effective dose levels. As with other new drugs, tranquilizers are often poorly selected, used when not needed, or used unwisely. In serious psychosis, large doses of the drugs may be necessary, and patients may be continued on maintenance doses for many months or years. (Be alert for drug habituation). For some patients the price of psychotic symptom control may be lasting neurological symptoms (tardive dyskinesia).

In general the *major tranquilizers* are useful for the following conditions: (1) schizophrenia—aggressive outbursts, noisiness, and destructive behavior, particularly; (2) affective disorders— hypomanic and manic states, paranoid disturbance, and agitated states in involutional psychoses; (3) acute brain syndrome—states of intoxication, delirium, and hallucinations; and (4) chronic brain syndrome—restlessness, violent outbursts, and destructive behavior. (See Table 7.)

ANTIANXIETY AGENTS (anxiolytics, minor tranquilizers)

These drugs are used primarily to control daytime tension and anxiety in patients with neuroses and as an adjunct in psychiatric and depressed patients with agitation. They have largely replaced the barbiturates and other sedatives, which are more appropriate for night-time sedation. These agents are commonly used by many persons facing situations of unusual stress. They are subject to abuse and hence should be administered with caution. In addition to demonstrable chemical action these drugs have a strong placebo effect.

They produce a mild sedation without impairing psychomotor performance. Skeletal muscle relaxation also occurs. Optimal doses vary widely, and these drugs should often be given intermit-

Table 8. Anxiolytics (minor tranquilizers)

Drug	How supplied	Dosage
Benzodiazepines		
Chlordiazepoxide HCl		
Librium	5, 10, 25 mg. caps (oral) I.V./I.M. 100 mg./5 ml.	15-100 mg. 100 mg. (x3/day)
Chlorazepate		
Tranxene	3.75, 7.5, 15 mg. tabs, (oral)	15-60 mg.
Tranxene SD	22.5 mg. time-release caps	
Diazepam		
Valium	2, 5, 10 mg. tabs (oral) I.V./I.M. 5 mg./ml.	4-40 mg. 5-10 mg. 30 mg./8 hr.
Oxazepam		
Serax	10, 15, 30 mg. caps, 15 mg. tabs	30-120 mg.
Prazepam		
Verstran	10 mg.	20 mg.
Lorazepam		
Ativan	1 & 2 mg.	1-10 mg./day
Clorazepate monopotassium		
Azene	3.25, 6.5, 13 mg. caps	6.5 mg., t.i.d.; 13 mg. h.s.
Antihistamines		
Hydroxyzine HCl		
Atarax	10, 25, 50, 100 mg. tabs	225-400 mg.
Vistaril	25, 50, 100 mg./ml. (I.M.)	
Hydroxyzine pamoate		
Vistaril	25, 50, 100 mg. caps 25 mg./5 ml. susp.	225-400 mg.
Carbamates		
Meprobamate		
Equanil	200, 400 mg. tabs; 400 mg.	200-1200 mg.
Miltown	caps; 200, 400 mg. caps,	
Others and generic	time-release	
Tybamate		
Tybatran	125, 250, 350 mg. caps	750-200 mg.
Miscellaneous		
Chlormezanone		
Trancopal	100, 200 mg. tabs	100-400 mg.

tently in accordance with fluctuations in intensity of anxiety. Tolerance develops with continued use.

Drowsiness is the most common side effect, and patients should be cautioned about driving a car or working around machinery. Ataxia, dizziness, headache, dry mouth, nausea, and hematological, allergic, renal, hepatic, and, at times, paradoxical hyperactive and rage reactions may occur. These drugs are widely prescribed and are commonly overdosed by patients with suicidal intent. (See Table 8.)

SEDATIVES AND HYPNOTICS

These drugs produce varying degrees of generalized depression of the central nervous system, ranging from sedation through hypnosis to anesthesia, respiratory depression, and death. Generally used for the treatment of night-time insomnia and severe daytime anxiety, these agents carry a high abuse potential and are commonly taken with suicidal intent. Effort should be made to identify patients who are prone to chemical dependency and not to yield to their demands for a chemical remedy for life's problems.

These drugs should be administered cautiously; and because their effectiveness is commonly reduced by the second week of use, an overall plan for counseling and management by other means is important. Although lacking analgesic activity themselves, they are helpful in alleviating the anxiety associated with pain, the anticipation of pain, and also adjunctively in the relief of muscle spasm.

For many years bromide salts and the barbiturates were prescription favorites for sedation, along with chloral hydrate and paraldehyde as hypnotics. The recent introduction of flurazepam and other benzodiazepines with a high therapeutic index (lethal: hypnotic dose) has minimized the hazard of overdosing.

The barbiturates vary in their degree of hynotic power and rapidity of action. Those with a phenyl radical, including the long-acting phenobarbital, possess anticonvulsant activities, whereas those with only aliphatic substituent groups do not.

Barbiturates with shorter duration of action include amobarbital (Amytal), butabarbital (Butisol), pentobarbital (Nembutal), and secobarbital (Seconal). The ultra-short acting barbiturates thiopental (Pentothal) and methohexital (Brevital) are given intra-

Table 9. Sedatives and hypnotics

Drug	How supplied	Dosage
Barbiturates		
Phenobarbital		
Eskabarb, Luminal, Sulfton, generic	15, 30, 60, 100 mg. tabs	100-320 mg.
Amobarbital		
Amytal, generic	15, 30, 50, 100 mg. tabs	50-300 mg.
Butabarbital		
Butisol sodium, Butazem, generic	15, 30, 50, 100 mg.	50-120 mg.
Pentobarbital		
Nembralin, Nembutal, generic	30, 50, 100 mg. tabs; 90, 100 mg. time-release caps	30-250 mg.
Secobarbital		
Seconal, generic	30, 50, 100 mg. tabs	50-300 mg.
Benzodiazepine		
Flurazepam		
Dalmane	15, 30 mg. caps	15-30 mg.
Chloral derivatives		
Chloral hydrate		
Aquachloral, Notec, Somnos, generic	225, 250, 450, 500 mg. caps; 60, 120, 300, 460, 500, 600, 900 mg. supp.	250-2000 mg.
Chloral betaine		
Beta-Chlor	850 mg.	
Triclofos sodium		
Triclos	750 mg.	
Piperidinedione derivatives		
Glutethimide		
Doriden	125, 250, 500 mg. tabs; 500 mg. caps	125 mg.-1 Gm.
Methyprylon		
Noludar	50, 200 mg. tabs. 300 mg. caps.	50-400 mg.

Continued.

Table 9. Sedatives and hypnotics—cont'd

Drug	How supplied	Dosage
Miscellaneous		
Ethchlorvynol		
Placidyl	100, 200, 500, 750 mg. caps.	500 mg.-1 Gm.
Ethinamate		
Valmid	500 mg. tabs.	500 mg.-1 Gm.
Methaqualone		
Quaalude, Sopor	150-300 mg.	
Methaqualone hydrochloride		
Parest, Somnafac	200-400 mg.	75-400 mg.
Paraldehyde		
Generic (May be given rectally in olive oil)	30 ml. containers	10-30 ml.
Mixtures		
Tuinal	Caps with 25, 50, or 100 mg. each of amobarbital sodium and secobarbital sodium	
Carbrital	Pentobarbital sodium, 90 mg., Carbromal, 240 mg.	
Carbrital demi	Pentobarbital sodium, 45 mg., Carbromal, 120 mg.	

venously to produce anesthesia and commonly prior to ECT. Pentothal is commonly used in 2.5% and Brevitol in 1% freshly prepared solution.

Periods of apnea or laryngospasm may be avoided by slow induction, but experience is required before the correct dosage and rate of administration of the quick-acting barbiturates will be clear to the physician. Very anxious or overactive patients will require rapid administration of Pentothal, which might lead to serious complications in normal or retarded individuals. Special caution should be used in elderly patients (smaller dose).

As an adjunct to certain phases of psychotherapy, a sufficient intravenous dose of Amytal, Pentothal, or other fairly rapidly acting hypnotic to produce mild drowsiness and release of inhibitions* has a number of uses during an interview. Instead of hypnosis, or as an adjuct thereto, the drug may be used with suggestion to remove hysterical conversion symptoms; greatest success appears with conversion symptoms of recent onset. In the treatment of acute combat anxiety or hysterical reactions, these drugs (often with hypnosis) enable patients to abreact hidden terrors and to face and accept the traumatic situation by repeatedly reliving it during narcoanalysis. In any such situation where strong catharsis of feeling results, the therapist must play the role of a powerful, understanding being who actively points out reality and suggests alternate ways of handling these matters. In addition, this method of producing relaxation and release of inhibitions has been used to help patients recover forgotten but disturbing memories and commonly as a diagnostic adjunct where the differential diagnosis of such conditions as hysteria, early psychosis, malingering, or epileptic seizures is in question. (See Table 9).

CENTRAL NERVOUS SYSTEM STIMULANTS

This classification includes drugs whose effects on mood are usually short-term. Although they decrease fatigue and produce varying degrees of insomnia, they cannot be considered as true antidepressants. They lead to restlessness and agitation rather than normalization of mood. Xanthene derivatives such as caffeine, theophylline, and theobromine belong in this group, as do the anorexient drugs, although in these latter the amphetamine-like effects may be minimal and viewed as side effects to the therapeutic purpose. Most important of these drugs are the amphetamines, with their sympathomimetic action. Since the advent of the monoamine oxidase inhibitors and tricyclics these drugs are little used in the treatment of affective disorders. Two drugs closely related in action, methylephenidate HCl (Ritalin) and pemoline (Cylert), are widely used in the management of hyperkinetic children. Methylphenidate is also used to potentiate the action of the tricyclics. Both the amphetamines and methyphenidate are useful in the treatment of narcolepsy.

---

*Methamphetamine hydrochloride (Methedrine, Pervitin, Desoxyn, Desoxyephedrine) has also been used to release inhibitions through excitement of the central nervous system.

Table 10. CNS stimulants

Drug	How supplied and dosage
Amphetamines	
Dextroamphetamine HC1	Time-release 15 mg. caps. (max. 40 mg./day); 5 mg. tabs.
Dextroamphetamine sulfate	Time-release 5, 10, 15 mg. caps.; 5 mg. tabs.; 5 mg./5 ml. elixir
Dextroamphetamine tannate	Time-release 17.5, 26.25 mg. tabs.
Amphetamine sulfate (Benzedrine)	Time-release 15 mg. caps. (max. 40 mg./day); 5 and 10 mg. tabs.
Methamphetamine HC1 (Desoxyn)	2.5, 5 mg. tabs.; Time-release 5, 10, 15 mg. caps.
Dexosyephedrine HC1 (Obedrin-LA)	10 mg. tabs. (generic)
Combinations	
Dexamyl	
Time-release capsules #1	Dextroamphetamine sulfate 5 mg., amobarbitol 32 mg.
Time-release capsules #2	Dextroamphetamine sulfate 10 mg., Amobarbital 65 mg.
Eskatrol	
Time-release capsules	Dextroamphetamine sulfate 15 mg., prochlorpenazine maleate 7.5 mg.
Other stimulants	
Methylphenidate HC1 (Ritalin)	5, 10, and 20 mg. tabs. (max. 60 mg./day)
Pemoline (Cylert)	18.75, 37.5, 75 mg. tabs. (max. 12.5 mg.)

Action

Typically euphoria, a decreased sense of fatigue, and increased alertness, initiative, and ability to concentrate with increased motor activity. Larger doses produce nervousness, restlessness, tremors, insomnia, tachycardia, hypertension, anorexia, GI disturbances, and mydriasis.

Adverse reactions

These drugs should be used with caution, as susceptible persons may develop psychic and occasionally physical dependence upon them. As they are readily absorbed, they should be prescribed in small quantities. Their continued use to allay fatigue is unjustified. Toxic features of chronic abuse result in a distinctive psychosis characterized by paranoia, stereotyped behavior, picking of the skin, and inner preoccupation with auditory and visual hallucinations. They should never be given to patients receiving MAO inhibitors.

Poisoning

Overdose results in an accentuation of sympathomimetic symptoms leading to hyperpyrexia, chest pain, acute circulatory failure, convulsions, and coma. Chlorpromazine may be useful in blocking the CNS stimulant effects. (See Table 10.)

ANTIMANIC AGENTS

Lithium carbonate is considered the only specific antimanic drug for use in manic-depressive illness. Because it requires 7 to 10 days to achieve a threshold level in body tissues, however, other antipsychotic agents are generally used, especially in severe cases to bring the motor hyperactivity under control. These agents are then tapered off, leaving lithium to control the mood change without producing sedation.

Long-term maintenance is reported effective in many patients (50 to 80%) in preventing the recurrence of manic attacks. Its effectiveness for the prevention of recurrent depression is less clear in those cases where there is not also a history of recurrent attacks of mania. For these latter the term "lithium deficiency" has been suggested, along with lifelong lithium prophylaxis. The use of lithium for a wide variety of other psychiatric conditions is still controversial.

Precautions

Careful monitoring of blood levels is essential, initially in the acute phase two to three times weekly, tapering to monthly during long-term maintenance. Commonly a serum level of 0.5-1.5 mEq./L. is considered therapeutic. As there is evidence that serum levels do not necessarily reflect true tissue levels, careful clinical observation with dosage adjustment is essential until better methods for detecting effective levels are found. Failure of good clinical response may well result from inaccurate detection of tissue levels. Lithium is contraindicated in patients with renal, hepatic, or heart disease or when electrolyte alterations occur with low sodium intake. Extreme dietary changes, vomiting, and diaphoresis can produce changes in lithium level with untoward results. Care should be observed with elderly patients in whom excretion rates may be slowed. Asymptomatic thyroid enlargement as well as hyperthyroidism has been reported with long-term administration, especially when tricyclics are also given. Concurrent administration of diuretics can markedly increase lithium to toxic levels. Adverse reports of lithium on fetal development have not been well substantiated, but because lithium crosses the placental barrier, the effect on neonatal electrolytes should be considered at the time of delivery.

Toxicity

Transient mild effects include nausea, diarrhea, malaise, thirst, polyuria, polydipsia, fatigue, and fine hand tremor. Such are commonly seen at levels of 1.5-2 mEq./L. As the level approaches 2 mEq./L. or above, drowsiness, vomiting, muscle weakness, ataxia, dryness of the mouth, abdominal pain, lethargy, dizziness, slurred speech, and nystagmus may occur. As the level moves upward blurring of vision, fasciculations, clonic movements, hyperactive tendon reflexes, choreoathetoid movements, epileptiform convulsions, toxic psychosis, syncope, and paroxysmal changes in the EEG may be seen. Circulatory failure, stupor, coma, and death have been reported at levels above 2.5 mEq./L.

Treatment of toxicity is fluid and electrolyte replacement therapy. Excretion of lithium is facilitated by osmotic diuretics (urea, amnitol), and alkalinization of the urine (infusion of sodium lactate and biocarbonate). If kidney function is impaired, hemodialysis or peritoneal dialysis may be used.

Lithium carbonate (Eskalith, Lithonate, Lithane, and generic) is supplied in 300 mg. caps and tabs. Initial dose is 300-600 mg. t.i.d. until serum level of 1-1.5 mEq./L. As attack subsides dosage can be decreased. Usually 300 mg. t.i.d. will maintain a level of 0.7-1.2 mEq./L. Elderly and children require reduced doses and caution.

Synthetic anticholinergics

These agents are used to control drug-induced parkinsonism and spasticity. They reduce akinesia, rigidity, tremor, masklike

Table 11. Anticholinergics

Drug	How supplied	Dosage
Drugs inhibiting structures innervated by postganglionic cholinergic nerves		
Atropine sulfate		0.5-1.0 mg. (hypo)
Belladonna tincture		0.6 ml. (oral)
Extract of belladonna		0.015 Gm. (oral)
Scopolamine hydrobromide		0.5 mg. (oral or hypo)
Synthetic anticholinergic agents		
Biperiden (Akineton)	2 mg. tabs. 5 mg./1 ml. ampules	2 mg., 1-3 times daily 2 mg. I.M.; repeat p.r.n. up to four doses in 24-hour period
Trihexyphenidyl HC1 (Artane)	2 and 5 mg. tabs. 5 mg. sequels (sustained release) 2 mg./5 ml. elixir	1-15 mg. daily
Methanesulfonate (Cogentin)	2 mg. tabs. 1 mg./2 ml. ampules	1-4 mg., 1-2 times daily 2 ml. I.M.
Procyclidine HC1 (Kemadrin)	5 mg. (scored) tabs.	2.5-5 mg. t.i.d. (max. 30 mg. daily)
Caramiphen HC1 (Panparnit)	12.5 and 50 mg. coated tabs.	12.5-50 mg., five times daily

facies, inertia, and propulsive gait; they control excessive flow of saliva and oily skin; and they lessen frequency and intensity of oculogyric crises.

Side effects include dry mouth, blurred vision, mild transient hypotension, nausea, and constipation. There is rarely a transient decrease in urinary flow, and occasionally short periods of euphoria or disorientation. Doses must be individually and gradually adjusted. Observe caution in patients with glaucoma. (See Table 11.)

ANTIDEPRESSANTS

These compounds are used for the treatment of depressive illnesses of all types, psychotic or neurotic, endogenous or reac-

Table 12. Antidepressant medication

Drug	How supplied	Dosage
Tricyclics		
Imipramine HC1		
Imarate, Janimine, SK-Pramine	10, 25, 50 mg. tabs. (oral)	75-350 mg./day
Presamine, Tofranil	10, 25, 50 mg. tabs. (oral) 12.5 mg./ml. in 2 ml. ampules (IM)	up to 100 mg./day divided doses
Tofranil-PM	75, 100, 125, 150 mg. caps. (oral)	75-350 mg./day
Amitriptyline HC1		
Elavil, Endep	10, 25, 50, 75, 100 mg. tabs. (oral)	75-300 mg./day
Elavil	10 mg./ml. in 10 ml. vials (IM)	80-120 mg./day divided dose
Desipramine HC1		
Norpramine	25, 50, mg. tabs. (oral)	75-200 mg./day
Pertofrane	25, 50 mg. tabs. (oral)	75-200 mg./day
Doxepin HC1		
Adapin	10, 25, 50 mg. tabs. (oral)	75-300 mg./day
Sinequan	10, 25, 50, 100 mg. tabs. (oral) 10 mg./ml. oral concentrate	75-300 mg./day
Nortriptyline HC1		
Aventyl	10, 25 mg. caps; 10 mg./5 ml. liquid (oral)	75-100 mg./day

tive, bipolar or unipolar. As a group they elevate mood, increase physical activity and mental alertness, improve sleep and appetite patterns, reduce morbid preoccupation, and lower the risk of suicide.

Psychostimulants were replaced by monoamine oxidase inhibitors, which in turn have been succeeded by the tricyclic compounds as the most effective and widely used antidepressant agents, although drugs from all three categories are still in use.

It is widely accepted that depressive psychosis results from

Table 12. Antidepressant medication—cont'd

Drug	How supplied	Dosage
Tricyclics—cont'd		
Pamelor	25 mg. caps. (oral)	
Protriptyline HC1		
Vivactil	5, 10 mg. tabs (oral)	15-60 mg. oral
Mixtures (antidepressant and antipsychotic for depression mixed with anxiety or agitation)		
Etrafon 2-10, Triavil 2-10	2 mg. perphenazine, amitriptyline 10 mg. tabs.	
Etrafon 2-15 Triavil 2-25	2 mg. perphenazine, amitriptyline 25 mg. tabs.	
Etrafon "A", Triavil 4-10	4 mg. perphenazine, amitriptyline 10 mg. tabs.	Max. 9 tabs.
Etrafon "Forte", Triavil 4-25	4 mg. perphenazine, amitriptyline 25 mg. tabs.	Max. 9 tabs.
Monoamine oxidase inhibitors		
Phenelzine sulfate		
Nardil	15 mg. tabs.	60-90 mg./day divided in 3 doses
Isocarboxazid		
Marplan	10 mg. tabs.	10-30 mg./day
Tranylcypromine sulfate		
Parnate	10 mg. tabs.	10-30 mg./day

decreased efficacy of the central adrenergic pathways. Both the tricyclics and the monoamine oxidase inhibitors produce a potentiation of central noradrenergic function although this is accomplished by different mechanisms. Tricyclic compounds inhibit the reuptake of norepinephrine and serotonin by the neurone terminals. Monoamine oxidase inhibitors block intracellular metabolism of biogenic amines, resulting in increased amine concentrations in the terminals. It has appeared that the tricyclic compounds are not entirely interchangeable in their actions; thus, patients failing to respond to one compound may react favorably to another. This has produced speculation that different depressive illnesses may have different underlying biochemical disorders. Thus, for example, it has been postulated that in one group the primary disorder lies with norepinephrine (NE) but not with serotonin (5-HT) or dopamine (DA), this group responding to treatment by imipramine, nortriptyline, and desimipramine; while another group, in which alteration is primarily in the 5-HT systems, shows better response to amitriptyline and doxepin. There is much research activity in this area and it seems likely that there will be further delineation of biochemical subgroups with an attendant specificity of drug prescription.

With all these compounds, however, there is a delay in symptom control for from 1 to 3 weeks and hence for acute and suicidal patients and for the severely depressed early ECT is indicated. Judicious combinations of antidepressants and ECT may, however, permit fewer ECT treatments with consequently less mental confusion and an earlier release from the hospital.

Imipramine is the standard against which other drugs of this class are usually measured. All may have some sedative effect, although this is less true of protriptyline, which has the most rapid onset (5 to 10 days) of action and may produce agitation in some patients. Doxepin is perhaps the most sedative and anxiolytic of this group.

TRICYCLICS

DOSAGE. Generally starting with small divided doses, the amount given is increased gradually until satisfactory improvement is noted. This may take 1 to 4 weeks. For maintenance the total dose should be given at one time, preferably at bedtime. Treatment should be continued for 6 to 8 months, at which time the maintenance dose can be gradually lowered over many weeks if there are no signs of recurrence. With the same oral dose given there are wide variations in plasma level occurring from patient to patient. For this reason the drug should be pushed to maximum tolerance level and then lowered. Some clinicians believe that the optimal response is not seen until the equivalent of 300 mg. of imipramine has been given.

SIDE EFFECTS. Side effects usually consist of dry mouth, constipation, blurred vision, and hyperhidrosis. Increased appetite and weight gain have been commonly reported. Less frequent are tachycardia, anorexia, anxiety, insomnia, increased ocular tension, orthostatic hypotension, toxic delirium, urinary retention, and adynamic ileus.

PRECAUTIONS. These compounds have been reported to aggravate the symptoms of schizophrenia and may convert depression into mania. They should be used with caution in patients with angle-closure glaucoma.

POISONING. Poisoning occurs within 1 to 4 hours of overdose. Symptoms are of anticholinergic toxicity. Respiratory and cardiac shock may be accompanied by ventricular arrhythmias. Agitation, coma, and a variety of neurological signs may occur. Early gastric lavage, attention to cardiac arrhythmia, and administration of physostigmine (1 to 3 mg. in divided doses, repeated as necessary) will be helpful.

DRUG INTERACTIONS. Beware of interactions with drugs used to lower blood pressure. Tricyclics block guanethedine and clonidine. The effects of alcohol, anticholinergic compounds, adrenergic agents (epinephrine, cold remedies, nasal decongestants), and thyroid preparations may be potentiated. Methylphenidate may inhibit the metabolism of tricyclic antidepressants and hence potentiate their action.

MONOAMINE OXIDASE INHIBITORS

Probably less effective than the tricyclic antidepressants, these drugs are usually tried after failure with tricyclics or ECT or in those patients who have previously shown a good response to them (MAO inhibitors). In addition, the MAO inhibitors have the serious disadvantage of producing hypertensive reaction with certain foods. Usually the joint administration of tricyclics and MAO inhibitors is not recommended, although more recently some good reports of the cautious use of these drugs simultaneously has helped treatment-resistant depressions. L-tryptophan, the amino acid precursor of 5-HT, has been suggested as increasing the efficacy of MAO inhibitors when given in doses of 5 to 9 Gm. per day.

DOSAGE. Initial dose is usually larger than the anticipated maintenance dose. The amount that relieves sumptoms should be

Table 13. Nutrients (vitamins, minerals, etc.)

Nutrient	Suggested daily supplement	Megadose	Precautions
Vitamins			
A (retinal*)	5,000 U		Toxicity with overdose
B_1 (thiamine)	2.5 mg.	100-500 mg.	
B_2 (riboflavin)	2.5 mg.	10-75 mg.	
B_3 (niacin)	30 mg.	3 Gm.	After meals to avoid flush; no flush with niacinamide
B_5 (pantothenic acid)	15 mg.	150 mg.	Large doses increase joint and tooth sensitivity
B_6 (pyridoxine)	3 mg.	150-1000 mg.	Large doses enhance dream recall
B_{12} (cyanocobalamine)	9 μ.	1000 μ. IM	
C (ascorbic acid)	250 mg.	3-10 Gm.	With large doses beware kidney stones in women taking calcium; may destroy B_{12} if given simultaneously by mouth
D (calciferol*)	400 μ		Toxicity with overdose
E (tocopherol*)	45 mg.	200-800 mg.	
K (menedine*)			20-25 mg. daily only if needed
Biotin	0.45 mg.	300 mg.	
Folic acid	0.4 mg.	1-5 mg.	Should accompany B_{12} administration
Major minerals			
Calcium	1 Gm.		

Magnesium	600 mg.		
Sodium			
Phosphorous	1.5 Gm.		Leg cramps with excess
Trace elements			
Cobalt			
Chromium	1 mg.		
Copper	2 mg.		
Fluoride			
Iron	25 mg.		Overdose from excess multivitamins
Iodine	225 μ.		
Manganese	5 mg.	6 mg.	
Molybdenum	0.1 mg.		
Selenium	0.2 mg.		
Zinc	20 mg.	45 mg.	
Choline	250 mg.	750 mg.	
Other			
Linoleic acid			
Para-aminobenzoic acid (PABA)	30 mg.	1,200 mg.	
Inositol	250 mg.	1 Gm.	
Rutin			
Bioflavinoids	50 mg.	200 mg.	

*Fat-soluble.

continued, given in divided doses. If a single dose is used it should not be given in the evening because of a generalized sympathomimetic (stimulating) effect.

ADVERSE REACTIONS. Hypertensive crises, particularly precipitated by the eating of foods with high tyramine content. Such crises are characterized by tachycardia, headache, palpitation, nausea, and vomiting. Occasional subarachnoid or intracranial hemorrhage can occur. Other treating physicians should be alerted that patients are taking these drugs. A card with this information and statement of drug interaction should be carried by the patient. Orthostatic hypotension may also occur, as well as dizziness, vertigo, headache, abnormal cardiac rates and rhythms, weakness, fatigue, dryness of mouth, blurred vision, constipation, and rashes.

PRECAUTIONS. These drugs should be avoided in schizophrenic patients. They can swing depression into mania. Patients should not concurrently take drugs containing sympathomimetic compounds such as cold remedies, decongestants, etc. Foods with high tyramine content should be strictly avoided, such as strong, aged cheeses, red wines, kippered and pickled herring, chicken livers, canned figs, broad beans (fava beans), chocolate, beer, yeast, meat extracts, game, and yogurt.

POISONING. Symptoms may be delayed for 12 hours or longer and are largely adrenergic and include agitation, increased respiration and heart rate, dilated pupils, increased tendon reflexes, weakness, tremors, ataxia, convulsions, sweating, hyperthermia, heart block, hypotension, delerium, and coma. Treatment consists of hemodialysis, forced diuresis, acidification of the urine, and administration of chlorpromazine. Phentolamine and propanolol have been used to counteract the hypertensive crises.

DRUG INTERACTIONS. Avoid adrenergic agents. Do not use meperidine (Demerol) and related agents. Withdraw levodopa 2 to 4 weeks prior to using these drugs. Use furazolidone with extreme caution. A 2-week interval after MAO inhibitor withdrawal is generally recommended prior to the use of tricyclics.

NUTRIENTS

There is increasing concern about the need to supply proper nutrients to the body, including its most sensitive organ the brain.

Orthomolecular medicine and orthomolecular psychiatry have been recently founded upon the proposition that individual differences include widely varying biochemical needs for some forty growth and maintenance chemicals, including both minerals and vitamins. The latter are used empirically in megadoses (megavitamin therapy). The appearance of psychiatric symptoms with deficiencies of niacin (dementia of pellagra), thiamin (Wernicke-Korsakoff syndrome), and ascorbic acid (scurvy) are prototypes. Seven subtypes of the schizophrenias have been attributed to such nutrient deficiencies. Sensitivity to certain food substances (food allergy) has also been delineated and supported by a considerable literature outlining a host of emotional and cognitive symptoms. With the advent of cytotoxic food testing, clinical management of such patients has become increasingly possible.

While these concepts are new and often controversial, it seems plausible that a brain supplied with adequate nutrients is better able to respond to other therapies concurrently given. (See Table 13).

SUGGESTED READINGS

American Medical Association: AMA Drug Evaluations, AMA Council on Drugs, ed. 3, Chicago, 1977, The Association.

Avery, G. S., editor: Drug treatment: principles and practices of clinical pharmacology and therapeutics, Acton, Mass., 1976, Publishing Sciences Group.

Baldessarini, R. J.: Chemotherapy in psychiatry, Cambridge, Mass., 1977, Harvard University Press.

Barchas, J. D. editor: Psychopharmacology: from theory to practice, New York, 1977, Oxford University Press.

Jarvik, M. editor: Psychopharmacology in the practice of medicine, New York, 1977, Appleton-Century-Crofts.

Jefferson, J.W., and Greist, J. H.: Primer of lithium therapy, Baltimore, 1977, The Williams & Wilkins Co.

Lipton, M. A., DiMascio, A., and Killam, K.: Psychopharmacology, a generation of progress, New York, 1978, Raven Press.

Pfeiffer, C.: Mental and elemental nutrients, New Canaan, Conn., 1975, Keats Publishing Co.

Shader, R. I., editor: Manual of psychiatric therapeutics: practial psychopharmacology and psychiatry, Boston, 1975, Little, Brown & Co.

Silverstone, T., and Turner, P.: Drug treatment in psychiatry, Boston, 1974, Routledge and Kegan Paul.

Simpson, L. L., editor: Drug treatment of mental disorders, New York, 1976, Raven Press.

Ulett, G. A.: Food allergy—cytotoxic testing and the central nervous system, Psychiat. J. Univ. Ottawa 4:April, 1979.

Usdin, E., Hamburg, D., and Barchas, J., editors: Neuroregulators and psychiatric disorders, New York, 1977, Oxford University Press.

26

Management of suicidal patients

INCIDENCE

In the United States, suicides account for 22,000 deaths a year. This is the tenth leading cause of death. There are about 10 attempted suicides for each 1 that is successful. Suicide is not a product of modern civilization but is influenced by social factors. Anthropologists have found it to be completely absent in some cultures, very common in others. The suicide rate decreases in time of war and in prosperity. Ireland, Chile, New Zealand, and Norway are among countries with low suicide rates; Sweden, Denmark, and Japan, among the highest. Suicide depends, however, not only upon broad social factors but also upon immediate environmental pressures and differences in individual personality structure.

Recent studies show that suicide occurs almost exclusively in persons clinically ill and that two-thirds of these suffer from either manic-depressive psychosis or alcoholism. Over 80% are older than 40 years and men outnumber women two to one. Seemingly more vulnerable are persons who live alone (single, divorced, or widowed) and those concerned over the death of a loved one or about personal ill health. Less serious attempts may occur after drinking and marital quarrels. The number of attempted suicides far exceeds the number of completed suicides.

Two-thirds of successful suicides communicated their intent to someone prior to the act. A smaller number of unsuccessful ones communicated such intent. One-fourth of all attempted suicides and over one-half of successful suicides have made previous attempts. One in ten has a family history of successful or attempted suicide. Most successful suicides have received medical or psychiatric care prior to the act.

Attempts to explain the dynamics of suicide include Freud's suggestion that anger toward others is turned inward against the self; that suicide is only a further step for a patient already "emotionally dead"; that the patient feels he will be reunited with loved ones after death; that he gains a feeling of omnipotence by destroying a life, though it be his own; or that suicide is welcomed as a form of punishment for feelings of worthlessness. Much that has been written about a "death instinct" was neatly summarized by Zilboorg (1937): "To say the death instinct gains the upper hand over the life instinct is merely an elaborate way of saying that man does die or kill himself." Hendin says it is worthwhile to inquire of everyone who attempts suicide concerning his attitudes toward death, about presumed events after death, and about his thoughts regarding the suicidal act.

The most common methods of attempting suicide in the United States include drug ingestion, cutting, and gas inhalation. In other countries favorite methods vary. The most common methods used in *successful* suicides are hanging, shooting, drug ingestion, and asphyxiation by gas. Drowning, shooting, and hanging are more commonly seen in men and poisoning in women. More subtle methods of suicide are the physiological such as, for example, the coronary patient who refuses to reduce his work schedule and the diabetic who suddenly is unable to balance his insulin and diet. Another form of "chronic suicide" is exhibited by alcoholics and addicts. Delirious patients, seen most often on medical and surgical wards, present a different type of suicidal risk in that they may take their lives in a state of anxious confusion, in which, for example, they can mistake a window for a door.

It has been found that suicide is rare among neurotics who show predominately an anxiety reaction. The hysteric's attempts at environmental manipulation through suicidal gesture may, however, perhaps from misjudgment, have a fatal outcome. The whole problem of evaluating the suicidal danger in neurotics is complicated by the frequent mislabeling as neurotic of those persons suffering from mild degrees of manic-depressive disorder. Commonly, however, a psychoneurotic (with obsessive-compulsive reaction, hysteria, etc.) may experience symptoms of depression as an episode of his basic neurosis.

PREVENTION

In evaluating suicidal danger, one must remember that suicidal thoughts or ideas, considered in more than a passing manner, have been found in as many as 50% of normal persons by some investigators. Hysterical and psychopathic individuals use attempted suicide as a means of revenge or spite, or to achieve their own way. In the chronic psychoneurotic or other unstable personality, acute alcoholism may release inhibitions and arouse strong feelings of guilt, fear, or aggression—with consequent suicide. The psychoneurotic with whom suicide is an obsessive rumination or in whom the suicidal thought is in the form of a fear instead of a desire presents less danger. In the case of persons who act out their problems it must be remembered that what is begun as merely a suicidal gesture may result in a successful attempt.

Even here, however, there is awareness of the possibility that the attempt may be successful; this action, in fact, has the nature of a gamble with death. The depressed patient is a potential suicide, and no suicidal talk is to be considered lightly. The agitated depressive who admits no delusions is a likely candidate, as is the patient with delusions of worthlessness, guilt, and need for punishment. It should not be forgotten that suicide is an important cause of death among chronic alcoholics. Feelings of futility in adolescence and in old age should be heeded as warning signals. Marked insomnia should also place the physician on his guard; early morning hours are a favorite time for suicide. A history of previous attempts or of suicides in the family may be important, and suicidal desire may yet lurk behind the smiling countenance in a rapidly recovering patient with depression. Evidence of bodily tension such as hand wringing may be the only warning sign that remains. The Rorschach and other tests can sometimes reveal suicidal intentions.

Many communities have organized suicide-prevention centers with 24-hour telephone coverage and available consultants. Although such centers appear very worthwhile in assisting persons with various types of emotional trouble, it would appear that persons calling in are not always those who have made suicidal attempts. A real focus of effort should be upon the high-risk patients who have been identified as making serious suicidal attempts.

Immediate hospitalization of the acutely depressed or suspected suicidal patient on a closed ward may be a lifesaving measure. But do not leave the patient alone while you step out to call the hospital! Adequate suicidal precautions can be observed only on a psychiatric division. A well-meaning companion is often little better than no preventive measure. In a general hospital setting, delirious patients should be evaluated when at their worst (during the evening hours) and should be kept on the ground floor and near the nurses' station. The use of antidepressant drugs is an effective tool to combat depression. As there is some delay in achieving an effective level with these drugs, electroconvulsive therapy is often necessary during the early stages of drug therapy.

Often the psychiatrist takes a calculated risk and follows the mild depressive as an outpatient. Here psychotherapy is not only of remedial benefit but also permits the psychotherapist to repeatedly evaluate the current suicidal risk. Adequate chemical sedation at night combined with dextroamphetamine sulfate (Dexedrine) in the morning has long been a useful routine. The antidepressants are extremely useful for cases of depression followed in the outpatient clinic. In selected cases ECT is also an outpatient procedure.

SUGGESTED READINGS

Avery, D., and Winokur, G.: Mortality in depressed patients treated with electroconvulsive therapy and antidepressants, Arch. Gen. Psychiatry **33**:1029, 1976.

Beck, A. T., Weissman, A., and Kovacs, M.: Alcoholism, hopelessness and suicidal behavior, J. Stud. Alcohol **37**(1):66, 1976.

Farberow, N. L., editor: Suicide in different cultures, Baltimore, 1975, University Park Press.

Farberow, N. L., Schneidman, E. S., and Leonard, C. V.: Suicide among general medical and surgical hospital patients with malignant neoplasms, Med. Bull. Veterans Admin. MB-**9**:1, 1963.

Fawcett, J.: Suicidal depression and physical illness, J.A.M.A **219**:1303, 1972.

Jacobziner, H.: Attempted suicides in adolescents by poisoning, Am. J. Psychother. **19**:245, 1965.

Miles, C. P.: Conditions predisposing to suicide: a review, J. Nerv. Ment. Dis. **164**:231, 1977.

Murphy, G. E.: The physician's responsibility for suicide. I. An error of commission, Ann. Intern Med. **82:**301, 1975.

Murphy, G. E.: The physician's responsibility for suicide. II. Errors of omission, Ann. Intern Med. **82:**305, 1975.

Nelson, S. H., and Grunebaum, H.: A follow-up of wrist slashers, Am. J. Psychiatry **127:**1345, 1971.

Petit, J. M., Biggs, J. T.: Tricyclic antidepressant overdoses in adolescent patients, Pediatrics **59:**283, 1977.

Reich, P., and Kelly, M. J.: Suicide attempts by hospitalized medical and surgical patients, N. Engl. J. Med. **294:** 1976.

Robins, L. N., West, P. A., Murphy, G. E.: The high rate of suicide in older white men: a study testing ten hypotheses, Soc. Psychiatry **12:**1, 1977.

Rosen, D. H.: The serious suicide attempt, J.A.M.A. **235:**2105, 1976.

Schmidt, C. W., Jr., and others: Suicide by vehicular crash, Am. J. Psychiatry **134**(2):175, 1977.

Shaffer, D.: Suicide in childhood and early adolescence, J. Child Psychol. Psychiatry **15:**275, 1974.

Shepherd, D. M., and Barraclough, B. M.: The aftermath of parental suicide for children, Br. J. Psychiatry **129:**267, 1976.

Weissman, M. M.: The epidemiology of suicide attempts, 1960 to 1971, Arch. Gen. Psychiatry **30:**737, 1974.

Wetzel, R. D.: Hopelessness, depression, and suicide intent, Arch. Gen. Psychiatry **33:**1069, 1976.

27

Sleep disorders

After Berger constructed the electroencephalograph in 1924-1929, five patterns of EEG activity during sleep were described by Loomis, Harvey, and Hobart in 1935. In 1953, Aserinsky and Kleitman described rapid eye movements (REM) during sleep using the electro-oculogram (EOG). When a subject was awakened during REM sleep, he was dreaming 74% of the time; whereas, during non-REM (NREM) sleep he was dreaming only 7% of the time. Temperature, metabolic rate, and electrical patterns of the brain of REM sleep approximated those of arousal. Pulse, respiration, and blood pressure varied widely during REM sleep in contrast to small changes during non-REM sleep. Non-REM sleep was studied further and normal sleep was divided into stages 1, 2, 3, and 4.

Almost one-third of one's life is spent asleep. Normal sleep proceeds in 90-minute cycles of REM and NREM sleep. Slow-wave sleep (SWS) predominates in the first part of the night, and REM sleep predominates in the last part of the night. Patterns are consistent night after night. Typical values for males in their twenties are: total time in bed, 442 minutes; sleep period time, 425 minutes; total sleep time, 419 minutes; sleep efficiency index, 95%; sleep latency, 15 minutes; number of stages entered, 41; number of awakenings, 3; REM period length, 30 minutes; number of REM periods, 4; 1% in stage 0 (wakefulness, predominantly alpha activity); 4% in stage 1 (light sleep, mixed low-voltage fast activity; 46% in stage 2 (spindle and K-complex activity and some delta activity); 6% in stage 3 (moderate amounts of delta activity);

15% percent in stage 4 (predominantly delta activity; and 28% in stage REM (stage 1 EEG activity with rapid conjugate eye movements). During REM sleep, dreaming, autonomic activity, and penile erection occur. Deprivation (by waking subject and interrupting stage REM) is followed by a compensatory REM increase ("need"). Slow-wave sleep (SWS) during stages 3 and 4 is associated with growth hormone secretion. Deprivation is followed by a compensatory increase. Blood levels of prolactin and testosterone increase throughout the night.

Factors that affect sleep are age, sex, naps, drugs, and disease. Average sleep time decreases from 16 hours at birth to 9 hours at puberty and decreases further with old age. After age 20 SWS declines and may disappear completely. Aging males lose SWS more than females. REM predominates in morning naps and SWS in afternoon naps. Afternoon naps reduce SWS the following night. Most drugs, including hypnotics, reduce REM sleep. Many drugs reduce SWS.

REM sleep dream recall late at night is most likely to be vivid, detailed, and visual when REM periods are longer and sleep is lighter. NREM dream recall is more thought-like.

Deprivation of sleep for prolonged periods leads to disorders of thought and perception indistinguishable from schizophrenia. Dement found that there is a specific need for REM sleep and it must be made up at later time if deprivation of REM occurs.

Sleep disorders include somnambulism, sleep talking, bruxism, enuresis, night terrors, nightmares, narcolepsy, hypersomnia, and insomnia. Sleep disturbances occur in 20% of the normal population and are very frequent in psychiatric disorders such as depression and schizophrenia.

SOMNAMBULISM. Sleepwalking is estimated to occur in 1 to 6% of the normal population, more in males and children. Frequently there is a positive family history. It is often accompanied by night terrors and enuresis. It occurs only during NREM sleep in stages 3 and 4. If awakened, sleepwalkers are confused; if not awakened, they are amnesic for the episode. Children outgrow the disorder. Adult somnambulists often have psychiatric disturbances. Treatment consists of safety measures such as locking doors and windows, sleeping on the first floor, and removing potentially dangerous objects.

SLEEP TALKING. Sleep talking is very common, it occurs during REM or NREM sleep.

BRUXISM. Persistent grinding of teeth occurs in adults even during sleep; it is associated with pain and trismus of the jaw; occurs during stage 2.

ENURESIS. Bedwetting occurs mainly in men and boys and is not related to dreaming. It can occur during all stages of sleep, but usually in stage 4. Excessive bladder contractions and higher heart rates are noted, and it may be familial. Parental training and administration of imipramine may be helpful. Enuresis resulting from nocturnal epilepsy, diabetes mellitus, infection, urological obstruction, or neurological disorder should be excluded.

NIGHT TERRORS. "Pavor nocturus" in children and "incubus" in adults is characterized by extreme panic and extreme autonomic discharge, mobility, vocalization, and little recall. Night terrors occur early in the night in stage 4 sleep and last for a minute or two. Children outgrow the disturbance but adults often have psychiatric disturbances. Psychological evaluation of children is indicated.

NIGHTMARE. A nightmare is a frightening dream at any age, with detailed recall of an unpleasant and frightening experience occurring during REM sleep. If persistent, psychiatric evaluation is indicated.

NARCOLEPSY. The narcolepsy tetrad includes excessive daytime sleepiness, cataplexy (sudden decrease in muscle tone precipitated by laughter, anger, or surprise), sleep paralysis, and hypnagogic hallucinations. Sleep attacks go directly into state REM. Stimulants help sleep attacks and imipramine the other symptoms. There is danger in using both types of drugs at once.

HYPERSOMNIA. Sleep is extended although stages are normal. Symptoms include excessive daytime sleepiness, sleep attacks, naps, automatic behavior, fatigue, depression. Awakening is difficult and associated with confusion. Stimulant drugs are effective. Eighty-five percent of excessive daytime sleepiness is caused by narcolepsy syndrome and sleep apnea. In boys periodic attacks of sleepiness recurring about every 5 months accompanied by bulimia and sometimes by the absence of sleep spindles is called Kleine-Levin syndrome. Periodic attacks of hypersomnia associated with obesity and respiratory insufficiency is called Pickwickian syndrome. Chronic hypersomnia may be a symptom of head injury, brain tumor, cerebrovascular disorder, or hypothyroidism.

INSOMNIA. Nighttime insomnia complaints are expressed as nighttime insufficient sleep, frequent awakenings, difficulty falling asleep, and early morning arousal. Daytime complaints are sleepiness, fatigue, depression, anxiety, and inability to nap. Causes of chronic refractory insomnia are sleeping pills, nocturnal myoclonus, sleep apnea, and rhythm disturbance. Nocturnal myoclonus (restless legs) is twitching of the anterior tibialis muscle for 2 to 5 seconds at approximately 28-second intervals only during sleep. Sleep apnea (periodic cessation of respiration during sleep) is a newly recognized respiratory syndrome diagnosable only during sleep. Patients complain of excessive daytime sleepiness, snoring, gasping for breath at night, frequent movement in sleep, fatigue, difficulty remaining alert, and early morning headaches. Obesity may be present. Patients say they postpone sleep, whereas narcoleptics cannot. Short naps do not help. Ritalin, Dexedrine, Desoxyn, and Tofranil are ineffective. Weight reduction, removal of enlarged tonsils, adenoids, or soft palate tissue and/or use of permanent tracheal valve in cases of obstructive apnea may be helpful. Nocturnal diaphragm pacing is being tried in patients with central sleep apnea.

SECONDARY SLEEP DISTURBANCE. Schizophrenic patients show a defect in recovery of SWS after experimental deprivation, but no consistent evidence to date of other abnormalities. Patients in remission have normal or exaggerated REM compensation. No REM rebound occurs in the acute state. Depressed patients show great variability in sleep patterns, which improve when clinical condition improves. Pregnant patients show depressed SWS in third trimester.

SUGGESTED READINGS

Karacan, I., Moore, C. A., Dement, B., and Williams, R. L.: Disturbed sleep as a function of sleep apnea: too much sleep but not enough, Texas Medicine **73:**1, 1977.

Mariuz, M. J., and Watters, C. J.: Enuresis in non-psychotic boys treated with imipramine, Am. J. Psychiatry **120:**597, 1963.

Schneck, J. M., and Fuselli, H.: Nightmare and sleep paralysis, J.A.M.A. **20:**725, 1969.

Shapiro, B., and Spitz, H.: Problems in the differential diagnosis of narcolepsy versus schizophrenia, Am. J. Psychiatry **133:**1321, 1976.

Sours, J. A.: Narcolepsy and other disturbances in the sleep-waking rhythm: a study of 115 cases with a review of the literature, J. Nerv. Ment. Dis. **137:**525, 1963.

Vogel, L. W.: A review of REM sleep deprivation, Arch. Gen. Psychiatry **32:**749, 1975.

Yoss, R. E., and Daly, D. D.: Narcolepsy, Arch. Intern Med. **106:**168, 1960.

Zarcone, V.: Narcolepsy, N. Engl. J. Med. **288:**1156, 1973.

28

Forensic psychiatry

The psychiatrist, in dealing with persons whose chief symptom is deviation in behavior, must frequently testify in court; for this reason the therapist should be familiar with medicolegal procedures. In the courtroom, as a special witness, his sole job is to give scientific facts or psychiatric opinions, not to defend the psychotic or to bring a criminal to justice. On the witness stand he should use clear and concise language that a lay jury can understand. He should be prepared to undergo cross-examination, even endure cajolery or threat to his personal esteem, and behave always in a modest and unemotional manner. However, a psychiatrist with an adequate workup of the patient and convinced of his position will rarely be subjected to detailed cross-examination by an experienced trial attorney.

COURTROOM TESTIMONY

Although the psychiatrist is called into court as a scientist and expert, he may be asked to give opinions as well as facts. He would do well to prepare his testimony beforehand with the advice of the trial lawyer who has called upon him, in order to know the kind of question he may be asked. He can appear very foolish, and indeed be of little help to anyone if he cannot give the kind of information needed by the court. He should remember that the information needed from his mental status examination will be different from case to case. Most courts will not permit the psychiatrist to decide whether the patient knows right from wrong or is or is not competent. They merely want his *opinion* of how the patient is functioning mentally—his mental state at some designated time—and possibly a psychiatric diagnosis. A physician usually cannot quote history taken by himself or by someone else, as this is hearsay evidence and not admissible. Of most importance are the findings on examination of the patient, with careful note taking at the time of such examination. The court will be interested in the logic leading to the diagnosis. The court may require "yes" and "no" answers in order to arrive at its verdict; however, it is possible to ask the judge for permission to explain.

CRIMINAL RESPONSIBILITY

A psychiatrist is frequently called upon to testify in criminal cases. He may be asked to give opinions in accordance with rules laid down in 1843 in the famous *McNaughton case* where in Scotland in 1843 a paranoid patient, David McNaughton, shot and killed the secretary to Prime Minister Robert Peel. The rule that was established than asks: "Was the accused laboring under such a defect of reasoning from a disease of his mind as not to know the nature and quality of the act he was doing, and if he did it, he did not know that what he was doing was wrong?" The majority of American psychiatrists today, as well as enlightened jurists, feel that this test is unsatisfactory, yet frequently some answer to it must be given. More recently there has been introduced the concept of *irresistible impulse* as a criminal defense. Although in itself not a good term, it implies psychiatrically acceptable doctrine that some individuals are less able to adhere to the right, by reason of abnormal urges which they have little power to control. This problem is closely allied to the question of the existence of *temporary insanity,* which, although almost nonexistent from the medical point of view, is a concept with which the forensic psychiatrist should be familiar. Ideally, the psychiatrist should give evidence to show: (1) whether the individual was suffering from a medically recognized disorder and (2) whether the disorder had distorted his social judgment and interfered with the exercise of customary social control. Proof of a mental disorder may serve to reduce the degree of crime (e.g., from murder to manslaughter).

The Durham decision in the District of Columbia provided a most hopeful shift in the handling of psychiatric testimony. Under the *Durham Rule* the behavior of the accused is considered as to whether it is a product of mental disorder. If it is judged to be so, the individual is committed rather than sentenced. Whereas many legal minds have feared that this criterion would result in the community's being flooded with psychopathic characters, the fact is that a very small percentage of criminals have successfully proved their behavior to be the result of mental illness. The doctor's role is to give evidence relating to the presence of a mental illness, not to express an opinion that the accused should be restrained or imprisoned for his offense. His function is not to recommend punishment or even to express an opinion as to the defendant's potential for crime or that he "undoubtedly" would commit similar crimes in the future if unrestrained.

COMMITMENT PROCEDURES

The procedure for commitment of insane patients or mentally ill persons varies from state to state but in general three basic methods are used: (1) examination by one or usually two physicians appearing before a judge, with a jury hearing on demand of the patient or at the judge's discretion; (2) in a few states a hearing before a commission consisting of a judge and two physicians or a physician and a lawyer; and (3) commitment upon certification by a physician, with hearing only upon appeal by the person being certified.

The widespread use of court commitment procedure was instituted to protect the sane person from being railroaded into a mental hospital, in the days when institutionalization was considered a putting away, rather than a procedure for purposes of medical treatment. Such commitment procedures involving public hearings with the patient present are cumbersome, expensive, and heartless, and they place the patient under needless and possibly harmful stress. The procedure is analogous to that in conviction for a crime and with paranoid persons may dangerously involve those who give testimony. It is hoped that in a more enlightened future a court-appointed commission of physicians can commit directly by certification.

In many states *observation commitment* is permitted for a brief, stated length of time, as an emergency procedure. This is accomplished by permission of the relatives and a statement by two qualified physicians. Most states today permit *voluntary commitment,* or informal procedures in which the patient may seek hospitalization for himself, if there is room and if the hospital admitting authority feels the patient will benefit from such hospitalization. In most cases he can obtain release a few days after written request unless by that time he has been formally committed. Patients who feel they are being restrained illegally may request a hearing through a *writ of habeas corpus.*

The commitment of mental defectives and alcoholics is, in some states, provided for under separate statutes. Voluntary admission of alcoholics has not been entirely satisfactory, because of their early demand for release when they become sober. Recent legislation that frowns upon repeated arrest and incarceration in jail for public drunkenness will surely bring greater hospital admission rates of persons whose main symptom is alcoholism.

PRIVILEGED COMMUNICATION

Communications between a patient and his physician are, in the majority of the fifty states, held to be confidential and such information cannot be released without the written permission of the patient or unless the patient calls the physician to testify in court on his behalf. Although this rule applies only to information pertaining to litigation, yet there is the moral and professional ethical obligation against disclosure of such information to any person other than those concerned with the patient's immediate health care. Recently there has been concern over the accessibility of medical records stored in a computer. In actuality, it is more difficult to break into computer storage than into an ordinary medical record library; hence, if due precaution and some of the new user identification techniques are utilized, such fears are unwarranted.

SEXUAL OFFENSES

Because of emotion aroused in the public by the report of deviant sexual activities, legislation has been enacted from time to time dealing with such offenders. Although some states have laws dealing with exhibitionism, bestiality, homosexuality, adultery, and prostitution, those who commit such acts are usually not dangerous to others.

The "sexual psychopath" clause is directed mainly toward pedophilia (sex relations with children) and rape (including statutory rape [sexual intercourse below the age of consent], incest, or forced rape). Ideally the purpose of such laws is to permit a truly indeterminate sentence of from 1 day to life imprisonment with the ultimate aim that the patient be incarcerated as long as is deemed necessary to protect the public but with the intention that he might be rehabilitated by psychiatric treatment and be released whenever it appeared that he was a good risk on parole. The wording of such laws varies from state to state, and thus difficulties have arisen in their administration.

Actually we know little of the practical dynamics of sexual psychopathy that would lead to an efficient treatment or cure of such conditions, and one defect in a law of this type is that it implies that we can predict who is likely to demonstrate socially dangerous sexual behavior. Some states permit hospitalization only after a criminal offense has been committed. Studies have shown that sex offenders have no single category of mental pathology and that men who are sex offenders often commit other types of crime and vice versa.

As Guttmacher points out, there is as much difference between the average exhibitionist and a rapist as between a shoplifter and a safecracker. Also there is no evidence that sexual criminals progress from minor offenses such as exhibitionism to major offenses like rape.

MENTAL INCOMPETENCY

The psychiatrist is frequently called upon to judge a patient's testamentary capacity or mental competency and to help the family with the institution of *guardianship* proceedings. In such cases, the significance of emotional disability is often overlooked by the court. In deciding competency, one should consider the background and experience of the person and also whether competency for only a specific act is to be judged (e.g., executing a will or some particular business transaction). It is important that the psychiatrist not consider competence generally but understand that the question is, instead, "competence for what particular purpose." Therefore, his mental status examination should be tailored to throw light upon the specific question.

Guardianship proceedings in most states are, in some ways, similar to commitment procedures. A petition is made to the court by friends or relatives and the patient is notified. The case may be tried by the judge alone in a probate or county court, although in a number of states a jury trial is still used and the patient has the right of counsel.

The adjudication that a person is mentally ill does not establish that such a person is incompetent. Thus mental illness may coexist with good mental capacity. A patient committed without a decision about his competency enjoys all of his civil rights, including the right to contract, to transfer property, to sue, and to be sued. In some states, however, statutes expressly declare that persons committed to state institutions are legally incompetent to contract.

In the case of *competence regarding the making of a will*, the fact that the patient had to be prompted to recall his property is not sufficient to prove unfitness to make a will. For testamentary purposes it is sufficient that the testator understand the condition of his estate, his obligation toward his relatives, and the importance and effect of the provisions of his will. Because senile persons may have increased suggestibility, the court may deem it important to ascertain whether undue influence was used when the will was made. Courts have sometimes ruled that it takes less mind to make a will than to make a contract.

It is of increasing importance that the physician have the consent of the patient before proceeding with any treatment procedure. This is especially true in connection with electroconvulsive therapies. A patient's mere signing of a routine release form is not sufficient. In recent suits for malpractice it has been important that evidence be presented to show that the possible side effects and complications of the procedure were fully explained. Where competence of the patient is in doubt, informed consent should be obtained from the next of kin. For emergency practices and for research procedures, a human rights committee can stand in judgment that the patient's rights were not abused. Research procedures should be of value for the patient himself and not merely for the good of humanity.

MARRIAGE AND DIVORCE

About half the states have laws intended to prevent insane persons from marrying; but in many the responsibility falls on the license clerk, who can hardly be expected to judge mental competency. Marriages of such persons are considered void or voidable and thus open to annulment, although children born of such void marriages are not considered legally illegitimate. Incurable insanity is a ground for divorce in more than half the states.

SUGGESTED READINGS

Bazelon, D. L.: The perils of wizardry, Am. J. Psychiatry **131:**1317, 1974.

Cocozza, J. A., and Steadman, J. H.: The failure of psychiatric predictions of dangerousness. Clear and convincing evidence, Rutgers Law Review **29:**1084, 1976.

Diamond, B. L.: Isaac Ray and the trial of Daniel M'Naghten, Am. J. Psychiatry **112:**651, 1956.

Goldstein, A.: The insanity defense, New Haven, 1967, Yale University Press.

Guttmacher, M. S.: The role of psychiatry in law, Springfield, Ill., 1968, Charles C Thomas, Publisher.

Guze, S. B.: Criminality and psychiatric disorders, New York, 1976, Oxford University Press.

Henn, F. A., Herjanic, M., and Vanderpearl, R. H.: Forensic psychiatry: profiles of sexual offenders, Am. J. Psychiatry **133:**694, 1976.

Henn, F. A., Herjanic, M., and Vanderpearl, R. H.: Forensic psychiatry: anatomy of a service, Compr. Psychiatry **18:**337, 1977.

Henn, F. A., Herjanic, M., and Vanderpearl, R. H.: Forensic psychiatry: diagnosis and criminal responsibility, J. Nerv. Ment. Dis. **162:**423, 1976.

Herjanic, M., Henn, F. A., and Vanderpearl, R. H.: Forensic psychiatry: female offenders, Am. J. Psychiatry **134:**556, 1977.

Kopolow, L. E.: A review of major implications of the O'Conner v. Donaldson decision, Am. J. Psychiatry **133:**4, 1976.

MacDonald, J. M.: Psychiatry and the criminal courts, ed. 3, Springfield, Ill., 1976, Charles C Thomas, Publisher.

Martin, R. L., Cloninger, R., and Guze, S. B.: Female criminality and the prediction of recidivism, Arch. Gen. Psychiatry **35:**207, 1978.

Mesnikoff, A. M., and Lauterbach, C. G.: The association of violent dangerous behavior with psychiatric disorders: a review of the research literature, J. Psych. Law **415:**1975.

Ray, I.: A treatise on the medical jurisprudence of insanity, 1838, Boston, Charles C. Little and James Brown.

Roth, L. H., Meisel, A., and Lidz, C.: Tests of competency to consent to treatment, Am. J. Psychiatry **279:**1977.

Sadoff, R. L.: Forensic psychiatry: a practical guide for lawyers and psychiatrists, Springfield, Ill., 1975, Charles C Thomas, Publisher.

Stone, A. A.: Mental health and law: a system in transition, Washington, D.C., 1975, U.S. Government Printing Office.

Stone, A. A.: Psychiatry and the law. In Nicholi, A. M., editor: The Harvard guide to modern psychiatry, Cambridge, Mass., 1978, Belnap Press of Harvard University Press.

Tomelleri, C. J., Lakshminarayanan, N., and Herjanic, M.: Who are the "committed"? J. Nerv. Ment. Dis. **165**:288, 1977.

Wald, M. S.: Legal policies affecting children: a lawyer's request for aid, Child Dev. **47**:1, 1976.

Yochelson, S., and Samerow, S. E.: The criminal personality, New York, 1977, Jason Aronson.

29

The psychiatrist and community mental health

THE PROBLEM

Mental illness is a serious public health problem. Nearly half of all hospital beds in the United States are devoted to the care of the mentally ill. Estimates have been variously given that 1 in every 20 persons will spend some part of his life within a mental hospital and that many Americans (approximately 1 in 5) are afflicted with less serious emotional maladies requiring treatment. Suicide alone accounts for 22,000 deaths a year, and there are an estimated 5 to 6 million chronic alcoholics in the United States. Studies by Essen-Möller in Sweden, by Srole in midtown Manhattan, and by Leighton and Leighton in Stirling County, a Canadian rural area, indicate that from one-third to two-thirds of the population studied showed symptoms suggestive of psychiatric disorder. Such figures, large though they may be, give only a partial picture of the amount of mental and emotional disturbance—in terms of their cost as measured by work hours lost to industry and tax dollars spent for treatment and custodial care and the indirect cost—such as the personal and community tragedies of delinquency, crime, personal isolation, boredom with work, purposelessness in day-to-day living, alcoholism, and drug addiction. The characteristics of clinic outpatients which were studied by Rosen, Bahn, and Kramer in 1961 clarify which disorders are now receiving diagnostic and some therapeutic attention in the United States. Approximately 200 per 100,000 population received clinic attention that year. The highest rates were for boys 10 to 14 years of age and girls 15 to 17 years of age. The lowest rates were for children under 5 years and adults over 65 years. Rates of first admission to state mental hospitals increase steadily with age and are higher for men than for women in every age group. Married adults are less likely to receive clinic care than are unmarried adults. Rates for organic brain syndromes are relatively high during the first 10 years of life, low in adolescence and young adulthood, and high again toward the end of the life-span. Among adults, psychoneuroses account for more of the female rate, whereas personality disorders account for more of the male rate. There is also evidence that clinics tend to devote more of their resources to these disorders than to the mentally retarded or to the delinquent.

Introduction of psychotropic drugs in 1955 had a considerable impact on public psychiatry. Since then, and for the first time in the long history of public mental hospitals, there has been a decrease in the number of hospitalized patients, dropping from 558,922 in 1955 to 370,849 in 1970. President John F. Kennedy, speaking before Congess in 1963, predicted a 50% decline in the state hospital patients in a 10- to 20-year period. It is notable that the present reduction has occurred in the face of a 7% yearly increase in admission rate.

PREVENTIVE PSYCHIATRY

The concept of preventive psychiatry includes programs for reducing the incidence of mental disorders (primary prevention), reducing the duration of disorders (secondary prevention), and reducing the impairment resulting from disorders (tertiary prevention). Inasmuch as the etiology of most psychiatric illness is not known, primary prevention today refers to educational programs and other methods of giving help to individuals at naturally occurring transition points in their lives and when coping with crises. Secondary prevention deals with early case finding, with population screening, and with making more effective treatment facilities available for larger numbers of persons. Tertiary prevention or rehabilitation refers to programs aimed at strengthening the links between the hospital and the community to help and supervise the discharged patient. Good aftercare programs prevent hospital readmissions. Perhaps one of the most heartening functions of the psychiatrist or of other mental health workers who move into the community is case finding. Partly because of primitive social taboos against mental disturbance and partly because of internal anxiety which may be mobilized by the effort of beginning to face one's fears, emotional disorders tend to be diagnosed correctly only after months or years of suffering. As with other chronic illnesses, however, treatment is increasingly effective and economical the earlier the diagnosis is made. At present there exist no proved tests for mass screening comparable to the chest x-ray program for tuberculosis.

THE PSYCHIATRIST IN THE COMMUNITY

It is evident that the public health psychiatrist does not confine his interest to the medical setting as such but is concerned with the total course of lives of individuals living in the community. This concern becomes focused on a diversity of biological, socioeconomic, and cultural conditions ranging from the poor hydration and nutrition of working class pregnant women in the south during the summer (which has been shown to be associated with prenatal brain damage), to the legal precedents for judging a criminal to be insane, to the value systems in our culture which define acceptable or unacceptable family behavior patterns. On national and community levels, the psychiatrist becomes involved in educational campaigns which seek to remove the stigma of mental disease, to educate the public about existing facilities, and to create a greater demand for adequate treatment for the mentally ill.

These activities are conducted frequently by service-minded volunteers working in collaboration with social agencies, social workers, educators, clergymen, courts, and others. The psychiatrist is frequently sought out by these persons for information about mental health and illness and he should be aware of the fact that whereas it is relatively easy to describe the warning signs of definite psychiatric disorders it is most hazardous to be dogmatic about mental health. Yet it is true that certain psychotherapeutic-like principles are involved in establishing an enlightened school system, an enlightened penal system, or an enlightened personnel system for a large organization. The psychiatrist is beginning to bring to these areas methods directed at uncovering the causes of individual or group malfunction, as well as problem-solving attitudes and techniques.

Even if he is sought out or welcomed by lay groups, the psychiatrist may encounter difficulties once he is out of a traditional medical setting. One of the first tasks here is to make a kind of diagnosis of the real purpose, sometimes hidden, for which psychiatric guidance is sought. Not infrequently community groups have hopes that the psychiatrist in some magical way can dispatch a vexing social problem. Here clearly the consultant's role is to aid the group in mastering its anxiety and to provide orientation about psychiatric aspects of the problem; but at the same time he should keep clear with all concerned where responsibility belongs. For example, if the psychiatrist is called upon in desperation after an outbreak of delinquent behavior in a high school, it is obviously dangerous for him to let the school believe that any single simple remedy is available for the complex problems of which such an outbreak may be symptomatic.

In these situations a useful tool is group discussion, led in a nonauthoritarian manner, which focuses upon a few specific questions which are of genuine concern to the group and with which they have had firsthand experience. Excellent movies or plays now available through mental health associations can present a wide range of vital questions concerning childhood (discipline, tantrums, sex information), adolescence (gangs, dating, struggle for independence), young adulthood (courtship, marriage, pregnancy), or later life (parenthood, job adjustment, retirement). The psychiatrist here encourages maximal group participation—through proper program planning, limiting the size of the group, arranging the chairs in a circle, setting up a cheerful and relaxed group atmosphere. He keeps the focus of discussion clarified and sets limits for group members who wish to dominate or wander too far off the topic. At the end he summarizes for the group lest they leave this somewhat unusual educational experience with an anxious feeling that they have "done all the work without getting any answers." After such emotionally involving, sensitively led group discussions, individuals can sometimes move in the direction of defining a psychological problem close to their own lives in a more constructive manner and, where necessary, seek therapeutic assistance.

MANAGEMENT OF CIVILIAN DISASTER

As part of his community responsibility a psychiatrist may be called upon to assist with sudden community catastrophes.

Exposure to unexpected personal danger, the witnessing of threatened or actual gruesome damage to loved ones, and experiencing separation from family and friends can tax the strongest personalities. Whether or not disaster produces an acute emotional disorder seems to depend upon a variety of factors. Degree and duration of physical stress, geographical closeness to the area of greatest danger, and previous susceptibility to anxiety apparently influence the likelihood of breakdown.

Diaster can produce many of the acute syndromes usually observed in psychiatric practice. Most individuals will show some signs of stress and are best treated by a word of encouragement and assignment to a constructive relief job. *Individual panic (blind flight)*, while infrequent, is dangerous in a crowd because of its contagion. A few individuals who lose control completely can precipitate a mad mass flight and therefore should be quickly segregated with gentle firmness by two or more attendants and remain attended until self-control is regained. Punitiveness (using cold water, slapping the face) should be avoided. *Obtunded reactions* occur in some persons who suddenly seem devoid of emotional reaction and act dazed or as though there were no danger. *Manic-like reactions* with inappropriate joking, rapid speech, and overactivity may occur.

Chronic psychiatric disorders may develop after a disaster, and where supportive measures fail, removal to a psychiatric hospital is indicated.

During the days and weeks following a disaster, the psychiatrist may be helpful in various ways through supportive group meetings with teachers, parents, other relatives of patients, and community leaders by demonstrating that it is safe to admit emotional disturbance following trauma and that realistic appraisal of unpleasant adjustments is more constructive than is denial of upsetting feelings.

THE COMMUNITY PSYCHIATRY MOVEMENT

Concern over mental health problems resulted in passage of Public Law 182 by Congress in 1956. This law established the

Joint Commission on Mental Illness and Health, whose final report, *Action for Mental Health*, 1961,* pointed out major problems that exist in psychiatry in the United States today. Cited were the great professional manpower shortage, an overemphasis upon treatment techniques inappropriate to the economic and social aspects of the problem, and a low level of service in state public psychiatry that results in custodial care in large crowded facilities. The report stressed the need for early and adequate treatment in smaller units and for a strengthening of community resources in the mental health field.

In 1963 President Kennedy recommended, and Congress passed, Public Law 88-164, which enabled local communities to obtain matching federal funds to construct local community mental health centers. These centers combine a variety of services, both impatient and outpatient, for children and adults, partial (day/night) hospital services, 24-hour emergency care, consultation, education, and research. Each center is designed to service a population area of 75,000 to 200,000 persons. In 1965 Congress passed P.L. 89-105 appropriating funds to assist in the staffing costs for these units. Although specifically suited to the needs of more populous areas and those more plentifully supplied with mental health professionals, some aspects of this plan have been imaginatively implemented in most states. In some less populous areas the program has included a few beds of a local country hospital, in other areas psychiatric consultation needs have been met via closed circuit television, and in others an administrative sectioning of large state hospitals into smaller units has served to focus upon and better meet the needs of given regional geographic units of the community. The use of small communities as after-care centers, patterned after the town of Gheel, Belgium, has met with some success.

Such a nationwide effort to upgrade public psychiatric care was indeed impressive but like many public programs has recently failed to receive adequate continuing financial support. However, no such program can achieve great success without the training of

---

*In Canada, a committee of psychiatrists appointed by the Canadian Mental Health Association made a similar study. Their report, entitled *More for the Mind*, 1963, gives a summary of similar problems that exist in that country together with practical suggestions for their solution.

additional psychiatrists who are willing to accept careers in public service. Another major concern is the lack of continuity in the conduct of public health programs as a result of high turnover of top administrative personnel. The ultimate solution to the costly and vexing problems of mental illness must, however, await the development of more effective treatment methods.

Major improvements in the delivery of mental health care are being accomplished through the application of modern electronic data-processing techniques to both the administrative and the clinical areas of psychiatry. This gives promise of great assistance with problems about patient records, personnel, statistics, and communication. Such methods will permit an actuarial approach to diagnosis and the prescription of more effective treatments. Computerized patient data files foster research upon sufficiently large case samples to give more meaningful answers to questions that have long troubled psychiatrists. Through these methods, widely separated psychiatric centers can agree upon and participate in a standard system of psychiatry, and with the ever increasing substitution of facts for theory a major revolution within psychiatry will surely occur worldwide.

SUGGESTED READINGS

Beiser, M.: Personal and social factors associated with the remission of psychiatric symptoms, Arch. Gen. Psychiatry **33:**941, 1976.

Borus, J. F.: Neighborhood health centers as providers of primary mental-health care, N. Engl. J. Med. **295:**140, 1976.

Borus, J. F., and others: Coordination of mental health services at the neighborhood level, Am. J. Psychiatry **132:**1177, 1975.

Brown, G. W., Bone, M., Dalison, B., and Wing, J. K.: Schizophrenia and social care, London, 1966, Oxford University Press.

Caplan, G.: Support systems and community mental health. Lectures on concept development, New York, 1974, Behavorial Publications.

Caplan, R. B.: Psychiatry and the community in nineteenth-century America, New York, 1969, Basic Books, Inc.

Dunham, H. W.: Society, culture, and mental disorder, Arch, Gen. Psychiatry **33:**147, 1976.

Essen-Möller, E.: Individual traits and morbidity in a Swedish rural population, Acta Psychiat. Scand. Suppl. 100, 1966.

Farazza, A. R., and Oman, M.: Overview: foundations of cultural psychiatry, Am. J. Psychiatry **135:**293, 1978.

Frankel, F. H.: Psychiatric consultation for nursing homes, Hosp. Comm. Psychiatry **18:**331, 1967.

Garrison, J.: Network techniques: case studies in the screening-linking-planning conference method, Family Process 13:337, 1974.

Glasscote, R., Sussex, J. N., Cumming, E., and Smith, L. H.: The community mental health center: an interim appraisal, Washington, D.C., 1969, Joint Information Service.

Golann, S. F., and Eisdorfer, C.: Handbook of community mental health, New York, 1972, Appleton-Century-Crofts.

Grunebaum, H.: The practice of community mental health, Boston, 1970, Little, Brown & Co.

Holleb, G. P., and Abrams, W. H.: Alternatives in community mental health, Boston, 1975, Beacon Press.

Hollingshead, A., and Redlich, F. C.: Social class and mental illness, New York, 1958, John Wiley & Sons, Inc.

Ingham, J. G., and Miller, F. M.: The concept of prevalence applied to psychiatric disorders and symptoms, Psychol. Med. 6:217, 1976.

Keskiner, A., Zalcman, M. J., Ruppert, E. H., and Ulett, G. A.: the foster community: a partnership in psychiatric rehabilitation, Am. J. Psychiatry 129(3):283-288, 1972.

Lamb, H. R.: Community survival for long-term patients, San Francisco, 1976, Jossey-Bass Publishers, Inc.

Liberman, R. P., and Bryan, E.: Behavior therapy in a community mental health center, Am. J. Psychiatry 134:401, 1977.

Macht, L. B., Scherl, D. J., and Sharfstein, S. S.: Neighborhood psychiatry, Lexington, Mass., 1977, D. C. Heath, Lexington Books.

Masserman, J. H., editor: Social psychiatry, New York, 1976, Grune & Stratton, Inc.

Powell, B. J., Othmer, E., and Sinkhorn, D.: Pharmacological aftercare for homogeneous groups of patients, Hosp. Comm. Psychiatry 28:125, 1977.

Saslow, G., and Peters, D. D.: A follow-up study of untreated patients with various disorders, Psychiatr. Q. 30:283, 1956.

Sletten, I. W., Schuff, S., Altman, H., and Ulett, G. A.: A statewide computerized psychiatric system: demographic, diagnostic, and mental status data, Int. J. Soc. Psychiatry 18:30-40, 1972.

Srole, L.: Measurement and classification in socio-psychiatric epidemiology: Midtown Manhattan study (1954) and Midtown Manhattan restudy (1974), J. Health Soc. Behav. 16:347, 1975.

Task force on community mental health program components: Developing community mental health programs: a resource manual, Boston, 1975, United Community Planning Corporation.

Ulett, G. A., Schnibbe, H., Ganser, L. J., and Thompson, W. A.: Mental health director: bird of passage, Am. J. Psychiatry 127:126-130, 1971.

Zusman, J., and Lamb, R. H.: In defense of community mental health, Am. J. Psychiatry 134:887, 1977.

Contributors to psychiatric thought

Abraham, Karl (1877-1925): German psychiatrist and psychoanalyst. Theory of pregenital stages, character types, and manic-depressive psychosis. Symbolism.

Ackerman, Nathan Ward (1908-1971): American psychiatrist. Family therapy.

Adler, Alfred (1875-1937): Austrian psychiatrist. Neo-Freudian. Founded school of individual psychology. Inferiority complex. Overcompensation.

Aichhorn, August (1878-1949): Austrian educator and psychoanalyst. Directed two reformatories. Published "Wayward Youth" (1925). Unsatisfactory relationship with parent is at base of delinquency. Punishment useless.

Alexander, Franz Gabriel (1891-1964): Hungarian-American psychiatrist and psychoanalyst. Neo-Freudian. Brief analytic psychotherapy Psychosomatic medicine. Active rather than passive analytic techniques. Corrective emotional experience.

Alzheimer, Alois (1864-1915): German neurologist. Described a type of presenile dementia (Alzheimer's disease).

Beard, George Miller (1839-1883): American psychiatrist who first used the term "neurasthenia" in 1869.

Beers, Clifford Whittingham (1876-1943): A mental patient who recovered and published "A Mind that Found Itself" (1909). This led to the mental hygiene movement.

Bell, Luther Voce (1806-1862): American physician. Bell's mania (catatonic exhaustion syndrome). Bell's palsy (facial nerve palsy).

Bender, Lauretta (1897-   ): American psychiatrist. Developed the

Bender-Gestalt test for brain damage and contributed to the knowledge of childhood schizophrenia.

Benedek, Theresa (1892-   ): Hungarian psychiatrist and psychoanalyst. Psychosexual function in women.

Benedict, Ruth Fulton (1887-1948): American social anthropologist. Related culture to individual's behavior. Published "Patterns of Culture" (1934).

Berne, Eric (1910-1970): Canadian-American psychiatrist and psychoanalyst. Neo-Freudian. Founded school of transactional analysis. Individual and group therapy.

Bernheim, Hippolyte Marie (1840-1919): French physician. Revived interest in hypnosis and treatment by suggestion at the Nancy School in France. Opposed Charcot's view that only hysterical subjects could be hypnotized. Challenged that "will" was cause of crime and said mechanism of suggestion explained both normal and abnormal behavior.

Binet, Alfred (1857-1911): French psychologist. Research on childhood and adolescence. Binet-Simon and Stanford-Binet tests.

Binswanger, Ludwig (1881-1966): Swiss psychiatrist. Neo-Freudian. Founded school of existential analysis.

Blandford, George Fielding (1829-1911): British psychiatrist. Noted that schizophrenic patients had a "peculiar odour."

Bleuler, Eugen (1857-1939): Swiss psychiatrist. Introduced term "schizophrenia" for dementia praecox, because onset was not always early and course was not always deteriorating. He put emphasis on dysharmony or split (schizo) between associations (thoughts) and affect (emotion).

Breuer, Josef (1824-1925): Austrian physician. Collaborated with Freud on cathartic therapy, which was reported in "Studies in Hysteria" (1895). Concepts of primary and secondary process.

Brigham, Amariah (1798-1849): American psychiatrist. A founder of the American Psychiatric Association and first editor of its journal.

Brill, Abraham Arden (1874-1948): American psychoanalyst. First American psychoanalyst. Active in New York Psychoanalytic Society. Translator of Freud's works into English.

Briquet, Paul (1796-1881): French psychiatrist. Published treatise on hysteria (1859).

Burrow, Nicholas Trigant (1875-1951): American student of Freud and Jung. Founded phyloanalysis. Formed group who went to camp and analyzed interactions of the members of the group.

Charcot, Jean Martin (1825-1893): French neurologist. Salpêtrière school. Described hysteria and treated it with hypnosis. Charcot joint seen in tabes dorsalis.

Conolly, John (1794-1866): British psychiatrist. Abolished restraints at Hanwell Asylum.

Coué, Emil (1857-1926): French hypnotist and psychotherapist. Autosuggestion and positive thinking. "Every day in every way I am becoming better and better."

Cushing, Harvey William (1869-1939): American surgeon and neurologist. In 1932 called attention to mental symptoms in patients with Cushing's syndrome.

Darwin, Charles Robert (1809-1882): English naturalist. Began the study of personality development with "Biographical Sketch of an Infant." Influenced Freud with concepts of phylogenesis and ontogenesis.

Deutsch, Albert (1907-1968): American psychiatrist. History of psychiatry. Published "The Mentally Ill in America" (1937).

Deutsch, Helene (1884-   ): Austrian psychoanalyst. Published "Neuroses and Character Types" (1930) and "The Psychology of Women" in two volumes (1944, 1945).

Deutsch, Felix (1884-1964): Austrian psychiatrist. First clinic on organ neurosis. Published "Applied Psychoanalysis" (1949). Activation of autonomic nervous system to release emotion. Sector psychotherapy.

Dix, Dorothea Lynde (1802-1887): American retired schoolteacher. Persuaded state legislatures to remove mental patients from jails and almshouses by building mental institutions for their care.

Dollard, John (1900-   ): American psychologist. Attempted to correlate learning theory with psychoanalysis. Published with Neal E. Miller "Personality and Psychotherapy" (1950).

Dunbar, Flanders (1902-1959): American psychiatrist. Psychosomatic medicine. Personality profiles. Accident-prone individuals were impulsive, decisive, and resentful toward authority with accident expiating the unconscious guilt by self-punishment. Published "Emotions and Bodily Changes" (1947).

Dunham, Henry Warren (1906-   ): American sociologist. Pioneering study with Faris on "Mental Disorders in Urban Areas: An Ecological Study of Schizophrenia and Other Psychoses" (1939). Highest rates of schizophrenia found in central city in lower socioeconomic area. Pattern of manic-depressive illness was random. Postulated that social isolation was a factor.

Durkheim, Émile (1958-1917): French sociologist. Coined term "anomie" (1897) to describe decreased sense of community affiliation due to increasing industrialization and urbanization because of secularization and individualism. He believed suicide rates were index of anomie.

Earle, Pliny (1809-1892): American psychiatrist. Prominent in planning and construction of mental hospitals in the early days. Published "Curability of Insanity" (1877).

Eitingon, Max (1881-1943): Austrian psychoanalyst. First person to be analyzed by Freud (1907). Later associated with Berlin Psychoanalytic Clinic. Founder of Berlin Psychoanalytic Institute and of Palestine Psychoanalytic Society.

Ellis, Henry Havelock (1859-1939): British sexologist. Introduced term "autoeroticism."

Erikson, Erik Homburger (1902-   ): German-American psychoanalyst. Neo-Freudian. Psychosocial theory of ego development and psychosexual development combining social adaptation with Freud's formulations. Published "Childhood and Society" (1950). Eight stages of ego development.

Esquirol, Jean-Etienne Dominique (1772-1840): French psychiatrist. Pupil of Pinel. Described "hallucinations" and "monomania." Applied statistics to his clinical studies.

Federn, Paul (1871-1950): Austrian psychoanalyst. Neo-Freudian. Ego psychology. Dreams of flying. Ego feelings. Was last surviving member of Wednesday Evening Society. Saved minutes of the meetings of Vienna Psychoanalytic Society.

Ferenczi, Sandor (1873-1933): Hungarian psychiatrist and psychoanalyst. Neo-Freudian. Psychoanalytic techniques: active therapy, forced fantasies, and setting a termination date (retracted later). Alloplastic and autoplastic adaptation.

Fliess, Wilhelm (1858-1928): German nose and throat specialist. Corresponded with Freud. Concept of bisexuality and periodicity of sexual function.

Foulkes, Siegmund Heinz (1923-   ): English psychiatrist. Group therapy. Combines psychodrama and psychoanalytic concepts and stresses group-as-a-whole phenomena.

Frankl, Victor Emil (1905-   ): Austrian psychiatrist. Paradoxical intension (negative practise) and dereflection (change of center of attention from self to a goal). Emphasized search for meaning (existential analysis).

Freeman, Walter (1895-1972): American psychiatrist. Popularized lobotomy in the United States. Research on lobotomy.

French, Thomas (1892-   ): American psychiatrist. Neo-Freudian. Chicago School. Integration of behavior by ego. Goal structures.

Freud, Anna (1895-   ): Austrian psychoanalyst. Neo-Freudian. Published "The Ego and Mechanisms of Defense" (1946). Psychoanalysis of children and adolescents. Analytic play therapy.

Freud, Sigmund (1856-1939): Austrian psychiatrist. Founder of psychoanalysis. Concepts of libido, regression, transference, regression, sublimation, id, ego, superego, preconscious, unconscious, Oedipus complex, psychopathology of dreams, topographical (regions of unconscious, preconscious) and structural (id, ego, superego) models.

Fromm, Erich (1900-   ): German-American psychoanalyst and social philosopher. Neo-Freudian. Malaise of person aspiring to freedom but having to comply with collective system. Personality types (receptive, exploitative, hoarding, marketing, productive). Published "Escape From Freedom" (1941).

Fromm-Reichmann, Frieda (1899-1957): German-American psychiatrist. Promoted use of psychotherapy in treatment of psychosis. Therapist's role as "participant observer" in treatment. Published "The Principles of Intensive Psychotherapy" (1950).

Gesell, Arnold (1880-1961): American pediatrician. Growth is the key concept to account for individual differences. Intelligence measures of infants and preschool children.

Gildea, Edwin Francis (1898-1977): American neuropsychiatrist. Fostered medical school undergraduate training in psychiatry and residency training in research.

Griesinger, Wilhelm (1817-1868): German psychiatrist. Pupil of Pinel. Recommended non-restraint in Germany.

Hall, Granville Stanley (1844-1924): American psychologist and sexologist. Research on childhood and adolescence.

Harlow, Harry Frederick (1905-   ): American psychologist. Studies of social deprivation in animals. Terrycloth-and-wire surrogate mother experiments in monkeys. Published "Biological and Biochemical Basis of Behavior" (1958).

Hartmann, Heinz (1894-1972): American psychiatrist and psychoanalyst. Neo-Freudian. Focus changed from ego functions between instinctual demands and superego values to conflict-free adaptive functions (autonomous functions).

Havens, Leston Laycock (1924-   ): American psychiatrist. Existential psychoanalysis.

Healy, William (1869-1962): British-American psychiatrist. Pioneer in the child guidance movement. Began Institue for Juvenile Research in Chicago (1909). Published six-year study (1922) demonstrating relationship between delinquency and socioeconomic factors. Discredited defective genes or degeneracy hypothesis.

Hecker, Ewald (1843-1909): German psychiatrist. Student of Kahlbaum. Described hebephrenia in 1871.

Heidegger, Martin (1889-   ): German philosopher. Founder of contemporary existentialism. Pupil of Husserl. Concept of Dasein (being there).

Heinroth, Johann Christian (1773-1843): German psychiatrist. First psychiatrist to use the word "psychosomatic." Psychosomatic causes of insomnia (1818). Stressed unity of total personality. Conflict led to guilt to mental illness.

Hollingshead, August de Belmont (1915-   ): American sociologist.

Sociological investigation in New Haven, Connecticut, showed that upper and middle class used outpatient clinics and private practitioners and lower class used hospitals. Published with Frederick Redlich "Social Class and Mental Illness" (1958).

Horney, Karen (1885-1952): American psychiatrist and psychoanalyst. Neo-Freudian. Helped relate social science to psychiatry. Founded school of holistic analysis.

Hull, Clark (1884-1952): American psychologist. Pioneering study on hypnosis. Published "Hypnosis and Suggestibility, an Experimental Approach" (1933).

James, William (1842-1910): American psychologist and philosopher. James-Lange theory is that "The bodily changes follow directly the perception of the exciting fact, and our feeling of the changes as they occur is the emotion . . ." This theory was replaced by Cannon-Bard theory of emotion.

Janet, Pierre (1859-1947): French psychiatrist. Pupil of Charcot. Described hysteria, automatisms, subconscious, dissociation. Introduced term "psychasthenia." Interested in multiple personalities.

Jaspers, Karl (1883-1969): American psychiatrist and philosopher. Existential school of psychiatry. Rejected positivism for proceeding from parts to whole and idealism for proceeding from the unique to the whole. The whole is being and is knowable only through existence. The parts are knowable through reason.

Jones, Ernest (1879-1958): Welsh neurologist and psychoanalyst. Three-volume biography of Freud.

Jones, Maxwell (1907-   ): South African-English psychiatrist. Rehabilitative techniques (open ward, patient government, therapeutic milieu, social and community aspects of psychiatry). Published "The Therapeutic Community" (1952).

Jung, Carl Gustav (1875-1961): Swiss psychiatrist and psychoanalyst. Neo-Freudian. Founded school of analytic psychology. Used terms anima, animus, persona, collective unconscious.

Kahlbaum, Karl Ludwig (1828-1899): German psychiatrist. Described catatonia in 1868.

Kalinowsky, Lothar Bruno (1899-   ): German-born neuropsychiatrist, came to U.S. 1940. Extensive work on electroconvulsive therapy and other somatic treatments.

Kallmann, Franz Joseph (1897-1965): German-born psychoanalyst and geneticist. Genetics of schizophrenia and manic-depressive psychosis.

Kanner, Leo (1894-   ): American pediatrician. Kanner's disease is infantile autism.

Kasanin, Jacob Sergi (1897-1946): American psychiatrist. Added subtype schizo-affective psychosis (1933), opposing Kraepelin's idea of no emotional expression (flat affect). Published "Language and Thought in Schizophrenia" (1944).

Kinsey, Alfred Charles (1894-1956): American biologist. Contemporary data on human sexuality against which a given theory could be examined. Published "Sexual Behavior in the Human Male" (1948) and ". . . Female" (1953).

Kirchhoff, Theodor (1853-1922): German psychiatrist. Psychiatric historian.

Kirkbride, Thomas Story (1809-1883): American psychiatrist. One of thirteen founders of American Psychiatric Association. Noted for Kirkbride plan, a design for constructing mental institutions (1854).

Klein, Melanie (1882-1960): British psychiatrist and child analyst. Neo-Freudian. Theories of early childhood development. Anaclitic depression.

Kohler, Wolfgang (1887-1967): German psychologist. Gestalt psychology. Experiments on problems solving by monkeys with "insight" and not "trial and error" only.

Korsakoff, Syergey Syergeyvich (1854-1900): Russian neurologist. Korsakoff's syndrome due to alcoholism. Wernicke-Korsakoff's syndrome.

Korzybski, Alfred Habdank Skarbek (1879-1950): Polish-American scientist and writer. Study of general semantics, the meaning of signs or sets of signs, especially connotative meaning.

Kraepelin, Emil (1865-1926): German psychiatrist. Differentiated manic-depressive disease and dementia praecox (schizophrenia) by correlating basic symptoms with course of illness.

Kraft-Ebing, Richard von (1840-1902): German neuropsychiatrist. Concerned with noxious factors (sex, alcohol, infection, industrialization, and social progress) on personality. Classic 19th century work on sexual aberration, "Psychopathia Sexualis."

Kretschmer, Ernst (1888-1964): German psychiatrist. Related body types (pyknic, asthenic, athletic, dysplastic) to personality (cyclothymic, schizothymic). Asthenic type also called leptosome.

Langfeldt, Gabriel (1895-   ): Norwegian psychiatrist. Introduced concept of "reactive schizophrenia" and term "schizophreniform psychosis."

Leighton, Alexander Hamilton (1908-   ): American social psychiatrist, anthropologist, and sociologist. Relation of social pressures to mental health. Published "My Name is Legion" (1959) and "People of Cove and Woodlot" (1960). The latter described the Stirling County study of psychiatric disorder in Canada.

Lewin, Kurt (1890-1947): German-American psychologist. Concept of field theory useful in experimental study of human behavior. Published "Field Theory in Social Science" (1951).

Lewis, Nolan Don Carpentier (1889-   ): American psychiatrist. Compiled bibliography of research in schizophrenia.

Liebeault, Ambroise August (1823-1904): French psychiatrist. Hypnosis and suggestibility.

Linton, Ralph (1893-1953): American anthropologist. Published "The Cultural Background of Personality" (1945) and "Culture and Mental Disorders" (1956).

Lombroso, Cesare (1836-1909): Italian criminologist and psychopathologist. Found in criminals and the mentally ill "stigmata of degeneration" (low hairline, webbing of ear pinnae, eyebrows meeting at midline, extra nipples, congenital naevi, clubbed feet). This was not confirmed.

Malinowski, Bronislaw (1884-1942): British anthropologist. Published "Sex and Repression in Savage Society" (1927).

Masters, William Howell (1915-   ): American obstetrician and gynecologist. Sexual counseling. Research into sexual activity and sexual response. Females found not passive with less frequent or lower response. No evolution from clitoral to vaginal orgasm. Masters and Johnson published "Human Sexual Response" (1966).

May, Rollo (1909-   ): American psychologist. Anxiety considered as threat to existence. Published "The Meaning of Anxiety" (1950).

McDougall, William (1871-1938): British-American psychologist. Purposive or hormic psychology. Goal seeking behavior (striving, foresight). Stimulated field of social psychology. Published "Psychoanalysis and Social Psychology" (1936).

Mead, Margaret (1901-1978): American cultural anthropologist. Individual and family traits related to culture. Published "Coming of Age in Samoa" (1928), "Sex and Temperament in Three Primitive Societies" (1938), "Growing Up in New Guinea" (1940), "The Balinese Character" (1942), "Male and Female" (1949).

Meduna, Ladislas Joseph von (1896-1964): Hungarian psychiatrist. He noted relief of symptoms in some patients following a seizure. It was said that epilepsy and schizophrenia rarely occurred together. So he produced artificial seizures with camphor-in-oil and later with Metrazol. He also introduced carbon dioxide therapy.

Mendel, Gregor Johann (1822-1884): Austrian botanist and Augustinian monk. Studies of inherited characteristics in peas and honey bees. Father of genetics.

Menninger, Karl Augustus (1893-   ): American psychiatrist. Described psychoanalytic concepts in systems theory terms. Defense mechanisms are coping devices (internal information adjustment processes). Negative feedback maintains steady states (homeostasis, "vital balance"). Operated the Menninger Clinic with his brother, Dr. William Menninger.

Mesmer, Franz Anton (1734-1815): Austrian physician. Gave demonstration of animal magnetism (hypnotism) in Vienna in 1775.

Meyer, Adolf (1866-1950): American psychiatrist. Psychobiology (distributive analysis and synthesis). Emphasis on total life experiences rather than on symptoms alone. Common-sense psychiatry.

Mitchell, Silas Weir (1829-1914): American neurologist. After the Civil War he was outspoken in his criticism of the isolation of psychiatry from medicine and lack of interest in research and training. Described causalgia.

Moebius, Paul Julius (1853-1907): German neuropathologist and sexologist. Divided mental disorders into endogenous and exogenous types.

Moniz, Egaz (1874-1955): Portugese neurologist. Persuaded Dr. Almeidia Lima to perform the first leucotomy (lobotomy). Received Nobel prize with Hess for discovery of therapeutic value of leucotomy (1949).

Morel, Benedict Augustin (1809-1873): Belgian psychiatrist. Introduced term "demence précoce" (dementia praecox) in 1856.

Moreno, Jacob Levy (1882-   ): Rumanian-American psychiatrist. Neo-Freudian. Psychodrama. Patient's conflicts acted out on stage (auxiliary ego, mirror, double, role reversal).

Pavlov, Ivan Petrovich (1849-1936): Russian neurophysiologist. Classic conditioning. Law of reinforcement.

Piaget, Jean (1896-   ): Swiss psychologist, Neo-Freudian. Cognitive development in children from direct observation.

Pinel, Philippe (1745-1826): French physician. Abolished forcible restraint in the management of the mentally ill. Esquirol was his pupil.

Prince, Morton (1854-1929): American psychiatrist. Hysterical dissociative states. Multiple personalities.

Rank, Otto (1884-1939): Austrian psychoanalyst. Neo-Freudian. Will therapy. Basic source of anxiety is birth trauma.

Ray, Isaac (1807-1881): American physician. Alienist. A founder of American Psychiatric Association. Published "Treatise on Medical Jurisprudence of Insanity" (1837).

Reich, Wilhelm (1897-1957): German psychiatrist. Neo-Freudian. Published "Character Analysis" (1928). Orgone therapy.

Reik, Theodore (1888-1969): Austrian lay psychoanalyst. Contributions to psychoanalysis on religion, masochism, and techniques. Studies of the couvade, death rites, and circumcision.

Robertson, Argyll (1837-1909): Scottish physician. Described Argyll-Robertson pupil, which is usually miotic, reacts to accommodation but not to light, and is slow to react to mydriatrics. It is observed in neurosyphilis, traumatic brain injury, brain tumor, infectious diseases of the brain, and multiple sclerosis.

Rogers, Carl (1902-   ): American psychologist. Client-centered (non-directive) psychotherapy.

Rorschach, Hermann (1884-1922): Swiss psychiatrist. A projective psychological test using ink blots to interpret the individual's personality functioning.

Rosen, John Nathaniel (1902-   ): American psychiatrist. Direct analysis for schizophrenic patients. Published "Direct Analysis" (1953).

Rush, Benjamin (1745-1813): American physician and father of American psychiatry. Protested conditions at the Pennsylvania Hospital. Applied statistical methods to his clinical studies. Published "Medical Inquiries and Medical Observations Upon the Diseases of the Mind" (1812).

Sakel, Manfred (1900-1957): Polish psychiatrist. Reported the use of hypoglycemic coma in the treatment of psychosis in 1933. "Insulin shock" therapy (IST) refers to the vasomotor collapse induced.

Salmon, Thomas William (1876-1927): American psychiatrist. In charge of psychiatric services in the army in World War II. Established National Committee for Mental Hygeine which emphasized prevention, early treatment, and research.

Schilder, Paul (1886-1940): American neuropsychiatrist. Group therapy at Bellevue Hospital in New York City using social and psychoanalytic principles. Concept of body image.

Schneider, Kurt (1887-   ): German psychiatrist. First rank symptoms of schizophrenia (hearing of one's thoughts spoken aloud, auditory hallucinations that comment on patient's behavior, somatic hallucinations, experience of having one's thoughts controlled, spreading of one's thoughts to others, delusions, and experience of having one's thoughts or actions influenced from the outside).

Sechehaye, Marguerite Albert (1887-   ): Swiss psychologist. Psychoanalytically oriented psychotherapy of a schizophrenic girl. Published "Symbolic Realization" (1951).

Sheldon, William Herbert (1899-   ): American physician. Body types (ectomorphic, mesomorphic, and endomorphic). Published "Varieties of Human Physique" (1940).

Skinner, Burrhus Frederic (1904-   ): American psychologist. Study of learning in animals and humans using "Skinner box." Operant conditioning.

Slavson, Samuel Richard (1890-   ): American theoretician. Neo-Freudian. Orthodox psychoanalytic group psychotherapy. Activity group therapy. The collective experience. Published "Introduction to Group Therapy" (1943).

Stekel, Wilhelm (1868-1940): Austrian psychoanalyst. Neo-Freudian. Dreams. Symbolism. Wild analysis. Thanatos (death wish).

Southard, Elmer Ernest (1876-1920): American psychiatrist. Introduced

Contributors to psychiatric thought **385**

the concept of psychiatric social work with publication of "The Kingdom of Evils" (1922) with Mary C. Jarrett.

Sullivan, Harry Stack (1894-1949): American psychiatrist. Neo-Freudian. Washington Dynamic Cultural School of Psychoanalysis. Sociological events emphasized.

Szasz, Thomas (1920-   ): Hungarian-American psychiatrist. Contends that behavioral symptoms deviating from the norm are not necessarily signs of pathology, Published "The Myth of Mental Illness" (1961).

Thompson, Clara (1893-1958): American psychoanalyst. Neo-Freudian. Washington Dynamic Cultural School of Psychoanalysis. Published "Psychoanalysis: Evolution and Development" (1950).

Tredgold, Alfred Frank (1870-1952): British physician. Mental deficiency. Idiot savant. Published first "Textbook of Mental Deficiency" (1908).

Tuke, Daniel Hack (1827-1895): British psychiatrist. Editor of "Dictionary of Psychological Medicine." Humanitarian care of mentally ill. Historian.

Tuke, William (1732-1819): A Quaker (Society of Friends) who founded York Retreat at York, England, in 1776 for thirty patients who were treated as guests and without mechanical restraints.

Wagner von Jauregg, Julius (1857-1940): Austrian psychiatrist and neurologist. In 1917, instituted fever therapy for the treatment of general paresis by inoculating patients with malaria.

Watson, John Broadus (1878-1958): American psychologist. Founded school of psychology (behaviorism).

Wernicke, Carl (1848-1905): German neurologist. Aphasia. Wernicke-Korsakoff's syndrome.

Weyer, Johann (1515-1588): Dutch physician and first psychiatrist. Published "De Praestigiis Daemonum" (1563) after studying women who had been accused of witchcraft.

White, William Alanson (1870-1937): American psychiatrist. Encouraged the use of psychoanalysis in the United States.

Whitehorn, John Clare (1894-   ): American psychiatrist. A student of Adolph Meyer. Taught techniques for the initial interview. Studied effects of therapist attitudes on treatment of schizophrenics. Therapist, type A was active, firm, set limits, expressed personal attitudes. Therapist, type B, was passive and instructional.

Wiener, Norbert (1894-1964): American mathematician. Introduced term "cybernetics" (science of control mechanisms). He suggested electronic control mechanisms (thermostats) are similar to regulatory mechanisms (feedback) in human nervous systems, social groups, and machines.

Wilbur, Hervey Backus (1820-1883): American educator. Pioneer in field of mental deficiency.

Wittels, Fritz (1880-1950): Austrian psychoanalyst. Published biography of Freud in 1924.

Wolpe, Joseph (1915-   ): South African-American psychiatrist. Behavior therapy by reciprocal inhibition and systematic desensitization.

Woodward, Samuel (1787-1850): American psychiatrist. Founder of Hartford Retreat. First president of the Association of Medical Superintendents of American Institutions for the Insane (1884). This organization became the American Psychiatric Association. Published "Essays on Asylums for Inebriates" (1838).

Zilboorg, Gregory (1890-1959): Russian-American psychoanalyst. Ambulatory schizophrenia. Criminology. History of psychiatry.

Glossary

AA Alcoholics Anonymous.

ABEPP American Board of Examiners in Professional Psychology.

Abadie's sign Early sign of tabes (syphilis), in which pressure on the testis or Achilles tendon does not elicit deep pain. Described by Jean Marie Abadie (1892-1932), a French ophthalmologist.

abreaction The discharge of forgotten (repressed) and previously unexpressed painful emotions. This occurs in psychotherapy when painful memories are recalled and relived in the present. The patient may then reach a new understanding of his current unrealistic symptoms, attitudes, emotions, or behaviors (insight). Relief is experienced through this emotional decompression and the realization that the way one felt and evaluated experiences as a child was circumscribed and that it is no longer necessary as an adult to fear and to protect oneself in the same fashion.

abstinence syndrome (withdrawal syndrome) Physical signs and symptoms (nausea, vomiting, abdominal pain, yawning, "gooseflesh," photophobia, tremor, visual hallucinations, seizures) developing after stopping or reducing the dose abruptly in a drug-dependent individual.

abstraction A general characteristic of a set of particulars. Similarities are abstractions: "An apple and an orange are both fruits." Differences are not abstractions: "A tree is tall and a bush is not." The abstraction is that both are plants. An abstraction of two abstractions: "Reward and punishment are both incentives to learning." Abstraction is one of the most difficult mental operations and is one of the first to be impaired when disease attacks the brain. In evaluating abstracting ability, three levels of abstraction are used: the abstract level—"Apple and orange are both fruits"; the functional level—"Both are good to eat"; and the concrete level—"Both have peelings and are round." When abstracting ability fails, the progression is from abstract to functional to concrete

387

and, finally, only differences can be given by the patient. Even when told the answer, such as "Apple and orange are both fruits," the patient who has severe deterioration will repeat his answer, "An apple is red and an orange is round." The meaning of proverbs requires abstract thinking: "All that glitters is not gold" means "External appearances can be deceptive." Patient may respond with another proverb: "You can't know a book by its cover." The response "It could be silver" is a concrete response not given by a person functioning normally. Difficulty with abstraction is observed in organic brain disease, schizophrenia, and mental retardation.

acalculia Inability to perform simple arithmetic. Seen in learning disorder and mental retardation.

acarophobia Fear of mites or small objects such as worms, pins, or needles.

accident proneness Tendency to have repeated accidents due to personality factors.

achluophobia Fear of the dark.

acid Lysergic and diethylamide (LSD).

acromegaly Hyperpituitarism, often with acidophilic adenoma of anterior lobe. Acromegaloid personality shows impulsiveness, moodiness, angry outbursts, and somnolence.

acrophobia Fear of high places.

acting out Displacement of behavioral response of the past onto the current situation. The displaced behavior gives partial relief of the emotional tension.

acute brain syndrome Organic brain syndrome that is reversible. Chronic brain syndrome means an irreversible organic brain syndrome.

ADAMHA (Alcohol, Drug Abuse and Mental Health Administration) A governmental agency within the Department of Health, Education and Welfare responsible for administering federal grant programs to advance and support research, training, and service programs in the areas of alcoholism, drug abuse, and mental health.

addiction Strong dependence upon alcohol or a drug. When the drug is withdrawn, abstinence syndrome appears.

adiadochokinesis Inability to perform rapid alternating movements. Seen in disease of cerebellum.

Adie's syndrome (myotonic pupil) Abnormality of the pupil and absent deep reflexes. Direct or consensual reaction to light is absent or almost absent. After exposure to dark room, pupil dilates and on exposure to light slowly contracts. Not to be confused with findings in tabetic neurosyhphilis (tabes dorsalis).

adolescence Period of growth from age 12 to 20; that is, from appearance of secondary sexual characteristics until sexual maturity.

adrenergic Relating to sympathetic nervous system.

aerophagia The swallowing of air in large amounts. Patient may relate this to being pregnant.

affect Emotional tone. The feeling accompanying an object, idea, or thought.

affirmative action A planned management program aimed at providing equal employment opportunity by preventing discrimination and disparate practices in recruiting, selecting, appointing, promoting, training, and disciplining employees.

aftercare Outpatient care after a psychiatric hospital admission designed to continue necessary therapy and help rehabilitate the patient.

aggression Forceful motor behavior accompanying anger.

agitation Severe motor restlessness (pacing, wringing one's hands, picking holes in skin) with anxiety. Seen in psychotic depression.

akathisia Inability to sit still with constant moving of feet or getting up and pacing with muscle quivering. May be seen as side effect of phenothiazine medication.

alienation Feeling of detachment from self, society, or from one's own feelings.

alienist Obsolete term for psychiatrist (who offered expert opinion on insanity).

alliteration The repetition of the first letter (consonant and sound) in a series of words, such as, sob, sigh, sorrow, and sin, or big brown bear. Initial rhyming, as opposed to end rhyming as in clang association. Seen in flight of ideas.

alloplasty Adapting by changing the environment. Term used by Ferenczi.

alpha feedback A technique in which information on alpha waves (EEG) is given constantly to a patient who then attempts to relax and return his brain wave pattern to a resting condition which is characterized by alpha waves.

alpha state A person in the alpha state is awake, resting, relaxed, and peaceful, and his brain wave pattern has alpha waves (EEG).

altruism Concern for the welfare of others above that of self. Term originated by Auguste Comte, philosopher. Freud said community interest was based on altruism. Bleuler used it as synonym for morality.

ambivalence Term first used by Eugene Bleuler to describe simultaneous positive and negative feelings or attitudes toward a person, object, or goal.

amentia (mental deficiency, oligophrenia, feeblemindedness) Lack of development of the mind. Dementia refers to a normally developed mind that deteriorates.

American law formulation (insanity defense) In 1972 the United States Court of Appeals for the District of Columbia upheld Section 4.01 of the American Law Institute's Model Penal Code, which stated, "A person is not responsible for criminal conduct if at the time of such conduct as a result of mental disease or defect he lacks substantial capacity either to appreciate the wrongfulness of his conduct or to conform his conduct to the requirements of law."

American Psychiatric Association (APA) National professional organization of psychiatrists founded in 1844 as Association of Medical Superintendents of American Institutions for the Insane. Its name was changed to American Medico-Psychological Association in 1891 and to APA in 1921.

amnesia Loss of memory.

amnesic-confabulatory syndrome A syndrome following head trauma, with disorientation, impairment of perception, amnesia, and confabulation (falsification to cover memory gaps). A similar picture in chronic alcoholism was described by Korsakoff.

anaclitic Depending on others. Anaclitic depression results when infant lacks mothering.

anamnesis Literally, means recollection. Refers to patient's historical account of his life before period of illness. Catamnesis refers to his history following the illness.

angioneurotic edema (Quincke's disease) Acute swelling in various localized skin areas. Classified by some physicians as a form of allergy. Has been called a psychophysiological skin reaction.

anhedonia Inability to experience pleasure.

anima Jung's term for the person's inner self.

anticholinergic side effect Blocking of parasymphathetic and somatic nerves by phenothiazine (dry mouth, blurred vision).

antianxiety drug (anxiolytic drug) Used to alleviate anxiety (Librium, Valium).

antidepressant drug (thymolytic drug, psychic energizer) Used to alleviate depression. Tricyclic drugs (Tofranil, Elavil) and monoamine oxidase inhibitors (Nardil, Parnate).

antimanic drug Drugs used to alleviate mania (lithium, haloperidol, chlorpromazine).

antiparkinsonism drug Drugs used to alleviate Parkinsonian symptoms (pill rolling tremor, lack of associated movements, drooling, oculogyric crises). Drugs include cogentin, kemadrin, artane.

antipsychotic drug (neuroleptic, ataractic, major tranquilizer) Phenothiazines (Thorazine, Stelazine, Prolixin), thioxanthenes (Taractan, Navane), and butyrophenone derivative (Haldol).

antisocial personality (sociopathic personality, psychopathic personality) A disorder characterized by inability to get along with society, "lack of conscience," and impulsive behavior. May have history of truancy, being expelled from school, arrests for minor charges, repeated loss of jobs after only a few months.

apathy Lack of interest and feeling. Seen in simple schizophrenia and depression.

apoplexy Sudden loss of consciousness due to cerebrovascular accident. A stroke.

asterixis (hand-flapping tremor) A neurological sign of metabolic encephalopathy (hepatic encephalopathy, uremic encephalopathy, chronic pulmonary insufficiency, malabsorption syndrome, bromism, magnesium deficiency, primary hyperthyroidism). Involuntary movements are associated with electromyographic evidence of periodic electric inactivity resulting in patient's inability to maintain a fixed posture.

athetosis A more or less continuous, slow, worm-like, writhing movement. Seen in Lou Gehrig's disease (amyotrophic lateral sclerosis). A sign of organic disease of the brain.

aura A warning sensation felt by the person before an epileptic seizure.

autoeroticism Masturbation. Term introduced by Havelock Ellis.

automatism Automatic behavior not under conscious control.

autonomic nervous system A part of the nervous system that controls processes outside awareness, such as heart rate, breathing, digestion.

autonomic side effect Drug side effect from disturbance of autonomic nervous system (hypotension, hypertension, blurred vision, nasal congestion, dry mouth).

autoplasty Adaptation by changing one's self rather than altering the environment. Term used by Ferenczi.

average A central value in a frequency distribution. The mode is the most frequent value. The median is the value in the middle, with 50% above it and 50% below it. The mean is the sum of values divided by the number of values.

aversive therapy A form of conditioning where an unpleasant or painful experience becomes associated with an undesirable behavior. Ingestion of alcohol followed by ipecac causes the patient to associate vomiting with the desire for an alcoholic drink.

battered child syndrome Physical injury, such as fractures, bruises, and burns from repeated beating or maltreatment of a child, usually by a parent.

bedlam Pandemonium. The local term for the London "lunatic asylum" established in 1402 (Hospital of St. Mary of Bethlehem). Without modern treatments, conditions were very chaotic and tickets were sold to the public for viewing of the strange activities of the patients.

behavioral sciences Sociology, psychology, and anthropology.

bestiality Sexual relations with an animal.

biofeedback A technique using polygraph or EEG to give information to patient about his bodily process (blood pressure, pulse, alpha waves) during therapy so that he can reinforce certain reactions and avoid others.

bipolar depression Manic-depressive illness in which both manic and depressed phases have occurred.

bisexual An adult who is attracted to and has sexual relations with both men and women.

bisexuality Freud's concept that each human being differentiates from a common base, anatomically, physiologically, and psychologically, into a male or female, and that regression toward this undifferentiated base occurs in illness and under certain environmental conditions (incarceration with one sex for long periods, as in prison or war).

black-patch syndrome A psychosis with confusion and paranoid ideas following cataract surgery when black eye patches were used on both eyes and the patient experienced sensory isolation.

blocking (thought deprivation) Interruption of a chain of associated thoughts so that a blank occurs. In psychosis speech may cease after the verb. Complete blocking is mutism. In normals, blocking is sometimes described as, "The word is on the tip of my tongue and I can't think of it."

blunted affect The normal emotional tone and its modulations are absent. This lack of modulation is sometimes referred to as flat affect. Seen in catatonic schizophrenia.

body language The nonverbal language in which the body is used to express thoughts and feelings.

borderline state (borderline psychosis) On the border of psychosis. Psychotic or psychotic-like syndromes may appear briefly.

Bourneville's disease (epiloia, tuberous sclerosis) Adenomata of skin and viscera, convulsions, mental deterioration beginning in childhood, malformations and glia tumors of brain.

Briquet's syndrome Hysteria. Described by Paul Briquet (1859).

bromism Intoxication with bromides (salt of bromic acid, such as potassium bromide, used as a sedative).

bruxism Persistent grinding of teeth in adults even during sleep; associated with pain and trismus of the jaw.

buggery Insertion of the penis into the anus or rubbing it between the folds of the buttocks. When the penis is that of an adult and the anus that of a child, the perversion is called pederasty.

bulimia Hunger characterized by voracious appetite. A bulemic episode may be followed by intentional vomiting by some person.

burned-out schizophrenic A chronic schizophrenic with apathy and withdrawal, whose florid symptoms have abated, but whose thought disorder persists.

capgras syndrome (illusion of negative doubles) The individual feels he is confronted by a double and not the real person because of nonexistent differences. (When imaginery resemblances are perceived, the condition is called "illusion of positive doubles.")

castration complex A group of ideas involving castration by the father as punishment for boy's love of his mother and wish to get rid of the father during the Oedipal phase of development.

catalepsy (waxy flexibility, cerea flexibilitas) Molding of the limbs into any position where they remain for long periods.

cataplexy Sudden attacks of sinking to the ground from loss of muscle tone. May be precipitated by laughter, anger, or surprise. REM stage sleep may follow attack.

catastrophic anxiety Sudden overwhelming anxiety in person with organic brain syndrome when confronted with problem he cannot solve.

catatonia Decreased tension. A subtype of schizophrenia with two phases, catatonic excitement (hyperactivity, stereotypy) and catatonic stupor (withdrawal, blocking, mutism, negativism, muscle rigidity, waxy flexibility).

catatonic exhaustion syndrome (Bell's mania, Scheid's cyanotic syndrome) Deadly catatonia reported in 1832 by Calmeil. Sustained motor and mental excitement, hyperpyrexia to 112° F., rapid pulse, loss of body weight, profuse clammy perspiration, fall in blood pressure and pulse.

catch-22 An expression from the novel *Catch-22* by Joseph Heller (1955), meaning one is in a situation with two choices and loses either way. Similar to double-bind.

catchment area Literally, watershed. Defined in the federal law creating comprehensive community mental health centers (1963) as an area serving at least 75,000 people and not more than 200,000. The concept was an attempt to bring mental health services close to the people served.

catecholamine A substance with catechol group (epinephrine, norepinephrine, dopamine).

catharsis A cleansing, purification, or purgation. Term was introduced by Freud for the process of bringing forgotten memories and their painful emotions into consciousness with relief of symptoms. This occurred during hypnosis or during free association.

cathexis The psychic energy or charge attached to an idea or object.

central nervous system (CNS) The spinal cord and brain, as opposed to the peripheral nervous system.

cerea flexibilitas (waxy flexibility) Condition in which person will retain a position in which he is placed for long periods of time. Seen in catatonia. Also called catalepsy and molding.

character defense A rather stable set of defense mechanisms that appears as a personality trait, such as an obsessive-compulsive character trait. Called the "armor" by Wilhelm Reich.

character disorder A personality disorder characterized by habitual maladaptive inflexible behavior.

cholinergic Relating to parasympathetic nerve fibers.

chronic brain syndrome Irreversible organic brain syndrome. Symptoms include disorientation, recent and remote memory loss, loss of intellectual functions, poor judgment, and lability of affect.

circadian rhythm Variations in emotional and physiological functions in 24 hour-cycles due to evolution with a "biological clock" in every cell.

circumstantiality Unessential details precede the main thought. Seen in obsessive-compulsive disturbances and schizophrenia.

climacteric Menopause in women about age 45, in men about age 55.

clouding of consciousness Consciousness not clear because of faulty sensory perceptions. Degree of clouding varies during the day. Seen in subdural hematoma and toxic conditions.

cognition Psychologists have divided mental functioning into three categories: cognitive (perceptual or intellectual), emotional, and conative (instinctual drives, wishes, cravings). Cognition is thinking (comprehension, judgment, memory) and includes problem-solving, abstracting ability, logical thinking, and hypothetical thinking.

coitus interruptus (onanism) Incomplete sexual relations, with withdrawal just prior to ejaculation.

cold turkey Refers to the "gooseflesh" from chills following abrupt withdrawal from opiates, without methadone or other drug to alleviate the abstinence syndrome.

competency to stand trial test In order to be convicted, accused must at the time of his trial understand the nature of the charge and the consequences that may result from his conviction, and must be able to assist in his defense.

complex A group of ideas in the unconscious sharing a common affect.

compulsion A mechanism of defense. An uncontrollable urge to perform an act repeatedly keeping unacceptable ideas or desires out of consciousness. The individual knows the act is illogical.

compulsive gambling A neurotic character disorder in which a person continues to gamble until he finally loses everything. He proceeds compulsively, unaware that his aim is to become a victim of his impulse.

concordance In genetics, having similar traits. The highest rate of concordance for the development of schizophrenia is seen in monozygotic (one-egg), identical twins.

condensation A single word, a phrase, or a symbol represents a group of ideas or a series of similar experiences. Characteristic of most dreams.

confabulation The unconscious filling of memory gaps with imaginary experiences of fantasy. Seen in Korsakoff's psychosis and senile dementia.

confidentiality A principal of medical ethics whereby a physician may not reveal confidences entrusted to him in the course of treatment, unless required to do so by law or to protect the patient or the welfare of others in the community. The psychiatrist has no legal right to maintain confidentiality, but he may confine his response to that which is relevant to the given situation. Some states have laws which consider information obtained in the therapist-patient or doctor-patient relationship privileged communication. This privilege is the patient's right and he can prevent the doctor from testifying. If the patient sues and wants to introduce psychiatric testimony, he may waive the privilege.

conflict A mental struggle between opposing forces, such as the id with superego, ego, ego-ideal, and reality.

consensual validation Comparison of one's thoughts and feelings with those of others. Term first used by Trigant Burrow, later by Sullivan in the dyadic doctor-patient relationship for the reduction of parataxic distortions. Used as group therapy technique.

coprolalia Use of foul language, particularly words relating to feces. Seen in schizophrenia, Gilles de la Tourette's disease, and frontal lobe syndrome.

counterphobia Mastery of phobic anxiety by continually coping with the feared object symbolically. The lion tamer continues to put his head in the lion's mouth and is reassured when he escapes.

countertransference Conscious or unconscious feelings of the therapist toward the patient.

CPI Constitutional psychopathic inferior. Obsolete term for sociopathic personality.

criminal responsibility In order to be convicted, the accused at the time of the alleged crime must have been able to formulate an intent to do harm.

crisis intervention Brief therapeutic approach used in the emergency room of hospitals or in the community to ameliorate psychiatric symptoms rather than cure. Group, individual, family, or drug may be used for a few days or weeks.

cross-cultural psychiatry Comparative study of mental illness and health among various societies. Behavior patterns acceptable in one culture may not be in another.

cultural deprivation The individual is not allowed full participation in the culture, because of race, status, or poverty.

cunnilingus Use of mouth or tongue to stimulate female gentalia, usually the clitoris, until the female has orgasm.

Cushing's syndrome Weakness, easy fatigability, painful adiposity of body and face (moon facies) with limbs spared, amenorrhea, hypertrichosis in women, hypertension, purple striae, polycythemia, osteoporosis, frequent hyperglycemia. Mental symptoms include depression, paranoid ideation, and schizophrenic-like psychosis.

cybernetics The scientific study of messages and communication in humans, social groups, and machines, especially in reference to regulation and control mechanisms (thermostats, feedback). Norbert Wiener suggested a similarity between the human nervous system and electronic machines.

death instinct In psychoanalytic theory, two basic drives exist—life instinct (sexual instinct, libidinal instinct, erotic instinct, Eros) and death instinct (destructive instinct, aggressive instinct, Thanatos). Concept published by Freud in "Beyond the Pleasure Principle" (1920).

De Clerambault's syndrome A woman believes prestigious man is madly in love with her, although contact momentary or never at all.

decompensation Breakdown of defense mechanisms with abnormal functioning, such as psychosis. Analogous to cardiac decompensation.

déjà vu "Already seen." False recognition or familiarity with a visual experience that actually never happened before. Compare déjà extendu (already heard), déjà eprouve (already tried out), déjà fait (already done), déjà pensé (already thought), déjà raconte (already recounted), déjà voulu (already desired). False unfamiliarity is jamais vu.

delirium An acute organic brain syndrome with restlessness, disorientation, illusions, hallucinations (often visual), and fear. Delirium tremens is delirium combined with tremor (hands, tongue).

delusion A false belief that is fixed. If doubted, the individual will continue to offer further proof.

dementia Absence or reduction of intellectual faculties as a consequence of organic brain disease; as opposed to amentia (mental retardation), in which intellectual functions were never developed.

dementia praecox Premature deterioration. Term used by Morel in 1857 to describe patients with deterioration, incurability, and onset early in life (adolescence). Bleuler changed term to schizophrenia in 1911 because not all deteriorated and not all had early onset.

denial A defense mechanism in which external reality is rejected and is replaced by a wish-fulfilling fantasy or behavior. Also used when internal reality (wishes, affects, impulses) is not allowed in consciousness.

depersonalization Sensation of unreality of oneself or parts of oneself. A feeling of being dissolved, losing one's identity. Amnesia victims lose sense of identity and former interests, but retain reality of physical self and environment. One patient said "I see someone in the mirror but I can't feel it is me."

developmental disability A disability developing before age 18, expected to continue indefinitely, and constituting a substantial handicap. Included are mental retardation, cerebral palsy, autism, epilepsy, and other neurological diseases.

dipsomania Compulsion to drink alcohol.

disorientation Impairment of ability to judge one's relation to time, place, or person. The individual cannot recall the date, then the month, the year, and the season. If severe, the individual does not recognize the place. One said the hospital was a store and nurses were clerks selling lingerie. If very severe, person is affected. One individual could not remember her married name or her maiden name, and could give only her first name. When disorientation clears, time, place, and person return in reverse order.

displacement A defense mechanism in which the affect is transferred from an unacceptable idea or object to an acceptable one. Fear of father may be displaced as fear of dogs.

dissociation A defense mechanism in which a group of mental processes is split off from the rest of the personality anf functions on its own (fugue, multiple personality, somnambulism, automatic writing). Or, the group of processes may be split off from their affect, as in conversion hysteria with la belle indifference.

distractibility Inability to focus attention. Attention is continuously diverted from one object or one direction to another. Seen in mania.

DNA (deoxyribonucleic acid) A substance in the cell nucleus; found in the genes and responsible for inheritance. The DNA determines the type of RNA produced, which determines the synthesis of specific protein enzymes.

double bind Gregory Bateson postulated that schizophrenic patients are caught in a communication double-bind with the parent, in which two conflicting messages are given. The child may be told to do well in school if he wants to be loved. But when he gets ready to go to the library the mother says she needs him and will get sick if he leaves her alone.

double blind study A drug study with placebo, in which the patients and those involved in the study do not know which patients are on the drug. The drugs and placebo are coded to keep the two groups (double) blind.

Down's syndrome (mongolism) Mental retardation, thick tongue tending to protrude, epicanthal folds giving slant-eyed appearance, stubby fingers, simian creases on hands and feet, and short stature.

Durham rule (insanity defense) In 1954 the United States Court of Appeals for the District of Columbia ruled that "an accused is not criminally responsible if his unlawful act was the product of mental disease or mental defect." The word "product" allowed the psychiatrist to give relevant medical testimony.

dyslexia Reading disability unrelated to intelligence. Person is unable to understand the written word.

dyspareunia Pain experienced by women during sexual intercourse, often emotionally caused.

echolalia Imitation of another person's words. Seen in catatonic schizophrenia and Gilles de la Tourette's disease.

echopraxia Imitation of another person's movements. Seen in catatonic schizophrenia.

ecology The study of the symbiotic relationships between organisms and their environment. As applied to humans, it deals with effects on environment of human institutions. Ecological patterns of the city can refer to the distribution of crime, poverty, schizophrenia, and delinquency.

ego The Freudian structural framework of the mind includes the ego, the id, and the superego. It is both conscious and unconscious. It mediates between the individual and reality.

ego alien The individual sees a symptom (compulsion) as foreign to the ego and unrealistic. In neurotics, the symptom is usually ego alien, whereas in the psychotic the symptom is perceived as part of the self and not foreign.

ego ideal That part of the ego developed from parental substitutes (parental images) which emphasize what one should be and do rather than what one should not do (superego).

eidetic image Vivid visualization of objects previously seen as a memory, fantasy, or dream. The individual has a "photographic memory."

elopement Unauthorized absence of a patient from the inpatient unit of a mental health facility.

empathy Ability to put oneself in another's place and understand his feelings and behavior.

encopresis Involuntary defecation not caused by organic defect. In a child over 2 years of age, it is result of poor training, retardation, or psychogenic regression. Usually occurs at night or during sleep.

engram A memory trace. Richard Semon coined term "mneme" to denote memory that all cells have by means of the engram, a physical trace left by repetition of stimuli, and the way acquired habits may be transmitted to descendants. In neurology an engram designates a neuronal pattern of an acquired skilled act.

enuresis Involuntary discharge of urine; bed-wetting.

ergasia Adolf Meyer's term for the activity of the total person.

erotogenic zone (erogenous zone) An area of the body that responds to stimulation with sexual arousal, such as, oral, anal, and genital zones.

erotomania Abnormal preoccupation with erotic fantasies or activities.

EST, ECT Electroshock therapy; electroconvulsive therapy.

estrangement The sense of loss of the environment.

ethnology The branch of anthropology that studies racial groups (origin, history, customs, institutions).

ethology The study of animals in their natural habitat and their behavior. Knowledge of imprinting came from these studies.

euergasia Term by Adolph Meyer for normal mental functioning.

eunuch A man castrated before puberty who subsequently develops the secondary sexual characteristics of a woman.

euphoria Exaggerated feeling of well-being.

exaltation Intense elation and feelings of grandeur. Manic affect progresses from euphoria to elation to exaltation.

exhibitionism Compulsive exposing of genitals or whole body to opposite sex.

extrasensory perception (ESP) Obtaining knowledge outside the normal avenues of the five senses through mental telepathy (extrasensory perception of mental activities of another person) or clairvoyance (extrasensory perception of events).

extroversion The turning of one's energies and interest to external things outside the self.

fantasy Daydream. Thinking influenced by unconscious conflicts, wish-fulfillment, and proposed solutions for anticipated future events.

fellatio Oral contact to stimulate the penis.

fetishism Sexual deviation in which an inanimate object, the fetish (shoe, lock of hair, piece of clothing), serves as a substitute for a person and is necessary for orgasm.

fixation The concept of arrest of psychosexual development at the oral, anal, or phallic phase. Inordinate quantitites of psychic energy are fixated at these infantile levels and contribute to the type of psychiatric symptoms that are present.

flagellation The act of whipping oneself or another for the purpose of sexual arousal.

flight of ideas A "running away" or flight of thoughts. Thoughts are speeded up and may jump from topic to topic. This train of thought can be followed by the normal person and is not bizarre, disjointed, or symbolic as in tangential thinking. This increased ease of associations may lead to rhyming, punning, joking, or listing of items.

floccillation Aimless picking or plucking, usually at the bedclothes or clothing. Common in delirium and not uncommon in senile psychosis. Called "carphology" by Galen.

flooding A technique in behavior therapy in which the phobic object or a representation is presented in intense form. When successful, the symptom disappears after several trials.

folie á deux Insanity of two. Two closely associated individuals have psychoses with the same delusion. Has been called communicated insanity because one partner may recover if separated from the more dominant individual.

forensic psychiatry Public forum or court psychiatry. The branch of psychiatry dealing with legal aspects of mental illness.

forepleasure The sexual play that precedes sexual intercourse.

formication Sensation of ants (or other small insects) creeping into or running over the skin. Seen in cocainism, delirium tremens, and morphine addiction.

free association A technique used by Freud in which the patient tries to express all his passing thoughts without censorship. This material is used to arrive at interpretations in psychoanalytic therapy.

free-floating anxiety Severe generalized anxiety not attached to a specific idea, object, or event. Seen in anxiety neurosis.

frigidity Absence of sexual response in the female.

frontal lobe syndrome Lack of initiative and spontaneity, apathy, short-lived aggressiveness, Witzelsucht (facetiousness), poor judgment, lack of inhibitions (exhibitionism, urination in public, coprolalia). Headaches are common. Treatable frontal dementias are general paresis, normal pressure hydrocephalus, and meningioma. Untreatable are Pick's disease, Alzheimer's disease, Huntington's chorea, and Marchiafava-Bignami disease.

frotteur One who rubs. Sexual deviation in which orgasm is induced by rubbing up against the clothing of another person of the opposite sex, usually in a crowd or on a crowded public conveyance.

fugue A flight from one's home or ordinary environment for a prolonged period with amnesia for past life and past identity. The individual begins a new life with different conduct. Later the past is recalled and the period of the fugue is forgotten.

fundamental symptoms Bleuler (1911) described schizophrenia symptoms as fundamental (primary, pathognomonic) and accessory (secondary, seen in other diseases). Fundamental symptoms were loosening of associations, dysharmony between thought and affect, ambivalence, and autism. The accessory symptoms included hallucinations, mannerisms, catatonia, and pseudodementia.

GABA (gamma-aminobutyric acid) An inhibitory neurotransmitter. May be related to epileptic discharge and to tardive dyskinesia.

Ganser's syndrome (nonsense syndrome, syndrome of approximate answers, prison psychosis, hysterical pseudodementia) Responses to questions are beside the point (Vorbeireden, paralogia) but show the question was understood. "Two plus two equal five"; "the wall is orange" (actually blue). Seen following head trauma and in acute psychotic reactions.

GAS (general adaptation syndrome) Hans Selye's term for the body's response to stress along the pituitary-adrenal axis.

Gault decision In 1967 in the case of Gault, the Supreme Court rendered the decision that a juvenile must be given proper notice of the charges, represented by counsel, protected against self-incrimination, and be allowed to confront and cross-examine witnesses. This assures due process and fair treatment under the 14th Amendment.

general systems theory A theoretical framework that integrates all systems into a hierarchy from subatomic particles to whole societies. Emphasizes holism rather than mechanistic stimulus-response theories of personality. Has potential for integrating interdisciplinary understanding of human behavior.

genetic marker A specific pathognomonic biochemical defect established in mental retardation diseases. In studies of depression the trait of color-blindness has been used as a genetic marker.

Gerstmann syndrome Finger agnosia, right-left disorientation, acalculia, and agraphia. Seen in parietal lobe pathology.

Gheel colony A colony in Gheel, Belgium, existing since the 13th century for the treatment of mentally ill patients in private homes in the community.

globus hystericus A sensation of a lump in the throat; results from hysteria.

GPI General paralysis of the insane. Obsolete term for general paresis.

GSR (galvanic skin response) The resistance of the skin to the passage of a weak electric current changes in response to emotional stimuli. This is used in the lie detector test.

habeas corpus (writ of habeas corpus) A legal term for a writ (petition) asking the court to determine whether confinement or detention (prison, mental hospital, juvenile detention facility) has been accomplished with due process of law. The literal meaning is "you should have the body."

halfway house A residential facility for mental patients who no longer need 24-hour hospital care, but can live in a home with others under supervision, pending full discharge back to the community. This is a form of transitional·living.

hallucination A false sensory perception with no external stimulus. Esquirol introduced the term and called it perception without object. Hallucinations occur with any of the five senses: sight (visions), hearing (voices), smell (bad odors), taste (bad taste of poison), touch (bugs crawling on skin). A false perception of the size of objects is called micropsia or macropsia. A false perception of people being very small is called Lilliputian hallucination. Hallucinations are to be differentiated from illusions, which are false sensory perceptions with an external stimulus. The latter are usually toxic in origin.

hallucinogenic drug A drug capable of causing hallucinations in the presence of a clear sensorium (mescaline, psilocybin, lysergic acid-diethylamide). Many other drugs or poisons can cause hallucinations, but the sensorium is not clear (delirium).

hallucinosis The presence of hallucinations with a clear sensorium, as opposed to hallucinations in delirium with a clouded sensorium (acute brain syndrome).

haptic hallucination (tactile hallucination) False perception of touch.

hebephrenia A type of schizophrenia with silly and inappropriate mannerisms, often seen in the young. Hebe was the Greek goddess of youth. Delusions, hallucinations, word salad, and regression also accompany this clinical type. Inappropriate smiling is to be differentiated from the grimacing in Huntington's chorea.

hedonism Philosophy that pleasure (rather than pain) is the greatest good. A life or action based on this principle is hedonistic.

heroin An opiate made from morphine and even more addicting. The most common "street drug." Also called "horse."

heuristic Encouraging discovery or research.

holism Based on the idea that the sum is greater than the parts. The whole person is studied and treated as an entity and not as a collection of characteristics or parts.

homeostasis A tendency to approach an equilibrium. The concept that the body attempts to maintain a balance of its various processes and thereby a stable system.

homosexuality Sexual attraction between two persons of the same sex.

Hunter's syndrome (mucopolysaccharidosis II) Mental retardation, gargoyle features, dwarfism, marked skeletal abnormalities. X-lined recessive trait affecting males.

Hurler's syndrome (gargoylism, mucopolysaccharidosis I) Mental retardation, gargoylism, hepatosplenomegaly, spade-like hands, hyperteliorism. An autosomal recessive trait.

hypertensive crisis Sudden severe rise in blood pressure that can cause intracranial hemorrhage and stroke. Can be seen as a side effect of some antidepressant drugs.

hypothyroidism Lack of production of thyroxin, hormone of the thyroid gland. In childhood this leads to cretinism and in adults to myxedema. The gland may be unable to manufacture thyroxin if iodine is missing from the diet.

hyperventilation syndrome Breathlessness, palpitation, light-headedness, faintness, numbness in the extremities and around the mouth, and sweating. Due to excessive blowing off of carbon dioxide from overbreathing, which may have started with anxiety or fear of dying or of having a heart attack. Can be controlled by breathing less often or by breathing into a paper bag, so that carbon dioxide is returned into the body.

hypnagogic hallucination Hallucination occurring just before falling off to sleep.

hypnopompic hallucination Hallucination occurring just before waking up fully.

hypnosis The induction of a trance-like state resembling sleep by artificial means. The subject responds to suggestions during the trance and may carry out certain posthypnotic suggestions.

iatrogenic illness A disease accidentally caused or made worse by a physician.

id According to Freud's structural theory of mental functioning, the id is the segment containing the instinctual drives and seeks to discharge their energy continuously according to the pleasure principal.

idea of reference Misinterpretation of the activities of others or of events by assuming personal reference and meaning when there is none. This occurs through the mental mechanism of projection. A desire to steal is projected as a suspicion that others are attempting to steal one's belongings. If two people are seen talking and laughing at a distance, the paranoid invididual wonders if they are discussing and laughing at him. When he becomes unshakably convinced of this, he has delusions of reference.

idealization A defense mechanism in which a person overestimates an attribute of another and considers him more perfect than he is.

identification A defense mechanism in which a person takes into himself a mental picture of another and acts as he conceives of this person as acting. This process is unconscious and not conscious as in imitation. In identification with the aggressor, the male child identifies with the father and incorporates his image at the end of the Oedipal period.

idiopathic Without known cause, for example, idiopathic epilepsy, as opposed to secondary epilepsy resulting from head injury or brain tumor.

idiot Obsolete term for mentally retarded individual with I.Q. of 0 to 25. Mental age of about 3 years. Custodial care is required and the individual is unable to dress himself or count money.

idiot savant A mentally retarded individual capable of remarkable feats of calculation or problem solving, such as remembering numbers of a series of railroad cars or of calculations based on calendar dates.

illusion False sensory perception with external stimulus. A misinterpretation of a shadow as an animal. Common in delirium and at dusk. Illusions suggest toxic psychosis; medication is a frequent cause.

imago Jung's term for an unconscious mental image of an important person during the early life of the child, such as the parent. The imago is usually idealized.

imbecile Obsolete term for mentally retarded individual with I.Q. of 25 to 50. Mental age is 3 to 7 years. May be seen in phenylketonuria.

impotence Inability to maintain an erection and engage in sexual intercourse.

implosion A behavior therapy technique in which patient closes eyes and is told to imagine feared conflict situations (aggression, rejections, sexual scenes, guilt); therapist adds more imaginations of similar kind. The anxiety or guilt is reproduced without the feared event and extinction of the affect occurs.

imprinting Learning based on early environmental experiences. A term used in ethology. A duck is "imprinted" and follows the individual it sees in the short period after hatching, whether it is a human or a duck.

incest Sexual intercourse between family members such as father-daughter, brother-sister, mother-son, or cousin-cousin.

incoherence Disconnected speech that is incomprehensible.

incorporation A defense mechanism in which an object is symbolically ingested orally.

individuation Term by Jung for the process of differentiating the individual personality.

informed consent The physician will describe (to the patient) the treatment, giving benefits and risks, discomforts, side-effects, long-term results if treatment fails, and consequences if no treatment is given. This will be done without coercion. Written consent is obtained for electrotherapy and for psychosurgery.

insanity A legal term meaning "of unsound mind."

insanity defense A legal concept that the accused is not criminally responsible by reason of insanity, as defined by law (McNaughten Rule, irresistable impulse test, Durham Rule, American Law Institute Formulation).

insight Recognition by a patient that his symptoms are caused by illness. On a deeper level, psychodynamic understanding of the origin and meaning of the symptoms.

instinct An inborn drive. The primary or basic instincts are self-preservation (aggressive drive) and procreation (sexual drive).

intake The initial interview at a psychiatric facility between a patient and a member of a psychiatric team.

intellectualization A defense mechanism in which lengthy reasoning is used to avoid confrontation by an unpleasant impulse or affect.

interpretation The therapist suggests to the patient the possible meaning of his symptoms and behavior based on resistances, defenses, transferences, and symbols.

introjection A defense mechanism in which a psychic representation of a loved or hated object is taken into one's ego system.

introversion A turning inward, with lack of interest in the outside world.

I.Q. (intelligence quotient) Mental age (measured by psychological tests) divided by chronological age multiplied by 100.

irresistible impulse test In 1922, some states added this test to the ability to know right from wrong test under the McNaughten Rule. The accused might know his act was morally wrong and against the law but still not have the "freedom of will" to resist the act and be held criminally not responsible.

isolation A defense mechanism in which an unacceptable impulse, idea, or act is set apart from its emotional charge or feeling tone.

Jacksonian epilepsy The convulsion begins with clonic movements in the thumb or great toe and marches up the limbs to the face without consciousness being lost. The seizure may also begin in the corner of the mouth. Described by John Hughlings Jackson. Indicates organic disease of precentral cortex.

jamais vu A false feeling of unfamiliarity with a situation that has happened.

jargon aphasia The patient utters a stream of unintelligible words; caused by a neurological disease.

judgment The capacity to draw correct conclusions and act accordingly. Judgment is impaired if the act is not consistent with reality— for example, walking out into a cold night in pajamas is poor judgment.

kinesthetic hallucination False perception of muscular movement, such as feeling of movement in an amputated limb (phantom limb).

kinesthetic sense Perception of one's own movement from sensory receptors located in the muscles, bones, and joints.

kinky hair syndrome Mental retardation, deficient growth, pili torti, hypothermia, blood vessel degeneration. Serum ceruloplasmin and copper content of organs low, possibly because of copper malabsorption.

Kleine-Levin syndrome Episodic hypersomnia, excessive eating, and absence of sleep spindles that occurs only in adolescent males.

kleptomania Compulsion to steal. Objects often have little value.

Klinefelter's syndrome Tall, thin male, breast enlargement, underveloped testes, mental retardation, genetic abnormality of chromosomes (XXY, XXXY, XXXXY).

Kluver-Bucy syndrome Bilateral temporal lobe ablation, characterized by loss of recognition of people, loss of fear, rage reactions, hypersexuality, excessive oral behavior, memory defect, and overreactivity to visual stimuli.

Korsakoff's syndrome Confusion, disorientation, anterograde amnesia, confabulation, polyneuritis, and alcoholism.

la belle indifference A calm mental attitude out of keeping with the degree of disability. Called "the beautiful indifference" by Janet.

labile Unstable. Labile affect changes every few moments.

lapsus linguae A slip of the tongue due to unconscious factors. Slip of the pen is called lapsus calmi.

latency phase Stage of psychosexual development from age 5 to 12, with cessation of sexual preoccupation and period of having friends and group of own sex.

latent content The hidden meaning behind the symbols in fantasies and dreams, as opposed to manifest content.

learning disability Inability to learn reading, writing, or arithmetic because of disorder in brain functioning and not because of lack of intellect, as in mental retardation.

lesbianism (sapphism) Female homosexuality. About 600 BC on the island of Lesbos, Sappho encouraged young women to engage in mutual sex practices.

Lesch-Nyhan syndrome Mental retardation, self-mutilating behavior, and elevated blood uric acid. X-linked recessive trait.

libido The energy associated with the sexual instinct.

lilliputian hallucination (microscopic hallucinations, micropsia) Hallucination of people in minature form. Term is derived from Lilliput, an imaginary kingdom of 6-inch people in *Gulliver's Travels*. This type of hallucination has been reported in intoxication from alcohol, chloral, ether, and trichlorethylene and in cholera, typhoid, scarlet fever, and cocainism.

litiginous The tendency to file law suits or to litigate. Seen in some paranoid patients.

logotherapy Frankl's term for his form of existential analysis.

loosening of associations A thought disorder in which connections are uneven, not relevant, symbolic, tangential, or paralogical Seen in schizophrenia.

LSD (lysergic acid diethylamide) Hallucinogenic drug discovered in 1942.

magical thinking The idea that thinking something is the same as doing it. Seen in children's thinking, dreams, and schizophrenia.

malingering Simulation of illness with intent to deceive.

mania Usually refers to one phase of manic-depressive psychosis, in which there is acceleration of ideas, emotions, and motility, such as flight of ideas, distractibility, clang association, joking, rhyming, punning, elation, exhaltation, and psychomotor hyperactivity. Mania is also used as a suffix to indicate preoccupation, obsession, or compulsion with: drinking alcohol (dipsomania), thinking about self (egomania), having erotic fantasies or activities (erotomania), stealing (kleptomania), power or wealth (megalomania), one idea (monomania), death or dead bodies (necromania), sexual relations in females (nymphomania), setting fires (pyromania), and pulling out hairs (trichotillomania).

manifest content The disguised conscious part of a dream that is remembered and reported, as opposed to the latent content, which is the unconscious, unsymbolized true meaning of the dream.

mannerism A repetitive involuntary gesture or activity peculiar to an individual, such as a rotary motion with the hand or taking a short step every third step.

mantra In transcendental meditation, a word or syllable used repeatedly to relax in order to return to the alpha state.

marathon group session (accelerated interaction) Group meeting (8 to 72 hours) with open expression of feelings ending in excitement or elation. Developed by George Bach and Frederick Stoller.

masculine protest The need to move from the passive feminine role to the active masculine role in order to overcome the inferiority complex, according to Adler.

masochism A sexual deviation in which the preferred mode of producing sexual excitement is by experiencing suffering through humiliation or by being bound and beaten. First described by an Austrian novelist, Leopold von Sacher-Masoch (1836-1895).

masturbation Self-manipulation of genitals for the purpose of sexual stimulation.

maximum security unit A specialized unit in a psychiatric hospital designed to avoid elopement and to control patients considered dangerous to others. The majority of the patients are in the process of pretrial evaluation or have been committed as not guilty by reason of insanity.

menarche The beginning of menstruation at puberty. Menopause is the end.

mens rea A legel term meaning "criminal mind." A criminal offense requires an intent to do harm (malice, to steal, negligence, a guilty knowledge). The accused must have the ability to form an intention to do harm.

mental mechanism A generic term for a variety of psychic processes that are functions of the ego and largely unconscious. Includes perception, memory, thinking, and defense mechanisms.

mental status The mental state. Cross-sectional rather than longitudinal (history) examination of the mind at a point in time. Six components are evaluated: general appearance and behavior, flow of thought, emotional reaction, sensorium and content of thought, and insight and judgment.

microcephaly Small head due to lack of development of the brain and premature closure of the sutures of the skull.

micropsia False visual perception with miniturization of objects.

migraine Severe headache on one side, with nausea and visual symptoms.

milieu therapy Therapeutic socioenvironmental influences created in the hospital for benefit to the patient.

minimal brain dysfunction (MBD) Behavior syndrome of children with irritability, hyperactivity, short attention span, and learning problems due to organic dysfunction in the diencephalon.

MMPI (Minnesota Multiphasic Personality Inventory) A psychological test administered by questionnaire to the adult patient individually or in groups; fourteen scales describe the personality.

M'Naghten Rule (insanity defense) In 1843 the English House of Lords ruled that the accused is not responsible for a crime if he "was laboring under such a defect of reason from disease of the mind as not to know the nature and quality of the act, or, if he did know it, that he did not know that what he was doing was wrong."

mood Feeling tone that is a longitudinal evaluation and exists over time, as opposed to affect, which is cross-sectional and at a single point in time.

moron Obsolete term for mentally retarded individual with I.Q. of 50 to 70. Mental age is 8 to 12 years, with ability to do routine work. Unable to multiply 7 × 8 but may be able to multiply 3 × 4. Above I.Q. of 50 the individual is educable and may reach fourth- to fifth-grade level and become self-supporting.

motivation In psychoanalytic theory symptoms, dreams, and slips of the tongue have an unconscious need or motive causing them to appear. They are not random mental phenomena that merely surface from time to time.

Nalline test Injection of Nalline (nalorphine HC1), a narcotic antagonist, will precipitate opiate withdrawal symptoms.

narcissism Self-love. In Greek mythology, Narcissus looked into a pool of water and fell in love with his own reflection. In psychoanalytic theory, primary narcissism is an early phase of infantile development when child has not differentiated between himself and the outside world and feels all pleasure derives internally; this leads to a feeling of complete control and omnipotence. Secondary narcissism results when external object love is redirected to the self.

narcolepsy (Gelineau's syndrome) A sleep disorder characterized by periodic sudden brief sleep attacks with falling due to loss of muscle tone. The narcolepsy tetrad includes excessive daytime sleepiness, cataplexy, sleep paralysis, and hypnagogic hallucinations.

narcotic blockade Treatment by the use of a drug (methadone) to inhibit the effects of a narcotic (heroin).

negative hallucination Something present is perceived as being absent. Seen in hysteria and under hypnosis.

negativism Resistance to outside suggestions or commands with refusal to eat, talk, or move a body part. Seen in catatonic schizophrenia.

neologism New word. A condensation of several words and concepts. For example, "sexmerized" was derived from sexual feelings thought to be controlled by mesmerism (hypnosis). Occurs in schizophrenia.

neurosis A minor mental disorder (no distortion of reality but impairment of functioning) with anxiety or converted anxiety symptoms (hysterical, phobic, obsessive-compulsive, depersonalization, hypochondriacal, neurasthenic). Delusions or hallucinations point to major mental disorder (psychosis).

nihilism Belief that oneself or a part of oneself does not exist. Nihilistic ideas or delusions include belief that one is dead, that one's family is dead, or that the world does not exist. Occurs in depression and schizophrenia.

nondirective approach An individual or group psychotherapeutic technique in which the therapist echoes the patient's ideas and does not direct the process by inserting his own ideas or questions. Other approaches to psychotherapy are supportive, directive, and interpretive.

nosology The science of classification of diseases.

nuclear family Includes the individual's parents and children. The extended family includes relatives closely associated with the family. The network includes the nuclear family, the extended family, other relatives, friends, work contracts, and recreational contacts. Foulkes believes the social network has a significant effect in the production of mental illness in the patient.

null hypothesis No difference exists between two groups (experimental and control) and any difference between the means is due to chance. In a scientific experiment, an "alternative hypothesis" is adopted which predicts a difference will exist beyond chance (.05 statistical significance or better), and that this is due to the variable being manipulated. If a statistically significant result is obtained, the null hypothesis is "rejected."

nymphomania In women, excessive desire for sexual intercourse.

obsession Idea that persistently thrusts itself into consciousness and is recognized as illogical.

Oedipus complex A pattern of repressed ideas from age 3 to 6. The child attaches sexual interest to the parent of the opposite sex and wishes to get rid of the parent of the same sex. The child then fears that the same sex parent wishes to harm him (castration). (In the Greek myth, Oedipus unknowingly killed his father, Laius, and married his mother, Jocasta; When he discovered this he blinded himself.)

oligergasia Mental retardation. Term used by Adolph Meyer.

oligophrenia Mental retardation. Oligo- means small, few, scanty.

oneirophrenia Dream mind. Confusion present in acute schizophrenic episode. Glucose tolerance test positive. Once thought to have better prognosis.

operant conditioning Term used by B. F. Skinner for the procedure of rewarding the subject when the desired behavior appears spontaneously. Behavior is shaped by reinforcement.

oral character Character traits are described by Abraham as optimistic, carefree, and generous, if first-stage sucking period is pleasurable. If not pleasurable, then character traits are pessimistic, apprehensive, demanding, and never satisfied. The second stage or biting stage of oral development is said to lead to the traits of tendency to hate and to destroy.

oral phase The first stage in psychosexual development with the mouth as the center of the child's needs, pleasure, and expression.

ordinal position Birth rank order.

organic brain syndrome (OBS) See acute brain syndrome. Exists with or without psychotic disorder.

orgasm The climax of sexual excitement, accompanied by a release of sexual tension. In men ejaculation occurs. Spasmodic contractions occur in the genital area in both sexes.

orientation One's awareness of time, place and person. Interfered with in organic brain syndrome.

orthostatic hypotension Sudden reduction in blood pressure on rising from a recumbent to an upright position. May be seen as side effect of medication.

overcompensation Feelings of inferiority are masked by extraordinary and exaggerated efforts to reach a goal of dominance.

paranoia Extremely rare. Gradual development of circumscribed paranoid system based on single idea or event which was misinterpreted. The rest of the personality remains intact. The term was used by Vogel in 1764.

paranoid Overly suspicious.

paraphrenia A chronic paranoid state with persecutory or grandiose well-systematized delusional system without deterioration or splitting of psychic functions as seen in paranoid schizophrenia.

parapraxis Misaction, such as slip of the tongue, slip of the pen, or mislaying of an article. Freud said these acts were caused by unconscious.

parasympathetic nervous system That part of the autonomic nervous system that controls the life-sustaining organs, such as the heart, under normal conditions. When danger threatens, the sympathetic nervous system takes over.

parataxic distortion A defense against anxiety, in which an individual perceives objects and interpersonal relationships in a distorted manner based on earlier experiences.

parens patriae The doctrine of parens patriae allows the state to intervene and act as a surrogate parent for those unable to care for or likely to harm themselves.

paresthesia Strange sensation in the skin (tingling, burning, tickling).

parkinsonian syndrome A pattern in disease of the basal ganglia, such as Parkinson's disease (involuntary tremors at rest, rigidity of muscles, lack of associated movements, shuffling gait). May be seen as side-effect of psychotropic drugs.

partial hospitalization One of the five essential services provided by a mental health center. Included are day, evening, and weekend hospital services on a part-time basis.

pavor nocturnus Night terror. A type of sleep disturbance. It differs from a nightmare in that the child does not remember the incident. He is found sitting up or running about screaming.

pecking order Hierarchy of authority in an organization or social group; in feeding behavior of chickens, a "pecking order" enforces the sequence for approaching the feeding tray.

pederasty Anal intercourse between a man and a boy.

pedophilia A sexual deviation in which a child is used for sexual purposes.

penis envy Freud's concept that the woman envies the man because he has a penis.

perseveration Persistent repetition of the same response to different questions, to a series of short stories, or to a series of ink blots.

persona Jung's term for the personality an individual shows to the world, as opposed to his inner self, or anima.

personality Habitual pattern of behavior, in terms of attitudes and mental and physical activities. Various ones described are anacastic, asthenic, compulsive, cyclothymic, explosive, histrionic, hysterical, inadequate, multiple, obsessive-compulsive, passive-aggressive, and schizoid.

perversion Sexual practice that deviates from the normal.

phallic phase The third stage of psychosexual development, ages 2 to 6. Interest centers in the phallus (penis) and the clitoris.

phenotype The outer appearance and attributes of a person which are changed by external conditions, as opposed to the genotype (set of genes received at conception).

phobia Unrealistic fear of an object or situation.

pluralism Multicausal factors affect behavior.

priapism The persistent abnormal erection of the penis, which usually occurs without sexual desire. May be side effect of a drug.

primal scene A child's real or fantasied observation of sexual intercourse between his parents.

primary process In psychoanalytic theory, primary process thinking is unconscious and id-related. It is nonverbal, pictorial, symbolic, magical, vague, and not logical. Secondary process thinking is preconscious and conscious and ego-related and proceeds with words, logic, reality-testing, and postponement of immediate instinctual desires if they appear dangerous.

privileged communication In some states the laws of evidence provide that communications told in trust (confidence) to a physician, priest, or attorney may be withheld; these are referred to as privileged communications. This right is waived by the client in cases involving the insanity defense.

projection A defense mechanism in which one accuses another of one's own unacceptable desires.

propfschizophrenia (engrafted schizophrenia) Schizophrenia is superimposed on mental retardation.

pseudobulbar palsy Degeneration of the pyramidal tracts above the medulla is accompanied by dysarthria, dysphagia, spasticity of the muscles, and impaired voluntary control over the emotional reactions (exaggerated, explosive).

psychiatrist A medical doctor with specialization in study and treatment of mental diseases. After four years of training and passing a written and oral examination by the American Board of Psychiatry and Neurology, he or she becomes a Diplomate in Psychiatry and is a medical specialist.

psychic determinism Freud states that psychic events are not random happenings. All phenomena have causes that operate on an unconscious level and beyond voluntary control.

psychobiology Term used by Adolph Meyer to refer to the holistic study of human beings as an integrated psychological and biological unit.

psychodrama J. L. Moreno's psychotherapeutic method using dramatization on the stage to act out conflicts by using others (auxiliary egos) to play the various roles.

psycholinguistics The study of factors that affect communication and verbal information.

psychological test An instrument for measuring the functioning of the psyche (mind). The most commonly administered tests are projective tests (Rorschach, drawing tests, TAT), psychometric tests (WAIS), and personality inventory tests (MMPI).

psychologist An individual who takes special training in the science of the mind, both normal and abnormal, and obtains a master's degree (M.S.) or a doctor's degree (Ph.D.). A clinical psychologist serves an internship that provides experience in treating mental illness.

psychosis A major mental disorder with reality testing impaired, daily life markedly interfered with, and severe symptoms (affect disorder, hallucinations, delusions, deficient memory, disorientation).

psychotomimetic drug (hallucinogenic drug) A drug that produces a condition that mimics psychosis (Mescaline, LSD, psylocybin) with a clear sensorium.

psychotropic drug A drug that affects the psyche (mind). Subtypes are antipsychotic, antidepressant, antimanic, antianxiety, and hallucinogenic drugs.

pyromania A compulsion to set fires.

quadrangular therapy Marital therapy involving four people: the husband, the wife, and each one's therapist.

Quincke's disease Angioneurotic edema.

rape Sexual intercourse without the woman's consent. Rape is an unexpected sexual assault and the violence aspect of the attack accounts for much of the victim's suffering.

rapport A relationship characterized by harmony, such as confidence of a patient in his therapist, which is expressed by a willingness to cooperate.

rapture-of-the-deep syndrome A psychosis induced by sensory deprivation in scuba and deep-sea divers.

rationalization A defense mechanism in which irrational thought or behavior is explained as reasonable or rational. The term was introduced by Ernest Jones. (In the fable, the fox said he didn't want the grapes he couldn't reach because they were sour.)

reaction formation A defense mechanism in which an unacceptable wish or impulse in the unconscious is converted to its opposite. An interest in dirt (feces) is converted to excessive need for cleanliness.

regression A defense mechanism in which an individual returns to an earlier pattern of behavior—for example, a new sibling is brought home and the older child returns to sucking his thumb.

reliability The degree of consistency in measurement. If a clock is mistakenly set forward 20 minutes, and is a good timepiece, it will "reliably" measure time incorrectly. The time it tells will have high reliability but low validity. A psychological test has high reliability if the same result appears when administered repeatedly.

REM Rapid eye movements seen in deep sleep.

repetition compulsion The irresistible need to repeat early emotional experiences over and over until the conflict is brought to consciousness and resolved.

repression A defense mechanism in which unacceptable ideas or affects are "forgotten" and removed from consciousness. In the unconscious they are inaccessible to ordinary recall.

resistance Opposition encountered when unconscious id material is about to emerge into conscious awareness, because the ego is threatened and defenses appear.

retrospective falsification Distortion of previously true memories in the unconscious because of affective needs and later recalled as false memories.

right to treatment The right of an involuntarily committed patient to treatment which will improve or cure his mental condition.

rigidity An individual is said to be rigid if resistance to change is marked.

RNA (ribonucleic acid) A substance manufactured by DNA and found in the cell nucleus.

sadism A sexual deviation in which the preferred mode of producing sexual excitement is by producing suffering by humiliation and inflicting pain. First described by French writer, Donatien Alphonse Francois de Sade (1740-1814).

satyriasis In men, a sexual deviation with insatiable need for sexual intercourse.

Sanfilippo's syndrome (mucopolysaccharidosis III) Mental retardation, mild skeletal abnormalities, seizures, athetosis. Autosomal recessive trait. Mucopolysaccharidosis, I, II, and III are accompanied by mental retardation, but IV, V, and VI are not.

Schreber-case Freud published "Notes Upon an Autobiographical Account of a Case of Paranoia" (1911), based on the "Memoirs of a Neurotic" by Daniel Paul Schreber (1903). He expressed a psychoanalytic viewpoint about paranoid delusions and their relation to homosexuality.

scotoma A blind spot in awareness due to psychological defense mechanisms.

screen memory A false memory recalled as a cover-up of a painful memory.

secondary gain Advantage gained because one is ill, such as release from responsibility or special attention.

sedative A drug that produces a relaxed or calm state (barbiturates, chloral hydrate, bromide).

sensorium The hypothetical seat of sensation in the brain. Contrasted with the motorium. Clear awareness of one's surroundings is described as a clear or intact sensorium. If orientation and memory are impaired, the sensorium is said to be cloudy. Impairment is related to organic rather than psychic dysfunction.

sensory deprivation Absence of sensory stimuli with loss of usual input of sensory perceptions. May lead to panic with delusions and hallucinations.

sibling In genetics, one of two or more children born at different times to the same parents.

sibling rivalry The concept that children compete for the attention of the parents and have feelings of hatred and death wishes toward each other.

sixty-nine The number 69 is a slang expression for fellatio and cunnilingus by two individuals simultaneously. The head of each is near genitals of the other.

snow-bird A cocaine addict.

sodomy Anal intercourse. Legal use of the term includes bestiality.

somnambulism Sleepwalking.

stereotypy Continuous repetition of a speech or motor activity. Seen in catatonic schizophrenia.

sublimation A defense mechanism in which unacceptable impulses are transformed into socially acceptable activities. Anal desires are sublimated into finger painting, oil painting, or writing.

substitution A defense mechanism in which an unacceptable goal is replaced by a similar but more acceptable one.

succinylcholine chloride (Anectine) A muscle-relaxing drug used to avoid the motor manifestations of the seizure in electroconvulsive therapy.

suggestibility State of easy compliance with another person's desires and wishes. Seen in hypnosis and in individuals with hysterical traits.

supportive psychotherapy Treatment in which defense mechanisms are reinforced and the patient is given reassurance, as opposed to uncovering the motives behind the symptoms and probing into conflicts.

suppression Conscious inhibition of unacceptable impulse, emotion, or idea as opposed to the unconscious defense mechanism of repression.

symbolism A defense mechanism in which a word or object comes to stand for another because of similarity or association.

sympathetic nervous system The part of the autonomic nervous system that prepares an individual for fight or flight.

sympathomimetic drug A drug that mimics the action of the sympathetic nervous system (amphetamine, epinephrine).

syndrome An abnormal cluster of signs (on physical examination) and symptoms (history) frequently seen together, which represent several diseases or causes. The term is used when the cause (etiology) is unknown.

tabes dorsalis (locomotor ataxia, tabetic neurosyphilis) Syphilis of the nervous system with wasting, lightning pains, dysuria, ataxia, Argyll-Robertson pupils, absent deep reflexes, loss of proprioceptive sensibility, and abnormal spinal fluid.

talion principle Retaliation in kind—"An eye for an eye, and a tooth for a tooth."

tangentiality (derailment) A disturbance of thought (associations), in which thoughts flow away from the subject material, like a tangent. (In geometry, a tangent is a straight line that touches a single point on a curve and goes off into space.) A schizophrenic patient may avoid a direct answer to a question and slide off into a series of sentences tied together by their symbolic meaning. If the question is repeated, the patient may slide off from the point again. The examiner may sense vagueness at first and then realize his question has never been answered. Circumstantiality differs because the patient is clearly on his way to the answer but compulsively gives unessential detail.

tarantism An uncontrollable urge to dance occurred in Southern Italy in the 17th century, which was ascribed to the bite of the tarantula. In the middle ages, hysterical dancing epidemics may not have been psychological in origin but may have been poisoning due to ergot, a fungus on the rye, which was baked into bread and released LSD from the ergot molecule.

tardive dyskinesia A syndrome first reported in 1956, induced by neuroleptics and characterized by involuntary movements of the tongue, face, jaws, and lips and sometimes with choreoathetoid movements of extremities or trunk.

TAT (Thematic Apperception Test) A projective test based on interpretation of a series of drawings.

therapeutic community A hospital ward environment with staff trained to encourage the resocialization and rehabilitation of the patient. Maxwell Jones published "The Therapeutic Community" in 1953.

third ear Introduced by German philosopher Nietzsche and later used to entitle a book called *Listening with the Third Ear* by Theodor Reich. The therapist with sensitivity intuitively hears the real or concealed meaning of patient's communications. Analogous to the expression "reading between the lines."

tic A twitch. Involuntary repetitive spasmodic motion of group of muscles, such as involuntary winking or looking over one's shoulder. Usually psychogenic, but may be seen in chronic encephalitis and in Gilles de la Tourette syndrome.

tic douloureux (trigeminal neuralgia) Painful twitch. Severe facial pain caused by disease of fifth cranial nerve.

tinnitus Ringing in one or both ears. Occasionally is a drug side effect.

tolerance Lessening effect of the same dose of a drug when it is administered repeatedly over a period of time. As a result, it is necessary to increase the dose in order to obtain the original effect.

topography Freud's concept of mental topography describes the psyche (mind) as divided into regions (conscious, preconscious, unconscious), and relates the structural components (superego, ego, id) to these specific locations.

torticollis Twisted neck. Wry neck.

T-group (training group) A sensitivity training group that emphasizes the development of self-awareness. Groups began in 1947 at Bethel, Maine, with professionals training to lead groups.

transference The transfer or projection of attitudes toward important figures of the past (father, mother) onto a current person, such as the therapist.

transsexualism Disturbance of gender identity often with lifelong desire to be the opposite sex. Some have been treated by sex-changing surgical procedures, hormones, and psychotherapy.

transvestitism (transvestism) The impulse to dress in the clothing of the opposite sex, usually associated with homosexuality.

trichotillomania A compulsion to pull out one's hair.

tricyclic drug Imipramine (Tofranil), amitryptiline (Elavil), and others of this class of antidepressant drugs are usually more effective than monoamine oxidase inhibitors.

trisomy The presence of an extra chromosome (47 instead of 46) in Down's syndrome. The twenty-first chromosome pair is increased from two chromosomes to three.

tumescence Congestion and swelling—for example, of the penis during sexual excitation.

Turner's syndrome A syndrome in females due to nondysjunction with only one X chromosome and no Y chromosome, called the XO variant. Secondary female sex characteristics do not develop.

uncinate fit A seizure (hallucination of smell or taste with chewing motions of the jaw) due to a tumor or lesion in the uncinate gyrus of the temporal lobe.

unconscious A hypothetical division of the mind which is not in awareness and contains drives, impulses, and memories. Some of these are easily remembered and referred to as in the preconscious. Others can be brought to consciousness by techniques such as free association or hypnosis.

undoing A defense mechanism in which a thought or action cancels out a previous thought or action. An unacceptable thought of wishing the mother to die is repressed and then expressed verbally as, "I wish you good health." This is then undone by a symbolic gesture of the hands of putting the words back into the mouth. This undoes the wish for health. The wish for death then threatens to break through again into consciousness and the statement, "I wish you good health," is repeated. This is undone again by the gesture of the hands. This occurs again and again, and demonstrates why the obsessive-compulsive patient cannot stop his repetitive activity.

unipolar depression An illness marked by repeated depressive episodes without manic episodes.

universalization A therapeutic technique whereby guilt is reduced and self-esteem is increased, when an individual in group therapy discovers others experience the same (universal) forbidden thoughts and impulses.

vaginismus Spastic contraction of vagina during intercourse.

validity The degree to which an instrument measures what it claims to measure. A psychological test has high validity if it can be shown to measure what it is attempting to measure. A comparison is made with another instrument (a standard, another psychological test, a specific behavior).

verbigeration The same phrases or words are repeated over and over in a stereotyped fashion. Seen in catatonic schizophrenia.

vertigo Dizziness.

voyeur A "peeping Tom," who derives pleasure from repeatedly seeking out opportunities to watch an unsuspecting woman, who is disrobing, naked, or engaged in sexual activity. Further sexual contact does not occur. Only men "peep," and one-fourth of those arrested are married. Another term is scoptophiliac.

WAIS Wechsler adult intelligence scale.

waxy flexibility (cerea flexibilitas, catalepsy, molding) A person placed in an unnatural position (arm upraised, finger bent) will retain this position for long periods. Seen in catatonic schizophrenia.

Wednesday Evening Society A meeting of Freud and his followers for the purpose of learning more about psychoanalysis. The group began in 1902 and became the Vienna Psychoanalytic Society in 1910.

Wernicke-Korsakoff syndrome Eye muscle weakness, nystagmus, pupillary changes, anterograde amnesia, polyneuritis, confabulation, hallucinations, no tremor. Seen in chronic alcoholism due to nutritional deficiency, especially vitamin B.

wet dream Seminal ejaculation during sleep.

white-out syndrome Psychosis occurring in Arctic explorers after continued monotonous experiencing of white snow.

WISC Wechsler Intelligence Scale for Children.

witzelzucht Facetiousness. Seen in frontal lobe tumor.

word salad (verbigeration) Speech consisting of disconnected words and phrases. Seen in hebephrenia or advanced stages of schizophrenia. May be composed of a series of neologisms.

working through Part of the treatment in psychoanalysis whereby free association brings conflicts into consciousness repeatedly until patient not only has insight but changes his personality into more mature character defenses.

WPPSI Wechsler Preschool and Primary Scale of Intelligence.

xenophobia Fear of strangers.

xerostomia Dry mouth.

zoophilia The use of animals as preferred to exclusive method of producing sexual excitement. Animal may be object of intercourse or trained to sexually excite the human partner by licking or rubbing.

zoophobia Fear of animals.

zygosity The state of being paired. Dizygotic means the product of two fertilized eggs (fraternal twins). Monozygotic means the product of a single fertilized egg (identical twins). Twin studies are used to separate genetic from environmental influences.

Index

A

AA (Alcoholics Anonymous), 198-199, 387
Abadie's sign, 387
ABEPP, 387
Abraham, K., 7, 375
Abreaction, 274, 291, 387
Abscess, EEG, 36
Abstinence syndrome
  alcohol, 109
  barbiturate, 206-207
  morphine, 205, 387
Abstract thinking, 44, 57, 105, 165, 387
Abstraction, 16, 387
Acalculia, 388
Acarophobia, 388
Accelerated interaction, 406
Accessory symptoms, 156, 164
Accident proneness, 235, 388
Acetylcholine, 216
Achluophobia, 388
Acid, 388
Ackerman, N., 375
Acrocephaly, 257
Acromegaly, 388
Acrophobia, 388
ACTH (adrenocorticotropin), 215
Acting out, 388
Action for Mental Health, 9
Active therapy, 7
Actual neurosis, 176

Acupuncture, 219, 226, 231, 297-300
Acute brain syndrome, 100-103, 388
ADAMHA, 388
Addiction, 197-209
Addicts Anonymous, 206
Adiadochokinesis, 388
Adie's syndrome, 388
Adjunctive therapists, 266-267
Adjustment reactions, 239-244
Adler, A., 6, 280-282, 375
Adolescence
  adjustment reaction, 241
  behavior disorders, 245-253
  compulsions, 185
  early, 63, 66, 388
  late, 63, 66, 388
  turmoil, 241
Adrenergic, 388
Adrenochrome, 158
Adrenolutin, 158
Aerophagia, 389
Affect
  ambivalence, 76
  anhedonia, 141, 390
  anxiety, 76
  apathy, 391
  blunting, 392
  depersonalization, 76
  depression, 76
  disharmony, 376
  ecstasy, 76

419

Affect—cont'd
  elation, 76
  equivalent, 200
  euphoria, 76
  exhaltation, 76
  fear, 110
  flat, 76
  grief, 141, 187
  inappropriate, 76
  lability, 99, 405
  panic, 76
  pleasurable, 76
  sadness, 76
  shallowness, 99
Affective disorders
  agitated depression, 142
  anhedonic states, 141
  atypical, 141, 147, 191
  bipolar depression, 141-142
  chronic, 141, 146
  depressive episode, 141
  endogenous depression, 5, 141
  episodic, 141-142
  exogenous depression, 5
  hypomania, 145
  involutional melancholia, 142
  manic episode, 143
  manic-depressive illness, 141,
    375
  postpartum depression, 142
  pseudo-dementia, 144, 146
  reactive depression, 141
  retarded depression, 141
  stuporous depressions, 142
  unipolar depression, 142
Affirmative action, 389
Aftercare, 374, 389
Aggression, 6, 222, 389
Agitated depression, 142
Agitation, 144, 389
Agnosia, 30
Agorophobia, 183
Agraphia, 29, 31
Aichhorn, A., 375
Akasthesia, 389
Akerfeldt test, 158
Al-Anon, 199
Alcohol, Drug Abuse and Mental
    Health Administration, 388

Alcoholics Anonymous, 198-199,
    387
Alcoholism, 198
  absenteeism, 198
  complications
    blackouts, 198
    cardiac decompensation, 109
    convulsions, 109
    death, 109
    delirium tremens, 109
    fractures, unrecognized, 109
    head injuries, 109
    hepatic coma, 111
    pathological intoxication, 110-
      111
    pneumonia, 109
    subdural hematoma, 120
    suicide, 198
  definition, 197
  diagnosis, 197-198
  incidence, 197-198
  life expectancy, 198
  psychoses
    alcoholic paranoid state, 110
    delirium tremens, 109
    deterioration, 110
    hallucinosis, 109-110
    Korsakoff's, 109
    Marchiafava's disease, 110
    pathological intoxication, 110-
      111
    Wernicke-Korsakoff's, 347, 418
  treatment, 198
Alexander, F., 214, 375
Alexia, 29
Algolagnia
  active (sadism), 195
  passive (masochism), 195
Algophobia, 183
Alienation, 389
Alienist, 389
Alliteration, 389
Alloplasty, 389
Alpha activity, 34-35
Alpha state, 389
Al-Teens, 199
Altruism, 389
Alzheimer, A., 375
Alzheimer's disease, 106-108, 375

Amaurotic idiocy (Tay-Sachs disease), 258
Ambivalence, 7, 77, 156, 160, 164, 389
Amenorrhea
  anorexia nervosa, 228
  depression, 142, 186
  false pregnancy, 232
Amentia, 389
American Law Institute Formulation, 389
American Psychiatric Association, 5, 390
Amnesia
  amnesic-confabulatory syndrome, 390
  anterograde, 74
  ECT, 311, 314
  generalized, 74
  head injury, 120
  hypermnesia, 74
  hysterical, 180
  organic, 74
  paramnesia (confabulation), 74, 394
  postconcussion, 119
  psychogenic, 74, 180
  retrograde, 74
  selective, 74
  sodium amytal treatment, 182
Amnestic syndrome, 109
Amok, 211
Amphetamines, 201-202, 206
Amytal interview, 182
Anacastic personality, 192
Anaclitic depression, 76, 249, 381, 390
Anal character, 176, 185
Anal phase, 66, 277
Anal sadistic phase, 185
Anemnesis, 390
Anectine; see Succinylcholine chloride
Anemia, 112-113
Angina pectoris, 225
Angioneurotic edema, 390
Anhedonia, 141, 390
Anima, 279, 390
Animus, 279

Anniversary reaction, 177
Anomie, 377
Anorexia, 165, 228
  nervosa, 228
Anosognosia, 30
Antabuse; see Disulfiram
Antisocial personality, 390
Anxiety, 76, 177, 400
  attacks, 224
  "free-floating," 76, 177, 400
  hysteria, 175, 183-184
  reaction, 175
Anxiolytic drug, 390
APA (American Psychiatric Association), 5, 390
Apathy, 391
Aphasia, 26-32
  agraphia, 29
  alexia, 29
  apraxia, 29
  examination for, 31-32
  formulation of, 31
  Freud's study, 32
  jargon, 26, 31
  motor, 29
  paraphasia, 31
  semantic, 31
  sensory, 29
Apoplexy, 391
Apperception, 73
"Approximate answers," 400
Aproxia, 30-31
Arachnodactyly, 257
Archetype, 279
Argot of addict, 201
Argyll-Robertson pupil, 383, 415
"Armor," 7
Arthritis, rheumatoid, 214
Association of Medical Superintendents of American Institutions for the Insane, 5
Associations, 277
Astereognosis (tactile agnosia), 30
Asterixis, 390
Asthenia, neurocirculatory, 177
Asthenic habitus, 165
Asthenic personality, 192, 411
Asthma, bronchial, 214
Ataxia, cerebellar, 110

Ataxic gait, 110
Athetosis, 391
Atropine (belladonna)
  coma treatment, 318, 321, 339
  with ECT, 309, 311, 322
  intoxication, 127
Attention, 71, 73, 192
Attitudes, 76
Atypical facial neuralgia, 235
Aura, 391
Autistic child, 162, 249
Autistic fantasy, 164
Autistic thought, 75
Autoeroticism, 378, 391
Autogenic training, 219
Automatic obedience, 77
Automatic writing, 291
Automatism, 6, 165, 391
Autonomic nervous system, 391
Autoplasty, 391
Autotopagnosia, 30
Auxiliary egos, 306, 412
Average, 391
Aversion, 77
Aversion therapy, 391
Avoidance, 176

B

Babinski, J., 6
"Bad trip," 209
Barbiturates
  chemotherapy, 332-333
  intoxication, 126-127, 206-207
  psychosis, 206
  withdrawal danger, 206
Battered child syndrome, 251, 391
Bayley Scales of Infant Develop-
  ment, 43
Beard, G., 177, 375
"Bedlam," 391
Bed-wetting, 241, 398
Beers, C., 375
Behavior
  disorders of children, 247
  modification, 259
  rating scales, 55-56
Behavioral sciences, 391
Behaviorism, 8, 385
Bell, L., 5, 375

Bell's mania, 393
Bender, L., 375
Bender-Gestalt test, 43, 376
Benedek, T., 376
Benedict, R., 376
Bereavement, 141, 146, 187, 217
Berger, 354
Berne, E., 295, 376
Bernheim, H., 6, 289, 376
Bernreuter Self-Sufficiency Ques-
  tionaire, 294
Bestiality, 195, 391
Beta activity, 34
Bicêtre, 4
Binet, A., 8, 376
Binet-Simon test, 376
Bini, 8, 308
Binswanger, L., 376
Biofeedback, 211, 219, 225-226,
  297, 391
Biogenic amine, 159
Bipolar depression, 141-142, 145,
  148, 392
Birth order, 280
Birth trauma, 6, 282
Bisexual, 392
Blackouts, 198
Black-patch syndrome, 392
Blandford, G., 375
Bleuler, E., 5, 156, 376
Blindness, hysterical, 181
Block design subtest, 42
Blocking, 75, 156, 159, 165, 392
Blood dyscrasias, 227-228
Blotchy skin, 165
Blunted affect, 392
Blushing, 220
Body image, 7, 215
Body language, 392
Body type
  asthenic, 5, 165, 381
  athletic, 381
  dysplastic, 381
  ectomorphic, 384
  endomorphic, 384
  mesomorphic, 384
  pyknic, 5, 149, 381
Borderline neurotic, 188
Borderline psychosis, 392

Borderline states, 194, 392
Bourneville's disease, 257, 392
Bowel training, 185
Bowlby, 249
Braid, J., 6, 289
Brain
    abscess, 36
    areas, 28
    damage, 255
    disorders, 99-140
    syndrome, 410
    trauma, 119-120
    tumor, 21, 36, 116
    waves, 34-35
Breuer, J., 6, 289, 376
Brigham, A., 5, 376
Brill, A., 376
Briquet, P., 376
Briquet's syndrome, 179, 376, 392
Broca's area, 28-30
Bromide intoxication, 123-124
Bromism, 392
Bronchial asthma, 214
Bruxism, 392
Buggery, 392
Bulimia, 165, 228, 234, 392
Burkhardt, 9
Burrow, T., 276
Butter, J., 5

C

Camphor-in-oil, 382
Cancer, 116, 235
    of pancreas, 21, 120
Cancerophobia, 144
Cannabis sativa, 207
Cannon, W., 215, 219
Capgras syndrome, 211-213, 392
Carbon dioxide therapy, 318, 382
Carbon monoxide intoxication, 124-125
Cardiospasm, 228, 229
Cardiovascular psychophysiological disorders
    essential hypertension, 224-225
    paroxysmal auricular tachycardia, 224
    vasodepressor syncope, 224
    vasomotor instability, 224

Cardiovascular psychophysiological disorders—cont'd
    Wolf-Parkinson-White syndrome, 224
Case history, 13, 16-20
Castration anxiety (fears), 176
Castration complex, 66, 183, 195, 393
Catalepsy, 165, 393, 418
Cataplexy, 393
Catastrophic anxiety, 393
Catatonia, 5, 156, 161, 165, 393
Catatonic exhaustion syndrome, 375, 393
Catatonic schizophrenia, EEG, 37
Catch-22, 393
Catchment area, 393
Catecholamine, 151, 159, 393
Catharsis, 6, 274, 393
Cathexis, 393
Catnip, 208-209
Causalgia, 236
Central nervous system (CNS), 393
Cerea flexibilitas, 77, 156, 393, 418
Cerebral arteriosclerosis (multi-infarct dementia) 103-106, 146
Cerebral dominance, 27, 38
Cerletti, U., 8, 308
Character
    analysis, 7
    "armor," 7
    defense, 7, 393
    disorder, 7, 190-191, 194, 393
    structure, 190
    types, 71, 191, 375
        anal, 176, 185
        oral, 409
Charcot, J., 6, 289, 376
Chemotherapy, 324-348
Child
    abuse, 251
    adjustment reaction, 241
    autistic, 249
    hyperactive, 100, 252
    minimal brain dysfunction, 249, 253, 407
    personality development, 62-66
    psychoanalysis, 245

Child—cont'd
  psychosis, 249
  with psychotic mother, 252
  "soft" neurological signs, 249
Childbirth 128-129
Childhood schizophrenia, 376
Chloral hydrate, 207
Cholinergic, 393
Chorea
  Huntington's, 37, 117, 257
  Sydenham's, 114
Chromosome
  nondysjunction, 256
  translocation, 256
  trisomy, 256
Chronic brain syndrome, 99-100, 394
Circadian rhythm, 142, 155, 394
Circumstantiality, 75, 394
Clang associations, 75, 149
Classification, 81-98
Claustrophobia, 183
Clear and convincing evidence, 365
Climacteric, 394
Cloetta's mixture, 318
Clouding of consciousness, 73, 394
Cocaine
  "bug," 72
  habituation, 207
  hallucinations, 72, 204, 207
  perforation of nasal septum, 207
  psychosis, 209
  "snowbird," 414
Cognition, 71, 394
Coitus interruptus (onanism), 394
"Cold turkey," 201, 394
Colitis, ulcerative, 230
Collective unconscious, 6, 380
Coma, 72, 119
Combat reaction, 239
Command automatism, 165
Commitment, 361-362
Community mental health, 367-374
Compensation, 67
Compensation neurosis, 180
Competency to stand trial, 394
Complex, 68, 159, 394
Compulsion, 77, 184, 394

Compulsion—cont'd
  fire-setting, 252
  gambling, 394
  handwashing, 185
  prolonged dressing, 185
  rituals, 185
  stealing, 193, 405
  touching of objects, 185
Conation, 71, 76
Concept formation, 71
Concordance, 394
Concrete thinking, 44, 57, 387
Concussion, 119-120
Condensation, 68, 164-165, 394
Conditioning
  classical, 383
  operant, 409
Confabulation, 74, 107, 125, 394
Confidentiality, 394
Conflict, 7, 67, 176, 179, 182, 395
Confusion, 73
Conolly, J., 156, 377
Conscious, 71, 277
Consciousness
  clouding of, 73, 394
  coma, 73, 119
  disorders of, 73
  stupor, 73, 165
Consent, informed, 404
Consensual validation, 395
Constitutional psychopathic inferior (CPI), 193
Constitutional types (body types), 5, 149, 165, 381, 384
Consultation, 275, 370
Continuous sleep therapy, 318
Conversion, 68
  hysteria, 176
  somatic, 220, 229
Convulsions, 36-38, 131-134, 202-203, 206-207
Convulsive therapy
  ECT, 308-313
  Metrazol, 315
  photoshock, 315
Coping mechanisms, 67-70, 72, 214, 240, 382
Coprolalia, 395

Coprophobia, 183
Coronary occlusion, 225, 227
Corrective emotional experience, 375
Cosmetic surgery, 221
Coue, E., 6, 377
Countercathexis, 277
Counterphobia, 233, 395
Countertransference, 274, 395
Courvoisier, 9
Cretinism, 256-257
Creutzfeldt-Jakob disease, 116
Crime, 376
Criminal responsibility, 395
Crisis intervention, 395
Cross-cultural psychiatry, 395
Cultural deprivation, 395
Culture and mental illness, 6, 157, 376, 382
Culture-specific syndrome, 211-213
Cunnilingus, 195, 395
Cushing, H., 377
Cushing's syndrome, 377, 395
Cybernetics, 395
Cyclothymic, 5, 191

D

Da Costa's syndrome (neurocirculatory asthenia), 177
Darwin, C., 8, 377
Daydreams, 75, 185, 191
Death
  bereavement, 141, 146, 187, 217
  dying, 187
  instinct, 396
  starvation, 228
  sudden, 226-227
  suicide, 228
  surgical patients, 226
De Clenambault's syndrome, 396
Decompensation, 396
Defense-mechanism, 67-69
Déjà entendu, 396
Déjà eprouve, 396
Déjà fait, 396
Déjà pensé, 396
Déjà raconte, 396
Déjà voulu, 396
Déjà vu, 16, 74, 165, 396

Delay, 9
Delinquency, 245, 375, 379
Delirium, 101-103, 109, 396
Delirium tremens, 109
Delmas-Marsolet, 9
Delta activity, 34
Delusion
  cancer, 144
  disease, 76, 144, 165
  fixed, 76
  grandeur, 76, 165
  guilt, 76
  hypochondriacal, 144
  inferiority, 165
  nihilistic, 144
  paranoid, 156
  pathological jealousy, 76
  persecutory, 75, 165
  poverty, 76
  reference, 80
  religious content, 143
  self-accusation, 76
  sexual content, 143
  sin, 76
  systematized, 76, 171
  unsystematized, 75, 165
Dementia, 4, 396
Dementia paralytica, 99
Dementia praecox, 5, 156, 376, 396
"Dementia precoce," 156
Denial, 68, 396
Deniker, P., 9
Depersonalization, 76, 180, 188, 396
Depression, 7, 76
  agitated, 142
  anaclitic, 76
  bipolar, 141
  childhood, 249, 390
  electroconvulsive therapy in, 308-309
  endogenous, 141, 187
  exogenous, 187
  involutional melancholia, 142
  manic-depressive, 144
  neurotic, 186-187
  postpartum, 142
  psychoneurotic, 176
  psychotic, 144

Depression—cont'd
  reactive, 141, 187
  retarded, 144, 149
  stuporous, 142, 150
  suicide and, 144-145
  symptom, 76
  syndrome, 186-187
  treatment of, 151-155
  unipolar, 141
Derailment, 147, 415
Dereistic thought, 75, 241
Dermatitis, 220, 330
Descriptive psychiatry, 5
Desensitization, systematic, 386
Deterioration, alcoholic, 104-105
Deutsch, A., 377
Deutsch, F., 377
Deutsch, H., 377
Developmental disability, 396
Diabetes mellitus, 233
Diagnostic procedures, 13-82
Dipsomania, 396
Disaster, civilian, 371
Disease
  Alzheimer's, 106-108, 375
  Bowineville's, 257, 392
  Creutzfeldt-Jakob's, 116
  Gilles de la Tourette's, 210, 212-
    213
  Graves, 234
  Huntington's, 37, 117, 357
  Hurler's, 402
  Kalischer's, 258
  Kanner's, 163, 249
  Marchiafava's, 110-111
  Parkinson's, 410
  Pick's, 106-108
  Tay-Sachs, 258
  von Recklinghausen's, 257
  Wilson's, 117-118
Disharmony, 156, 376
Disorientation, 396
Displacement, 68, 397
Disposition, 76
Dissociation, 6, 7, 68, 176, 397
Distractibility, 73, 193, 397
Distributive analysis, 7
Disulfiram, 198
Divorce, 364-365

Dix, D., 5, 377
DNA (deoxyribonucleic acid), 397
Doctor-patient relationship, 273
Dollard, J., 377
Dopamine, 151, 159, 215, 325, 342
Double bind, 158, 226, 251, 397
Down's syndrome (mongolism),
    255, 397
Dream analysis, 6
Dream state, 73
Dreaming, 68, 344, 354
Drinking
  episodic, 183
  habitual, 184
Drive
  hereditary, 71, 159
  instinctual, 71
Drivenness, 77
Drug
  antianxiety, 330-331, 390
  anticholinergic, 338-339
  anticonvulsive, 135-137
  antidepressant, 339-346
  antimanic, 337-338
  antipsychotic, 324-330
  anxiolytic (minor tranquilizer),
    330-331
  ataractic, 325, 390
  barbiturate, 332-333
  butyrophenone, 325, 329
  hallucinogenic, 201, 203, 208,
    401, 412
  hypnotic, 332-334
  monoamine oxidase inhibitor
    (MAO), 343
  neuroleptic (major tranquilizer),
    324-330
  phenothiazine, 325
  psychic energizer, 390
  sedative, 332-334
  stimulant, 335-336
  thymolytic, 390
  tranquilizer, 324-330, 330-331
Drug abuse, 200-209
Drug dependence
  alcohol, 184, 197
  amphetamines, 201-202, 206, 208
  barbiturates, 206-207, 209
  chloral hydrate, 207

Drug dependence—cont'd
chlordiazapoxide (Librium), 207
cocaine, 204, 207, 209
dextropropoxyphene (Darvon), 207
diazepam (Valium), 207
ethchlorvynol (Placidyl), 207
glutethimide (Doriden), 207
hashish, 207
heroin, 207
marijuana, 207
meprobamate (Miltown, Equanil), 207
methaqualone (Quaalude), 207
methyprylon (Noludar), 207
morphine, 205
opiates, 200-206
paraldehyde, 207
Drug intoxication
alcohol, 110
atropine, 127
barbiturate, 126
belladonna, 127
bromide, 123
chloral hydrate, 127
corticosteroid, 127
digitalis, 103
iproniazid, 127
isoniazid, 127
lithium, 338
paraldehyde, 127
psychedelics
banana peels, 208
catnip, 208-209
lysergic acid diethylamide (LSD), 208, 401
mescaline, 208, 401
morning glory seed, 208
nutmeg, 208
plants, 209
psilocybin, 401
stramonium, 208
"sniffing," 208-209, 414
Dunbar, F., 214, 219, 377
Dunham, H., 157, 377
Durham decision, 297, 360
Durkheim, E., 377
Dynamic psychiatry, 7
Dyslexia, 397

Dyspareunia, 180, 397
Dyspraxia, 31

E

Earle, P., 5, 377
Echolalia, 77, 164, 397
Echopraxia, 77, 165, 398
Ecology, 377, 398
Economic viewpoint, 277
Ecstasy, 76
EEG (electroencephalograph), 33
activation techniques, 37-38
alpha activity, 34
beta activity, 34
delta activity, 34
epilepsy, 35
examination, 33-39
Huntington's chorea, 37
hypnosis, 36-37
hysteria, 36
neurosyphilis, 37
schizophrenia, 37
sociopathic personality, 37
theta activity, 34
Effort syndrome, 177
Ego
alien, 398
boundaries, 166
definition, 277, 398
ideal, 277, 398
Eidetic image, 398
Eitington, M., 378
Elation, 76
Electroconvulsive therapy, 8, 151-152, 169, 186, 308-313, 398
consent, 364
contraindications, 312
EEG changes, 311
equipment, 313
indications, 308
memory changes, 311
mode of action, 312
technique, 309
Electrosleep, 314-315
Electrostimulation, focal, 27
Electrostimulation therapy, 8, 9, 314
Ellis, H., 378
Elopement, 398

EMG (electromyograph), 221
Empathy, 281, 285-286, 302, 398
Encephalopathy
  alcoholic, 110
  lead, 125
  Marchiafava's disease, 110
  nicotinic acid (niacin) deficiency, 347
  Wernicke's encephalopathy, 110
Encopresis, 230, 398
Encounter group, 303
Endocrine mechanisms, 216
Endocrine psychophysiological disorders
  acromegaly, 388
  Cushing's disease, 377, 395
  hyperthyroidism, 233-234
  hypoparathyroidism, 234
  hypothyroidism (myxedema), 233-235
  obesity, 234-235
Endogenous psychosis, 5
Endorphins, 299
End-setting, 284
Eneuresis, 241, 398
Engrafted schizophrenia, 411
Engram, 27, 31, 398
Epilepsy, 130-139
  EEG patterns, 35-39
  fetal hydantoin syndrome, 259
  nocturnal enuresis, 356
  psychosis with, 115-116
  temporal lobe, 140
Epiloria, 257, 392
Ergotrophic system, 215
Ergasia, 398
Ergasiology, 7
Erikson, E., 290, 378
Erotogenic zone (erogenous zone), 398
Erotomania, 398
ESP (extrasensory perception), 279, 399
Esquirol, J., 4, 378
Essential hypertension, 224-225
EST; *see* Electroconvulsive therapy
Estrangement, 398
Ethnology, 398

Ethology, 398
Euergasia, 398
Eunuch, 398
Euphoria, 399
Eutonia, 119
Exaltation, 399
Exhibitionism, 195, 399
Existential analysis, 376, 379
Existentialism, 379
Exogenous psychosis, 5
Extended family, 409
Extrapyramidal symptoms, 325
Extrovert, 3, 399

F

Fairy tales, 279
Falconer, W., 5
False pregnancy, 232
Falsification, retrospective, 74
Family, 409
  therapy, 244, 375
Fantasy, 68, 75, 164, 185, 399
Faris, 157, 377
Fatigue, 188, 192
Fava beans, 346
Fear, 110
Federn, P., 8, 378
Feeblemindedness (mental retardation), 254-259
Feedback (regulatory mechanism), 385
Feeling tone, 76
Fellatio, 195, 399
Fenichel, O., 189
Ferenczi, S., 7, 378
Fetal alcoholism syndrome, 111
Fetal hydantoin syndrome, 259
Fetishism, 399
Fever therapy, 8, 114
Field theory, 381
"Fight or flight," 215
Fire-setting (pyromania), 252
First rank symptoms, 384
Fixation, 399
Fixed ideas, 6
Flagellation, 195, 399
Flat affect, 76
Fleiss, W., 378
Flight of ideas, 75, 399

Floccillation, 399
Flooding, 184, 399
Folie á deax, 211, 213, 399
Forensic psychiatry, 359-366, 399
Forepleasure, 399
Formication, 204, 399
Foulkes, S., 378, 409
Frankl, V., 378, 406
Free association, 6, 27, 278, 400
"Free-floating" anxiety, 76, 177, 400
Free-floating attention, 278
Freeman, W., 9, 319, 378
French, T., 378
Freud, A., 7, 378
Freud, S., 6, 61, 65-66, 156-157, 174-176, 183, 195, 276-278, 289, 378
Friedman, 9
Friedreich's ataxia, 258
Frigidity, 180, 232, 400
Fromm, E., 379
Fromm-Reichman, F., 8, 167, 379
Frontal lobe syndrome, 116, 400, 418
Frotteur, 400
Fugue, 180, 400
Fundamental symptoms, 156, 164, 400

G

GABA (gamma-aminobutyric acid), 400
Gage, Phineas, 9
Gait, peculiarities, 77
Galen, 4, 399
Galvanic skin response (GSR), 401
Gambling, compulsive, 394
Ganser syndrome, 210, 213, 400
Garden therapy, 4
Gargoylism, 402
GAS (general adaptation syndrome), 215, 400
Gastrointestinal disorders, 228-230
Gault decision, 400
"Gedankenlantwerden," 72
Gelineau, tetrad of, 408
General adaptation syndrome, 215, 400

General paresis (general paralysis of insane), 37, 99, 111-114
General systems theory, 400
Genetic marker, 401
Genetic principle, 277
Genitourinary disorders, 232
Gerstmann syndrome, 401
Gesell, A., 8, 379
Gheel colony, 372, 401
Gildea, E., 379
Gilles de la Tourette's disease, 210, 212-213
Gjessing, 163
Globus hystericus, 401
Glue "sniffing," 208, 209
Goldstein, K., 273
"Goofballs," 208
"Gooseflesh" ("cold turkey"), 201, 203, 205
Grand mal, 133
Greisinger, W., 5, 379
Grief, 141, 187, 230
Grimaces, 77, 114
Group therapy, 234, 302-306, 376
GSR (galvanic skin response), 401
Guardianship, 363
Guilt, 77, 144, 379
Gustatory hallucination, 72, 164
Gyrectomy, 320
Gyri of Gratiolet, 30

H

Habeas corpus, 401
Halfway house, 401
Hall, G., 8, 379
Hallucination
  auditory (hearing), 72, 110, 116, 337
  body sensation, 165
  childhood, 73
  cocaine, 72-73
  colored, 109
  deep sensation, 72
  definition, 401
  derogatory, 171
  distancing, 135
  "Doppelgänger," 72
  elementary, 72
  extracampine, 72

Hallucination—cont'd
  functional, 72
  "Gedankenlautwerden," 72
  gustatory, 72, 164
  haptic, 401
  heautoscopy, 72
  hypnagogic, 72, 356, 402
  kinesthetic, 405
  Lilliputian, 72, 401
  macropsia, 72
  mass, 72
  micropsia, 72
  negative, 73, 408
  olfactory (smell), 72, 116
  persecutory, 164
  "phantom limb," 73, 405
  pleasant, 207
  pseudohallucination, 72
  sexual, 72
  small animals, 109
  smell, 72
  tactile, 72, 165, 401
  taste, 72, 164
  true, 72
  vestibular sensation, 73
  visual, 72, 109, 337
  voices, 72, 337
Hallucinogens, 201, 203, 208, 401,
    412
Hallucinosis, 109-110, 401
Hand wringing, 351
Handedness, 27
Hand-flapping tremor, 391
Handwashing, 185
Harlow, H., 379
Hartman, H., 379
Hashish, 207
Havens, W., 379
Head injury, 119
Headache, 221, 225-227, 407
Healy, W., 245, 379
Heath, 157
Hebephrenia, 161, 379, 401, 418
Hecker, E., 5, 156, 379
Hedonism, 193, 402
Heidegger, M., 379
Heinroth, J., 5, 379
Hematoma, subdural, 120
Hemocysteinuria, 257

Hemodialysis, 127, 338
Hemophilia, 228
Hepatic coma, 111
Hepatolenticular degeneration,
    117-118
Here-and-now approach, 283
Heredity, 158-159
Heroin, 402
Hexafluorodiethyl ether, 315, 322
Hippocrates, 4, 214
History of psychiatric thought,
    4-10
Histrionic, 192, 411
Holism, 402
Hollingshead, A., 379-380
"Holy seven," 214
Homeostasis, 215, 402
Homosexuality, 172, 195, 402
Horney, K., 8, 284-285, 380
Hull, C., 289, 292, 380
Humanitarian treatment, 4-5
Hunter's syndrome, 402
Huntington's chorea, 37, 117,
    257
Hurler's disease, 402
Hydrotherapy, 4, 319, 323
5-Hydroxytryptamine, 215-216
Hyperactive (hyperkinetic) child,
    100, 252
Hyperhydrosis, 178
Hypermnesia, 74
Hyperparathyroidism, 234-235
Hypersomnia, 356-357
Hypertelorism, 257
Hypertension, 224-225, 227
Hypertensive crisis, 346, 402
Hyperthyroidism, 233
Hyperventilation syndrome, 177,
    222-223, 402
Hypnosis, 6-7, 27, 182, 219, 289-
    292, 296, 376, 402
Hypnotic drugs, 332-333
Hypochondriacal neurosis, 188
Hypomania, 145
Hypoparathyroidism, 234
Hypotension, orthostatic, 410
Hypothalamus, 216
Hypothyroidism, 233-234, 402
Hysteria, 6, 179-182, 376

Hysterical personality, 192, 411
Hysterical symptoms, 179-182

I

Iatrogenic illness, 402
Id, 277, 402
Idealization, 403
Ideas
  death of, 164
  fixed, 6
  of poverty, 165
  of reference, 76, 80, 403
Identification, 68, 403
Idiopathic, 403
Idiot, 403
Idiot savant, 403
Illusion, 72, 392, 403
Imago, 403
Imbecile, 403
Implosion, 184, 403
Impotence, 232, 403
Imprinting, 398, 403
Impulse neurosis, 192
Inborn error of metabolism, 157
Incest, 195, 404
Incoherence, 404
Incontinence, 233
Incorporation, 404
Individual psychology, 6, 280, 375
Individuation, 62, 279, 404
Indoklon; *see* Hexafluorodiethyl
  ether
Industrial therapy, 266-267
Infancy, 62-65
Infantile neurosis, 277
Inferiority complex, 6, 280, 375
Informed consent, 404
Inhibition, 68
Insanity, 404
Insanity defense, 389, 397, 404, 407
Insight, 16, 404
Insomnia, 5
Instinct, 71, 404
Instinctual impulses, 277
Insulin coma therapy, 8, 169, 315-
  318
Intake interview, 404
Intellectualization, 75, 404
Intelligence, 8, 13, 41-44

Intelligence quotient (IQ), 404
Interpersonal relations, 8
Interpretation, 278, 404
Interview, amytal, 14, 164
Intoxication
  alcohol, 110
  barbiturate, 126
  bromide, 123
  carbon monoxide, 124
  drugs, other, 126-127
  heavy metals, 125-126
  insecticides, 127
  lithium, 338
  psychedelics, 208
  "sniffing," 208-209, 414
Introjection, 68, 404
Introvert, 6, 404
Involutional melancholia, 142
IQ (intelligence quotient), 404
Irresistable impulse, 360, 404
Isolation, 68, 404

J

Jackson, J., 405
Jacksonian epilepsy, 404
Jacksonian seizures, 133
Jacobsen, C., 9, 221
"Jags," 208
Jamais vu, 74, 396, 405
James, W., 380
Janet, P., 6, 183, 380
Jargon aphasia, 26, 31, 405
Jaspers, K., 380
Jaundice, 330
Jealousy, 76, 191
Jones, E., 380
Jones, M., 9, 380
Judgment, 16, 405
Jung, C., 6, 380

K

Kahlbaum, K., 5, 156, 380
Kalinowsky, L., 380
Kalischer's disease, 258
Kallmann, F., 148, 157, 380
Kanner, L., 249, 380
Kasanin, Jr., 380
Ketz, S., 158
Kinesthetic hallucination, 405

Kinesthetic sense, 405
Kinky hair syndrome, 405
Kinsey, A., 194-195, 381
Kirchhoff, T., 381
Kirkbride, T., 5, 381
Klein, M., 245, 381
Kleine-Levin syndrome, 405
Kleinfelter's syndrome, 405
Kleptomania, 193, 405
Kluver-Bucy syndrome, 405
Kohler, W., 381
Koro, 212
Korsakoff, S., 381
Korsakoff's syndrome, 109, 405
Korzybski, A., 381
Kraepelin, E., 5, 156, 381
Kraft-Ebing, R., 381
Kretchmer, E., 5, 381
Kussmaul, A., 8

L

La belle indifference, 180, 405
Labile, 405
Lability of affect, 233, 405
Lalophobia, 183
Langfeldt, G., 166, 381
Language disorder, 26-32
Lapsus calmi, 405
Lapsus linguae, 405
Latah, 197
Latency phase, 63, 405
Latent content, 405
Latent schizophrenia, 162
Lawrence-Moon-Biedl syndrome, 258
Lead poisoning, 125, 259
Learning disability, 405
Learning theory, 287-289
Leighton, A., 9, 367, 381
Leptosome, 381
Lesbianism, 405
Lesch-Nyhan syndrome, 406
Leukemia, 226, 235
Leukotomy, 319
Lewin, K., 381
Lewis, N., 382
Liberson, V., 9
Libido theory, 406
Liebault, A., 6, 289, 382

Life chart, 7
Life crisis, 218
Life stress scores, 236
Life style, 280
Life-space interview, 305
Lilliputian hallucination, 72, 406
Lima, A., 9, 319
Limbic system of brain, 216
Linton, R., 382
Lithium therapy, 150-151, 337-338
Litigious behavior, 76, 171, 406
Lobotomy (lobectomy), 9, 169, 186,
    319-332
Localization, 27
Locomotor ataxia, 415
Logorrhea, 75
Logotherapy, 378, 406
Lombroso, C., 382
Loosening of associations, 147, 156,
    406
Loss of ego boundaries, 166
Low back pain, 221
LSD (lysergic acid diethylamide),
    406
Lupus erythematosus, 120
Lysergic acid diethylamide (LSD),
    406
Lysozyme, 230

M

Macropsia, 72
Magical thinking, 75, 406
Mahler, 163
"Mainlining," 208
Major tranquilizer, 390
Malignancy, 235
Malingering, 180, 205, 211, 213,
    406
Malinowski, B., 382
Mandala, 279
Manganese poisoning, 125
Mania
    hypomania, 76
    kleptomania, 192
    monomania, 171
    nymphomania, 409
    pyromania, 193
    trichotillomania, 416
Manic-depressive psychosis, 5, 7

Manifest content, 406
Mannerism, 77, 165, 406
Mantra, 406
MAO inhibitor, 150-151
Marathon group session, 303, 406
Marchiafava-Bignami disease,
    110-111
Marijuana, 201, 207, 292
Masculine protest, 6, 280, 406
Masochism, 195, 407
Masters, W., 382
Masturbation, 185, 193, 196, 407
Maturity, 63, 67
Maximum security unit, 407
May, R., 382
Mayer-Gross, 162
McDougall, W., 382
Mead, M., 382
Mechanisms of defense
    acting out, 388
    compensation, 67
    condensation, 68, 394
    conversion, 68, 176
    denial, 68, 198, 396
    displacement, 68, 176, 397
    dissociation, 68, 397
    idealization, 463
    identification, 68, 403
    incorporation, 404
    inhibition, 68
    introjection, 68, 404
    introversion, 404
    isolation, 68, 404
    overcompensation, 6, 410
    projection, 68, 191, 411
    rationalization, 413
    reaction formation, 68-69, 229,
        413
    regression, 69, 195, 277, 413
    repression, 69, 413
    somatization, 69
    sublimation, 69, 414
    substitution, 414
    symbolization, 69, 415
    undoing, 69, 417
Meditation, 219, 225
Meduna, L. von, 8, 162, 308, 382
Megavitamin therapy, 347
Melancholia, 4

Memory disorders, 74, 180, 390
Memory recall (flashback), 27
Menarche, 407
Mendel, G., 382
Menninger, K., 382
Menninger, W., 382
Mens rea, 407
Mental hygiene movement, 375
Mental illness, 367-368
Mental mechanism, 407
Mental retardation, 63, 254-259
Mental status, 13, 15-16, 407
Mercury poisoning, 125-126
Mescaline, 401
Mesmer, F., 5, 383
Methadone maintenance treatment,
    206
Metrazol shock treatment, 8, 382
Meyer, A., 7, 156, 383, 409
MHPG, 151
Microcephaly, 257, 407
Micropsia, 72, 406-407
Migraine, 225-227, 407
Milieu therapy, 9, 407
Minimal brain dysfunction, 247,
    249, 253, 407
Minnesota Multiphasic Personality
    Inventory, 407
Mitchell, S., 383
MMPI, 407
M'Naghten, D., 360
M'Naghten rule, 407
Mode, 408
Moebius, P., 5, 383
Molding, 418
Mongolism, 255, 259, 397
Moniz, E., 9, 319, 383
Monoamine   oxidase   inhibitor,
    150-151, 186, 340-341, 343-
    346
Mood (sustained affect), 76, 408
Moon facies, 395
Moral treatment, 4
Morel, B., 5, 156, 383
Moreno, J., 383
Morning glory seeds, 203
Moron, 408
Morphine, 205, 324
Motivation, 408

Motor disorders 76-77
Mucopolysaccharidosis, 402, 414
Multi-infarct dementia, 103, 105, 106, 146
Multiple personality, 176, 180
Multiple sclerosis, 119
Munchausen syndrome, 210
Muscle relaxants, 305
Musculoskeletal disorders, 221-222
Music therapy, 4
Mutism, 165
Mydriasis, 336
Myotonic pupil, 388
Myxedema, 233

N

Nalline test, 206, 408
Nancy school, 6
Narcissism, 408
Narcolepsy, 408
Narcotic blockade, 408
Negativism, 73, 77, 165, 408
Neologism, 75, 408
Neoplasm, 116, 235
"Nervous exhaustion," 177
Neurasthenia, 188, 375
Neurocirculatory asthenia, 177
Neurofibromatosis, 257
Neuroleptic, 390
Neurological examination, 22-24
Neurosis, 6, 81, 174-189, 408
    "actual," 176
    anxiety, 175, 177-178
    conversion hysteria, 176
    depersonalization, 188
    depressive, 186-187
    hypochondriacal, 188
    hysterical, 179-182
    impulse, 192
    neurasthenia, 188, 375
    obsessive-compulsive, 7, 176
    phobic, 176, 183-184
    psychasthenia, 6, 183, 380
    traumatic, 189
Neurosyphilis, 111-114
Neurotransmitters, 151
Nevoid amentia, 257-258
Night terrors, 356, 410
Nightmares, 224

Nihilism, 141, 144, 408
Nondirective approach, 408
Nonrestraint, 4, 5
Nonsense syndrome, 400
Noradrenaline, 325
Norepinephrine, 151, 159, 215, 342
Normal pressure hydrocphalus
    (NPH), 101
Nosology, 409
Nuclear family, 409
Null hypothesis, 409
Nurse, 266
Nymphomania, 409
Nystagmus, 418

O

Obesity, 234
OBS; *see* Organic brain syndrome, 410
Obsession, 6, 184, 409
Obsessive-compulsive neurosis, 7, 176
Occipital lobe, 32
Occupational therapy, 168, 266
OD; *see* Overdose, 322, 337, 343
Odor, schizophrenia, 158, 165, 376
Oedipal phase, 61, 63, 66
Oedipus complex, 409
Old age, 61
Oligergasia, 409
Oligophrenia, 409
Onanism, 394
Oneirophrenia, 162, 409
Open ward, 9
Operant conditioning, 409
Opium addiction, 201-206
Oral character, 409
Oral eroticism, 7
Oral phase, 277, 409
Ordinal position, 410
Organ inferiority, 6, 282
Organ jargon, 6
"Organ language," 218
Organ neurosis, 81
Organic brain syndrome, 99-140, 410
Orgasm, 72, 410
Orientation, 16, 73, 99, 410
Orthomolecular psychiatry, 347

Orthostatic hypotension, 410
Osmond, H., 157
Overcompensation, 6, 375, 410
Overdose, 201, 322, 337, 343
Overgeneralization, 165
Oxycephaly, 257

P

Pain, 235, 297-300, 332
Panic, 76, 144
Panting, 204
Paraldehyde, 199, 207, 324
Paralogical thinking, 164, 171
Paralysis agitans, 121-122
Paramnesia, 74
Paranoia, 156, 171, 410
Paranoid personality, 171
Paranoid schizophrenia, 161, 410
Paranoid states, 171-172
Paraphasia, 30
Paraphrenia, 171, 410
Parapraxis, 74, 410
Parapsychology (extrasensory perception), 279, 399
Parasympathetic nervous system, 410
Parataxic distortion, 274, 410
Parens patriae, 410
Parietal lobe syndrome, 401
Parkinsonian syndrome, 410
Participant observer, 8
Passivity, 229
Pastoral counseling, 267
Pathological intoxication, 110
Pathological jealousy, 76
Pathological liar, 75
Patient government, 9
Pavlov, I., 8, 383
Pavor nocturnus (night terrors), 356, 410
Pecking order, 411
Pederasty, 195, 411
Pedophilia, 195, 362, 411
Pellagra, 122, 347
Penetrance, 157
Penfield, W., 27-28
Penis envy, 411
Pennsylvania Hospital, 4
Peptic ulcer, 229

Peptide releasor substances, 217
Perception, 71-72
Perforation of nasal septum, 207
Pernicious anemia, 121
Persecution, delusion, 75
Perseveration, 182, 411
Persona, 411
Personality, 411
Personality development, 8, 60-70
Personality disorders 190-194
  anacastic, 192, 411
  antisocial, 5, 82
  asthenic, 192, 411
  compulsive, 411
  cyclothymic, 191, 411
  epileptoid, 191
  histrionic, 192, 411
  hysterical, 192, 411
  inadequate, 193, 411
  obsessive-compulsive, 186, 192, 411
  paranoid, 191
  passive-aggressive, 193, 411
  pattern disturbance, 191
  psychopathic, 193
  schizoid, 191, 411
  sociopathic, 192, 201
  trait disturbance, 191
Personality profile, 220
Personality types, 215
Persuasion, 182
Perversion, 195, 411
Petit mal, 36
Phallic phase, 277, 411
"Phantom limb," 73, 236
Phenotype, 411
Phenylketonuria, 257, 259
Phenylpyruvic oligophrenia, 257
Phobias, 144, 183, 388, 411, 418
Phobic neurosis (anxiety hysteria), 183-184
Phonemes, 72
Photic stimulation, 37
Photoshock, 315, 323
Phrenology, 27
Physical examination, 21-22
Physical (somatic) therapies, 308-313
Piaget, J., 8, 383

Piblokto, 212
Pick's disease, 106-108
Pickwickian syndrome, 356-357
Pinel, P., 4, 383
Pituitary adrenocortical axis, 215
Pituitary dystrophy, 258
PKU (phenylketonuria), 257, 259
Placebo effect, 273, 330
Pleasure principle, 277
Pluralism, 411
Poisoning, 124-127
Polatin, P., 163
Polydactyly, 258
Polypharmacy, 169
Porphyria, 122-123
Posthypnotic suggestion, 291
Postictal clouded states, 131
Postoperative period, 101
Postpartum psychosis, 128-129
Posttraumatic constitution, 119
Poverty of ideas, 165
Power instinct, 6
Pratt, J., 302
Preadolescence, 63, 66
Precipitating factor, 187
Preconscious, 277
Prefrontal lobotomy, 319-332
Pregenital stages, 7, 66, 277, 375
Pregnancy, false, 232
Premenstrual tension, 232
Presenile dementia, 106-108, 375
Preventive psychiatry, 368-369
Preyer, W., 8
Priapism, 411
Primal scene, 176, 411
Primary anxiety, 6
Primary process thinking, 160, 277, 411
Prince, M., 7, 289, 383
Principle, 277, 415
Prison psychosis, 400
Privileged communication, 362, 411
Process schizophrenia, 166
Projection, 68, 171, 411
Projective tests, 13, 44-49
Propfschizophrenia, 411
Prototoxic behavior, 274
Proverbs, 57

Pruritus, 220
Pseudobulbar palsy, 411
Pseudocyesis, 232
Pseudodementia, 144
Pseudohallucinations, 72
Pseudologica fantastica, 75
Pseudoneurotic schizophrenia, 163
Psilocybin, 401
Psoriasis, 220
Psychasthenia, 6, 183, 380
Psychedelic drugs, 208-209, 401
Psychiatric examination, 15-22
Psychiatric interview, 14-15
Psychiatrist, 264, 412
Psychiatry
    community, 367-373
    cross-cultural, 395
    descriptive, 5
    dynamic, 277
    forensic, 359-365
    orthomolecular, 347
    preventive, 368-369
Psychic determinism, 412
Psychoanalysis, 6, 7, 276-278
Psychobiology, 7, 412
Psychodrama, 302-303, 306, 383, 412
Psychodynamics, 60, 64-75
Psychogenic amnesia, 74
Psycholinguistics, 412
Psychological tests, 40-59, 412
Psychologist, 265-266, 412
Psychomotor epilepsy, 36
Psychomotor retardation, 77, 150, 186
Psychomotor seizures, 38, 134
Psychoneurosis, 81, 174-176, 186
"Psychopath," 81, 190, 193
Psychopathic personality, 18, 37, 390
Psychopharmacology, 9
Psychophysiological disorder, 81, 214-238
Psychosexual development, 6
Psychosis, 81, 412
Psychosocial factors, 214
Psychosomatic illness, 5, 214-238
Psychosurgery, 319-321

Psychotherapy
  behavioral
    biofeedback training (Green), 296-297
    learning theory therapy (Dollard), 287-289
    Reciprocal inhibition (Wolpe), 292-295
  brief, 8, 221, 244, 301, 375
  doctor-patient relationship, 273-275
    active analytical therapy (Stikel), 384
    analytical psychology (Jung), 278-280, 380
    character analysis, 380, 383
    Chicago school (Alexander and French), 375, 378
    classical psychoanalysis (Freud), 276-278, 378
    cultural school (Fromm), 379
    direct analysis (Rosen), 167, 384
    ego analysis (Klein), 381
    hypnoanalysis (Wolberg), 290
    individual psychology (Adler), 280-282, 375
    intensive psychotherapy (Fromm-Reichman), 167, 278, 379
    interpersonal psychiatry (Sullivan), 385
    psychobiological therapy (Meyer), 274, 383
    sector therapy (Deutsch), 377
    transactional analysis (Berne), 295-296, 376
    will therapy (Rank), 282-284, 383
  experiential
    autogenic training (Luthe), 300
    client-centered therapy (Rogers), 274, 285-287
    existential analysis (Binswanger), 376
    logotherapy (Frankl), 378
  group, 302-307
  individual, 269-301
  supervision, 275-276

Psychotherapy—cont'd
    supportive, 415
    termination, 276
Psychotomimetic drug, 412
Psychotropic drug, 412
Puerperal psychosis, 128-129
Punishment, 4, 375
Punning, 143
Pyromania, 412

Q

Quadrangular therapy, 412
Quincke's disease, 390, 412

R

Rage, 192
Rank, O., 6, 383
Rape, 196, 362, 412
Rapport, 412
Rapture-of-the-deep syndrome, 413
Rationalization, 413
Ray, I., 5, 383
Raynaud's disease, 225, 227
Reaction formation, 413
Reality, 277
  principle, 277
  testing, 174, 191
Recall, 27, 74
Recent memory, 74
Recidivism, 194
Reciprocal inhibition and desensitization, 183, 186, 292-295
Recognition memory, 73
Recollection, 29
Redl, F., 247
Redlich, F., 380
Regression, 69, 195, 277, 291, 413
Regressive shock therapy, 169
Rehabilitation, 20
Reich, W., 383
Reik, T., 383
Relaxation techniques 221, 219, 225, 236, 296, 300
Reliability, 413
Religion, 6, 76
REM, 354, 413
Remote memory, 74
Repetition compulsion, 413

Repression, 413
Reserpine, 146, 325
Resistance, 278, 413
"Restitutis ad integram," 159
Reticular activating system, 27, 216
Retrograde amnesia, 74
Retrospective falsification, 74, 413
Rheumatoid arthritis, 214, 221
Rhyming, 143
Ribonucleic acid, 413
Right to treatment, 413
Rigidity, 165, 413
Ritual, 185
RNA (ribonucleic acid), 413
Robertson, A., 383
Rogers, C., 274, 384
Rope-climbing, 158
Rorschach, H., 351, 384
Rorschach test, 44-48, 149-150, 163,
    181, 213, 384
Rose, J., 167, 384
Rule of free association, 278
Rush, B., 4, 384

S

Sadism, 195, 413
Sakel, M., 8, 315, 384
Salmon, T., 384
Salpêtrière, 6
Sanfilippo's syndrome, 414
Sapphism, 405
Satyriasis, 413
Scheid's cyanotic syndrome, 393
Schilder, P., 7, 384
Schizophrenia
    accessory symptoms, 164
    borderline, 392
    "burned out," 392
    EEG, 37
    first rank symptoms of Schneider,
        384
    fundamental symptoms, 164
    "odor," 158, 165, 376
    oneirophrenia, 409
    origin of term, 376
    periodic relapsing, 163
    prepsychotic, 162
    primary symptoms (features), 160
    process, 166

Schizophrenia—cont'd
    propfschizophrenia, 411
    pseudoneurotic, 163
    pseudopsychopathic, 162
    reactive, 166
    secondary symptoms, 160
    types (DSM II), 160-163
"Schizophrenogenic" mother, 158
Schneider, K., 170, 384
School refusal (phobia), 144
Schreber case, 156, 172, 414
Scoptophiliac, 417
Scotoma, 414
Screen memory, 414
Scurvy, 347
Sebaceous adenoma, 257
Sechehaye, M., 384
Secondary gain, 180, 414
Secondary process thinking, 277
Sedatives, 332-333
Seizures
    akinetic, 36
    auditory, 134
    febrile, 132
    focal
        motor, 36, 133
        sensory, 134
    grand mal, 133
    hypothalamic, 134
    hysteria, 131
    infantile spasms, 132
    Jacksonian, 133
    myoclonic, 36, 133
    olfactory, 134
    petit mal, 132
    psychomotor, 36, 134
    temporal lobe spike, 36, 38, 134
    thalamic, 134
    visual, 134
Selye, H., 216, 220
Senile dementia, 103-106
Sensitivity training group, 303
Sensorium, 73, 414
Sensory deprivation, 414
Separation anxiety, 64, 144
Serotonin, 151, 342
Sexual deviation, 194-196
Sexual offender, 196
Sheldon, W., 384

Shock treatment, 169, 308-314
Sibling, 414
Sibling rivalry, 414
Side effects, 325, 326, 330, 332, 336-339, 342, 343, 390, 391, 411, 416
Sighing respirations, 178
Simon, J., 8
Skin disorders, 220-221
Skinner, B., 384, 409
Slavson, S., 384
Sleep, 354
Sleep disorders, 356-357, 410
Slurring of consonants, 112
"Sniffing," 208-209, 414
"Snowbird," 414
Social class, 379-380
Social Readjustment Rating Scale, 216-217
Social worker, 265
Sociopathic personality, 82, 390
Sodium amytal, 182
Sodomy, 414
"Soft" neurological signs, 249
Soldier's heart, 177
Somatic treatment, 308-313
Somatization, 69
Somnambulism, 180, 355, 414
Southard, E., 384
Speech, 27-29
Spider web-spinning, 158
Spitz, R., 249
"Splitting"
  of thoughts and affect, 376
  of psychic function, 159
Srole, L., 367, 374
Startle reaction, 73, 239
State hospital, 5
Status epilepticus, 139
Statutory rape, 362
Stekel, W., 384
Stereotypy, 77, 164-165, 414
"Stranger anxiety," 64
Stress, 177, 192, 215, 235, 239-240
Structural point of view, 277
Stupor
  catatonic, 165
  depressive, 142, 150
  organic, 73

Sturge-Weber syndrome, 257-258
Subdural hematoma, 120
Subdural hemorrhage, 120
Sublimation, 69, 414
Substitution, 414
Succinylcholine chloride, 309, 323, 414
Suggestibility, 73, 415
Suggestion, 6, 179, 182, 291, 376
Suicidal gesture, 181, 351
Suicide, 127, 186, 308-309, 332, 340, 349-353, 377
Suicide equivalent, 230
Sullivan, H., 7, 284, 385
Superego, 66, 277
Supportive psychotherapy, 415
Suppression, 415
Susto, 212
Sydenham's chorea, 114
Symbiotic psychosis, 163
Symbolization, 69, 176, 179, 182, 187, 229, 375, 415
Sympathomimetic drug, 415
Symptom formation, 69-70
"Synchronistic" relationship, 279
Syncope, 225
Syndromes
  abstinence, 109, 205-207, 387
  abused child, 251, 391
  acute brain syndrome, 100-103, 388
  Adie's, 388
  alcohol withdrawal, 109
  amnesic-confabulatory, 390
  barbiturate withdrawal, 206-207
  battered child, 251, 391
  black-patch, 392
  Briquet's, 179, 376, 392
  Capgras, 211-213, 392
  catatonic exhaustion, 375, 393
  chronic brain, 99-100, 394
  culture specific, 211-212
  Cushing's, 395
  Da Costa's (neurocirculatory asthenia), 177
  De Clerambault's, 396
  depressive, 144
  Down's, 255, 397
  effort, 177

Syndromes—cont'd
  extrapyramidal, 325
  false pregnancy, 232
  fetal alcohol, 111
  fetal hydantoin, 259
  fire-setting, 252
  frontal lobe, 116, 400
  Ganser's, 210, 213, 400
  Gelineau's, 408
  general adaptation, 215, 400
  Gerstmann's, 401
  Kinky hair, 405
  Kleine-Levin, 405
  Kleinfelter's, 405
  Kluver-Bucy, 405
  Korsakoff's, 109, 405
  Lawrence-Moon-Biedl, 258
  Lesch-Nyhan, 406
  minimal brain dysfunction, 253,
    407
  morphine abstinence, 205, 324
  Munchausen, 210
  normal pressure hydrocephalus,
    101
  occipital lobe, 32
  organic brain syndrome, 99-140,
    410
  parietal lobe, 401
  phobic, 183
  Pickwickian, 356-357
  rapture-of-the-deep, 413
  Sanfilippo's, 414
  Scheid's cyanotic, 393
  Sturge-Weber, 257-258
  tardive dyskinesia, 325, 415
  temporal lobe, 116, 134-135
  Turner's, 417
  Wernicke-Korsakoff's, 347, 418
  Wernicke's, 110
  white-out, 418
  withdrawal, 109, 205-207, 387
  Wolf-Parkinson-White, 224
Syphilis, 111-114
Systematic desensitization, 386
Szasz, T., 385

T

TA (transactional analysis) 295, 296
T group (training group), 303, 416

Tabetic neurosyphilis, 415
Tactile hallucination, 401
Talion principle, 415
Tangential thinking, 75, 159, 415
Tarantism, 415
"Taraxein," 157
Tardive dyskinesia, 325, 415
TAT (Thematic Apperception Test),
    44, 146
Tay-Sach's disease, 258
Team approach, 263-268
Temporal lobe epilepsy, 134-135
Temporal lobe tumor, 116, 417
Tension, 76, 330
  headache, 221
  insanity, 156
Tests and scales
  Bayley Infant Scales of Develop-
    ment, 43
  Bender-Gestalt, 43
  Binet-Simon Test, 376
  Block Design, 42
  Brief Psychiatric Rating Scale, 56
  Clyde Mood Scale, 56
  Comprehension and Similarities,
    56
  Concept Formation Test, 44
  Cornell Index, 55
  Draw-a-Person Test, 48
  General Information Subtest, 57
  Goldstein-Scheerer Tests of
    Abstract and Concrete
    Thinking, 44
  Guilford-Martin Temperament
    Profile, 55
  Inpatient Multidimensional Rat-
    ing Scale, 56
  Kent E-G-Y, 57
  memory for digits, 57
  Minnesota Multiphasic Personal-
    ity Inventory, 49, 55, 407
  Picture Frustration Study, 48
  proverbs, 57
  Psychiatric Rating Scale, 55
  Revised Stanford-Binet Scale, 40,
    43, 376
  Rorschach Test, 44-48, 149-150,
    163, 181, 213
  Saslow Screening Test, 55

Tests and scales—cont'd
  sentence completion test, 48
  Social Readjustment Rating Scale, 215-217, 220
  subtracting serial 7's, 16, 57
  Thematic Apperception Test, 416
  Vineland Social Maturity Scale, 56
  Ward Behavior Rating Scale, 55
  Wechsler Adult Intelligence Scale (WAIS), 42, 418
  Wechsler Intelligence Scale for Children (WISC), 43, 418
  Wechsler Preschool and Primary Scale of Intelligence (WPPSI), 418
  Willoughby Personality Schedule, 294
  word association test, 48
Thalamic seizures, 134
Thalamotomy, 320
Thalamus, 29
Thanatos, 384
Therapeutic community, 206, 416
Therapeutic milieu, 9
Theta activity, 34
Thinking
  autistic, 75
  concrete, 44, 57, 387
  dereistic, 75
  magical, 75
  obsessive, 184
  paralogical, 164
  primary process, 160, 277, 411
  rational, 74
  secondary process, 277
  slow, 148
  tangential, 75, 159, 415
Third ear, 416
Thompson, C., 385
Thought, 75
  disorders, 75, 166, 184, 389, 392, 399, 406
  dereistic, 75
Thymolytic drug, 390
Tic, 77, 416
Tic douloureux, 416
Tinnitus, 416
Tolerance, 416

Topectomy, 320
Topographical approach, 277, 416
Torticollis, 416
Training group (T group), 416
Trance states, 36
Transactional analysis, 295, 296
Transcendental meditation (TM), 296-297, 300-301
Transference, 6, 182, 274, 416
Transference neurosis, 277
Transient situational disturbance, 239-244
Translocation, 256
Transmethylation, 158
Transsexualism, 196, 416
Transvestism, 195, 416
Trauma, brain, 119-120
Tredgold, A., 256, 385
Treponema pallidum, 113
Tremor
  asterixis, 391
  at rest, 410
  coarse, 109
  fine, 338
  hand-flapping, 391
  intention, 117
Trephining, 9
Trichotillomania, 416
Tricyclic drug, 340-341, 416
Trigeminal neuralgia, 416
Trisomy, 256, 416
Trophotropic system, 216
Tuberous sclerosis, 257, 392
Tuke, D., 385
Tuke, W., 4, 385
Tumescence, 417
Turner's syndrome, 417
Twin studies, 148, 157, 169, 418
"Type A behavior," 225
Tyramine, 346

U

Ulcer, peptic, 229
Ulcerative colitis, 230
Uncinate fit, 116, 417
Unconscious, 6, 277, 417
  collective, 7
Undoing, 69, 417
Unipolar depression, 141-142, 417

Universalization of guilt, 417
Unsystematized delusions, 80
Urgency, 232
Urticaria, 220

V

Vaginismus, 417
Validity, 417
Vasomotor instability, 224
Vasomotor rhinitis, 223
Venesection, 4
Verbigeration, 165, 417, 418
Vertigo, 417
Visual finger agnosia, 30
Vitamin deficiency, 347
Volition, 76
Volubility, 75
Vomiting, 229, 257
von Wagner-Jauregg, J., 8, 385
"Vorveireden," 400
Voyeur, 417
Voyeurism, 195

W

Watson, J., 8, 383
Watts, J., 9, 319
Waxy flexibility, 165, 393, 418
Wednesday Evening Society, 418
Wepman, J., 29, 32
Wernicke, C., 385
Wernicke-Korsakoff syndrome, 347,
    418
Wernicke's syndrome, 110
Wet dream, 418
Wet palms, 178
Weyer, J., 385
White, W., 385
Whitehorn, J., 385
White-out syndrome, 418

Wiener, N., 385
Wilbur, H., 385
Wilcox, P., 9
"Wild analysis," 384
Will, 5, 71, 76
Will therapy, 6, 282-284
Wilson's disease, 117-118
Withdrawal reaction, 247
Withdrawal syndrome, 109, 205-
    207, 387
Wittels, F., 386
"Witzelsucht", 116, 418
Wolf-Parkinson-White syndrome,
    224
Wolpe, J., 386
Women, psychosexual function, 376
Woodward, S., 5, 386
Word salad, 75, 165, 418
Working through, 68, 272, 278, 418
Worthlessness, 144
Writ of habeas corpus, 362, 401
Writing, automatic, 291
Wry neck, 416

X

Xenophobia, 418
Xerostomia, 418
XO variant, 417

Y

Yawning ("the yaps"), 205
York retreat, 4

Z

Zilboorg, G., 350, 386
Zoophilia, 182, 418
Zoophobia, 183, 418
Zygosity, 418